Ethics
and Research
With
Children

A Case-Based Approach

OXFORD
UNIVERSITY PRESS

2005

OXFORD
UNIVERSITY PRESS

Oxford University Press, Inc., publishes works that further
Oxford University's objective of excellence
in research, scholarship, and education.

Oxford   New York
Auckland   Cape Town   Dar es Salaam   Hong Kong   Karachi
Kuala Lumpur   Madrid   Melbourne   Mexico City   Nairobi
New Delhi   Shanghai   Taipei   Toronto

With offices in
Argentina   Austria   Brazil   Chile   Czech Republic   France   Greece
Guatemala   Hungary   Italy   Japan   Poland   Portugal   Singapore
South Korea   Switzerland   Thailand   Turkey   Ukraine   Vietnam

Library of Congress Cataloging-in-Publication Data
Kodish, Eric.
Ethics and research with children : a case-based approach / Eric Kodish.
p. cm.
Includes bibliographical references and index.
ISBN-13 978-0-19-517178-5
ISBN 0-19-517178-0
1. Pediatrics—Moral and ethical aspects. 2. Medical ethics—Case studies. 3.
Children—Diseases—Treatment—Moral and ethical aspects. I. Title.
RJ47.K64 2004
174.2'8—dc22   2004008004

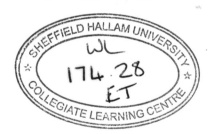

1 3 5 7 9 8 6 4 2

Printed in the United States of America
on acid-free paper

This book is dedicated, with honor, respect, and love
to my parents, JoEllen and Joseph S. Kodish

Preface

Putting together a book can best be described as a labor of love. This book has been a team effort from the start and has been a true pleasure to edit and assemble. The idea for the book emerged from the first meeting of our core research team in a project entitled "Pediatric Research Ethics: A Multidisciplinary Analysis." With generous funding from the Greenwall Foundation, we brought together a diverse and talented group of scholars to tackle the difficult issues raised by involving children in research. As we talked about a mechanism to disseminate our work, it quickly became apparent that a book-length treatment of the subject was needed. For this reason, the first thank you goes to Mr. William Stubing and the Greenwall Foundation, which made this project possible.

The members of the Greenwall project team and consultants, as well as other colleagues in the small world of pediatric ethics, quickly became the contributors to this book. The quality of the final product reflects the excellent scholarship, wonderful writing, and critical thinking of these outstanding individuals. I am personally grateful to each of the contributors for the effort and thoughtfulness that I know will be apparent to readers.

Several special people helped to make this book possible. Amy Harris-Yamokoski assisted with the formatting and editing process. Shlomit Zuckerman provided most of the questions for discussion that will help to make this a user-friendly teaching tool. Linda Robinson tolerated my countless requests for organizing the chapters and printing hard copies, helping me to keep track of just about everything. Finally, Michelle Eder directed the initial research project and quickly assumed many of the organizational and administrative responsibilities for bringing the book together. In addition to contributing an outstanding chapter, her dependable assistance, patience, and good judgment are highly valued and appreciated.

My colleagues at Rainbow Babies and Children's Hospital and Case Western Reserve University provided the fertile academic setting that makes the climate right for growing books. I am especially grateful to my research team and colleagues at the Rainbow Center for Pediatric Ethics for their insight and camaraderie. The children with cancer and blood diseases that I have had the privilege of caring for over the years, and their dedicated and courageous families, continue to inspire me and help me to recognize more clearly the need for better research to save lives and relieve suffering.

Joan Bossert, Lisa Stallings, and the team at Oxford University Press have helped me to understand the process of bringing this book from idea to reality. I appreciate their support and enthusiasm for this project.

Drs. David Sperling and Danny Kranitz provided squash, guitar, and friend-ship to help sustain me through this and other professional challenges. They are wonderful doctors and even better human beings. My brother Jeff Kodish was there for support, good humor, and perspective all along the way. In this year of his 90th birthday, my grandfather Milton Kodish continues to be a role model of graceful aging, zest, and love for life.

Finally, I cannot conclude the preface of a book about children without men-tion of my t(h)ree children, Tamar Aliza, Oren Moshe, and Elan Isaac Kodish. They have each helped me to understand what makes children so special and wonderful, and I am proud to have them call me Abba. They are a blessing. The biggest thank you and expression of my love is to my wife, Perach. Words cannot even come close.

Contents

Contributors

Jean Belasco, MD
Clinical Associate Professor of Pediatrics
Division of Oncology
Children's Hospital of Philadelphia

Jessica Wilen Berg, JD
Associate Professor of Law and Bioethics
Case Western Reserve University Schools
of Law and Medicine

Myra Bluebond-Langner, PhD
Distinguished Professor of Anthropology
Founding Director of the Center for
Children and Childhood Studies
Rutgers University

Jeffrey R. Botkin, MD, MPH
Professor of Pediatrics and Medical Ethics
Primary Children's Medical Center
University of Utah

Fabio Candotti, MD
Senior Investigator
Genetics and Molecular Biology Branch
National Human Genome Research
Institute

Donna T. Chen, MD, MPH
Assistant Professor of Health Evaluation
Sciences, Psychiatric Medicine, and
Biomedical Ethics
University of Virginia Health System

Christopher Church, PhD
Professor of Philosophy and Religion
Baptist College of Health Sciences

Susan E. Coffin, MD, MPH
Division of Infectious Diseases,
Department of Pediatrics
Children's Hospital of Philadelphia
University of Pennsylvania School of
Medicine

Lauren K. Collogan
Program Officer, Center for Urban
Bioethics
The New York Academy of Medicine

Amy DeCicco
Research Project Coordinator
Center for Children and Childhood
Studies
Rutgers University

Douglas S. Diekema, MD, MPH
Associate Professor of Pediatrics and
Medical History and Ethics
University of Washington School of
Medicine

Rebecca Dresser, JD
Professor of Law and Humanities in
Medicine
Washington University

Michelle Eder, MA
Program Coordinator
Department of Bioethics
Cleveland Clinic Foundation
and
Doctoral Candidate, Department of
Anthropology
Case Western Reserve University

Erin Flanagan-Klygis, MD
Assistant Professor of Pediatrics
Rush Medical College
Rush Children's Hospital

Alan R. Fleischman, MD
Senior Advisor, The New York Academy of
Medicine
Clinical Professor of Pediatrics,
and
Clinical Professor of Epidemiology and
Population Health
Albert Einstein College of Medicine

Joel E. Frader, MD
Professor of Pediatrics/Professor of
Medical Humanities and Bioethics
Feinberg School of Medicine
Northwestern University
and
Division Head, General Academic
Pediatrics
Children's Memorial Hospital

Gail Geller, ScD
Associate Professor
Johns Hopkins University
Department of Pediatrics
Phoebe Berman Bioethics Institute

Pamela S. Hinds, PhD, RN, CS
Director of Nursing Research
St. Jude Children's Research Hospital

Edwin M. Horwitz, MD, PhD
Associate Member of Hematology
Oncology
Divisions of Stem Cell Transplantation
and Experimental Hematology
St. Jude Children's Research Hospital

Eric Kodish, MD, FAAP
Chairman, Department of Bioethics
Cleveland Clinic Foundation
and
Professor of Bioethics and Pediatrics
Case School of Medicine

Gerald P. Koocher, PhD
Professor and Dean, School of Health
Studies
Simmons College

John Lantos, MD
Associate Professor of Pediatrics and
Medicine
Chief, General Pediatrics
Associate Director, MacLean Center for
Clinical Medical Ethics
University of Chicago

Stacy Laswell, MPH
Division of Reproductive Health
Centers for Disease Control and
Prevention

Molly Martin, MD
Department of Pediatrics
University of Chicago

Paul B. Miller, MA, MPhil, JD
Department of Bioethics
Dalhousie University

Robert M. Nelson, MD, PhD
Department of Anesthesiology and Critical
Care Medicine
Children's Hospital of Philadelphia
University of Pennsylvania School of
Medicine

Lainie Friedman Ross, MD, PhD
Department of Pediatrics
MacLean Center for Clinical Medical
Ethics
University of Chicago

Victor M. Santana, M.D.
Director, Solid Tumor Program
St. Jude Children's Research Hospital

John Santelli, MD, MPH
Chief, Applied Sciences Branch
Centers for Disease Control and
Prevention

Marjorie A. Speers, PhD
Executive Director
Association for the Accreditation of
Human Research Protection Programs
(AAHRPP)

Charles Weijer, MD, PhD
Department of Bioethics
Dalhousie University

Benjamin Wilfond, MD
Associate Investigator
Social and Behavioral Research Branch
National Human Genome Research
Institute
and
Department of Clinical Bioethics
Warren G. Magnuson Clinical Center
National Institutes of Health

Ethics
and
Research
With
Children

1

Ethics and Research With Children: An Introduction

Eric Kodish

A CASE STORY

The cure for childhood cancer will not be discovered without research. A new drug that targets the molecular trigger for malignant cell transformation is being studied in children with terminal cancer. I have been taking care of Abby, a twelve-year-old with metastatic osteosarcoma, for the past 18 months. Abby is dying. She is eligible for the drug study, but it holds only the most remote prospect of helping her. At the same time, the drug may be risky and could accelerate her death. Without the participation of children like Abby, knowledge about this new drug and others like it will never be obtained, and the cure for childhood cancer will not be found.

Abby looks at me and asks whether I think she should be in the study. How should I answer her question? Where do I begin to analyze the moral issues that emanate from Abby's story, and how do I balance the rational and emotional components of my human response to Abby and the dilemma we face? Do I owe it to all the children who will get cancer in the next several decades to say yes, or should I protect Abby from further suffering and say no? By asking the question, is Abby looking to me for hope, or is she seeking my permission to quit fighting? Should I defer this decision to her parents, or take responsibility and make a decision as her doctor? I do not know how to best respond to Abby, so I begin by creating this book.

CHILDREN AND RESEARCH

Children like Abby are both vulnerable subjects who need protection from research risks and therapeutic orphans who have been denied access to the benefits of research. In the United States, recent federal mandates have promoted the inclusion of children in clinical research and provided investigators and the phar-

3

maceutical industry with new financial incentives to study drugs in children (National Institutes of Health, 1998; U.S. Food and Drug Administration, 2004). This policy shift contradicts a long tradition of protecting children from the peril of research. Like all policy decisions, the move to conduct more research with children carries potential benefits and drawbacks. Despite years of debate and controversy, fundamental ethical questions about pediatric research persist. The twin goals of access and protection are not easily reconciled. The participation of children in research raises troubling questions that are not easily answered.

The goal of this book is to promote more thoughtful attention to the complex ethical problems that arise when research involves children. To that end, we have selected a wide range of cases in pediatric research ethics. Each chapter is based on a case, a story that relates to research with children. Following the case is an ethical analysis designed to provide insights and suggest answers to the questions raised. Each chapter concludes with a set of questions for further discussion that are intended to present a constructive challenge to the reader. The cases are grouped into three sections: Research Involving Healthy Children, Research Involving At-Risk Children, and Research Involving Children With Serious Illness. Within each section, chapters are arranged to begin with the case involving the youngest child-subject(s), with subsequent cases placed in ascending order of child-subject age.

This introductory chapter has three goals: to provide a review of the fundamental ethical issues raised by research involving children, to develop the rationale for the case-based approach to pediatric research ethics used in the remainder of this book, and to suggest ways that readers may find this volume most helpful. The reader is encouraged to begin with this chapter, which is designed to set the foundation for a better understanding of ethical issues in research involving children. Subsequent chapters may be of more or less interest to particular readers depending on the topics raised by the specific case that is discussed. Our purpose is to stimulate moral reflection on the most challenging, and sometimes controversial, issues in pediatric research ethics. Simple answers do not exist for the thorny questions raised by this topic and these cases, but this book, like the field of bioethics, can at least serve to ask the right questions. Rather than providing a dry summary of historical, policy, or legal considerations around pediatric research ethics, the goal in this volume is to work "up from cases," capturing the relevant ethical issues in the compelling real-life circumstances that present themselves to those engaged in making decisions. In other words, this book is written with the hope and belief that moral discourse about challenging cases can help us to do the right thing.

The arguments for and against the participation of children in research are compelling, and the stakes are high. Current and future children have much to gain and much to lose from the outcome of these debates. Children must, therefore, remain at the center of consideration. The development of lifesaving cures for lethal childhood diseases depends on advances in pediatric research, yet child-subjects are at risk for harm even when intentions are good. Worse yet, children may be exploited or abused in the course of unethical studies.

Children have often in the past been the victims of harmful medical experimentation (Lederer & Grodin, 1994). During the Nazi regime in Germany, children were used as human guinea pigs in research conducted by Dr. Josef Mengele. One gripping account by Eve Mozes-Kor, a survivor of the twin study at Birkenau, is a must-read narrative for anyone considering the ethical implications of any research involving children (Mozes-Kor, 1992). After describing her memories of "the smell of burning flesh, the medical injections, the endless blood taking, the tests, the dead bodies all around us, the hunger and the rats," this courageous woman implores scientists to "put themselves in the place of the subject and see how they would feel," and to "remember that the research is being done for the sake of mankind and not for the sake of science." In the aftermath of World War II, studies conducted at Willowbrook State School in New York engendered tremendous controversy about the ethics of pediatric research in this country (Ingelfinger, 1973, p. 425). Residents of Willowbrook experienced crowded and unsanitary conditions, and suffered from a high endemic rate of viral hepatitis. In the studies at question, mentally impaired children were deliberately infected with viral hepatitis in order to study the natural history of this disease and subsequently test therapy.

To this day, discussion of the Willowbrook studies elicits strong reactions from vigorous defenders and pointed critics alike.

Fifty years ago, in response to the Nazi atrocities, the Nuremberg Code was promulgated. Taken literally, the first principle of the code suggests an absolute prohibition on pediatric research. By requiring that "the voluntary consent of the human subject is absolutely essential. This means that the person involved should have legal capacity to give consent" (Levine, 1986, p. 425), the Nuremberg Code raises the possibility of a complete ban on research involving children. Twenty-five years ago, Paul Ramsey suggested a literal interpretation and strict compliance with the Nuremberg Code, asserting that children should be protected from the "violent and false presumption" that he characterized as the "alleged . . . implied consent of the child" (Ramsey, 1976). Importantly, Ramsey's position applied only to research without the prospect of direct benefit to the child. The current U.S. federal policy governing the conduct of research with children was directly shaped by Ramsey's ongoing debate over nontherapeutic pediatric research with Richard McCormick (Jonsen, 1998).

While Ramsey suggested an absolute prohibition on nontherapeutic pediatric research, McCormick took the position that research with children was not only morally acceptable but morally obligatory (McCormick, 1974). Their fascinating discourse outlined the contours of the debate for years to come and remains relevant as we consider pediatric research ethics in the 21st century. The current U.S. federal regulations, designed to provide explicit "additional protections" for children in research, were the result of the perceived need to categorize children as vulnerable research subjects but allow for limited pediatric research to proceed: a compromise between the positions of Ramsey and McCormick (Additional protections, 1983). In the words of Albert Jonsen, the current regulations are both "carefully restrictive and sensibly permissive" (Jonsen, 1988, p. 155).

The additional protections have been and will continue to be associated with a cost. The term "therapeutic orphan" was coined in 1963 to describe children as a class of individuals left behind in medical progress (Blumer, 1999). For several decades, research policy protected children but failed to provide incentives for the conduct of pediatric research. Coupled with the disincentives associated with the additional protections found in federal regulations (U.S. Department of Health and Human Services, 1983) and the lack of a substantial market for pediatric drugs relative to adults, children (as a class) were categorically denied access to research and its benefits. Only within the past decade has the pendulum begun to swing in the other direction. In 1998, a new National Institutes of Health (NIH) policy stipulated that "children must be included in NIH-conducted or supported research involving humans, unless there are sound ethical and scientific reasons to exclude them" (National Institutes of Health, 1998). The Office of Protection from Research Risks (now known as the Office of Human Research Protections), in a letter dated July 1, 1998, explained that "new NIH policy was developed because medical treatments applied to children are often based upon testing done only in adults, and scientifically evaluated treatments are less often available to children due to barriers to their inclusion in research studies" (Ellis & Puglisi, 1998).

Perhaps more important, the federal government (including Congress, the NIH, and the Food and Drug Administration [FDA]) have recognized the need to include children in medical research. The FDA has altered its policy to give the pharmaceutical industry a financial incentive to conduct pediatric research. To some extent, this policy shift attempts to compensate for the limited market in pediatric drugs. Effective April 1, 1999, the FDA required that new drugs and biologics be studied in pediatric patients (U.S. Department of Health and Human Services, 1997). The Food and Drug Modernization Act now provides a 6-month patent extension for pediatric labeling, the so-called exclusivity clause (Section 111), providing a very significant economic inducement to companies developing drug products. Speaking to the Society for Pediatric Research at its annual meeting in 2000, then FDA Commissioner Dr. Jane Henney cited several reasons for the historical reluctance of the pharmaceutical industry to study new drugs in children (Henney, 2000). The commissioner noted that these barriers include high costs, a relatively small market, and the "ethical dogma" that often precludes children from research participation. She reported that the FDA position on this issue has changed, and the dogma has been revised so that the goal is now to encourage pediatric research.

Even in the course of scientifically important and ethically designed studies, bad outcomes will inevitably occur. The fact that a child is harmed in the course of research participation does not automatically imply that the study was unethical. To hold all pediatric research to this unachievable standard would be to paralyze efforts to improve health care for children. Although it is critical that we learn from cases, we also must be cognizant of the fact that research will always involve risk, and tragedy cannot be completely prevented. In these tragic circumstances, the appropriate moral questions should center on what can be learned and how can future tragedies be prevented.

With the dramatic shift in policy goals, mandates, and incentives comes a need for attention to the ethics of pediatric research. The next section reviews fundamental ethical issues that provide a foundation for the ethics of research involving children, and explains best interests; risk, harm, and wrong; permission, assent, and consent; and the ethics of subject selection as they relate to children in research. These core concepts will provide the tools for discussion and serve as a guide for the reader in the case-specific ethical analyses that follow in subsequent chapters. Then follows a section on the value of cases and a discussion of how to best use this book, before returning to Abby to conclude this introductory chapter.

ETHICAL ISSUES

Terminology, Moral Roles, and Fundamental Ethical Principles

Accurate terminology is too often abandoned in discussions of research ethics. Unfortunately, this adds to the confusion in what is already an extremely complex set of moral questions. Because the duties and obligations of various individuals have a significant impact on reasonable expectations, ethical analysis is enhanced when the role of each individual is clearly defined. Because people with illness are most frequently called *patients* by those who provide professional health care services, it may be difficult to change nomenclature in the research context. However, the implications of being a *patient* are quite different from those of being a research subject. Patients expect to get medical care, and recruiting them for studies may lead to understandable confusion about direct medical benefit. In the past decade, advocacy groups and various communities have promoted the concept of active participation and partnership between those conducting and enrolling in research studies (Dresser, 2001). Although this has prompted a move away from the term research *subject* in favor of *participant*, the term *subject* is more appropriate for children. It may be ethically desirable to empower older children to become more active "participants" in the research decision, but such active participation is the exception in pediatric research. Because they are often not active in the decision about participation in research (Olechnowicz, Eder, Simon, Zyzanski, & Kodish, 2002) and, in many cases (i.e., research involving the newborn) they cannot possibly have a voice, the term *subject* is preferable to *participant* in pediatric research. For these reasons, this book on pediatric research ethics will in most cases use the term *subject* to describe children involved in research.

Based on analogous considerations, the book will call those who provide professional health care services *clinicians*, while those who conduct studies that involve children are termed pediatric *investigators*. Although *clinicians* have a clear fiduciary obligation to act in the best interest (see below) of their pediatric *patients*, the obligations of *investigators* are more complex and potentially in conflict.

Investigators embrace the goals of research, best defined as efforts that contribute to the development of generalizable knowledge (Levine, 1986). Many individuals, in the course of their day-to-day activities, routinely perform both *clinician* and *investigator* functions. However, the extent to which these individuals and other concerned parties (children, parents, Institutional Review Board [IRB] members) are able to distinguish these roles will dramatically enhance clear and careful analysis of complex ethical questions. Confusion about the patient-subject and clinician-investigator roles can exacerbate the "therapeutic misconception," which occurs when subjects believe that therapy and research are governed by the same primary goal: to advance the individual's best interests (Appelbaum, Roth, & Lidz, 1982). It is hoped that careful use of appropriate terminology in this book will help to dispel this common and potentially dangerous misconception (Dresser, 2002).

This is not to suggest that careful use of language will magically make all the ethical problems go away, and that then these problems will be easily solved. The inherent conflicts people face while playing more than one role in daily life are ubiquitous, whether it be juggling the adult role of parent and professional, or a sick child's role as student versus patient. Yet, a consistent understanding of the role each person plays in a particular moral dilemma will at least allow for a common starting place in efforts to discern the most ethical course of action.

Before turning to some of the key concepts in pediatric research ethics, it will be helpful to place the question of research ethics in a broader context. The *Belmont Report,* the most influential document in modern American research ethics, suggests that three key principles must be recognized as the moral foundation of human subjects research: respect for persons, beneficence, and justice. The report defines respect for persons as incorporating at least two ethical convictions: "first, that individuals should be treated as autonomous agents, and second, that persons with diminished autonomy are entitled to protection" (Belmont Report, 1978). Beneficence is "strongly" understood by the writers of the *Belmont Report* as "(1) do not harm and (2) maximize possible benefits and minimize possible harms." Justice, according to *Belmont*, requires "fairness in distribution."

Discussion of the following more specific concepts each relate to these three fundamental principles. Concern about best interests derives from the principle of beneficence, while the discussion of risk, harm, and wrong relates to both beneficence and respect for persons. Informed consent, parental permission, and assent are manifestations of the principle of respect for persons applied in practice. Subject selection issues primarily relate to concerns about the principle of justice. The *Belmont Report* articulates the framework for analysis of human subject research ethics and serves as an excellent platform on which to build a better understanding of ethics and research involving children.

Best Interests

As noted above, someone other than the child-subject will most often make decisions about the participation of a child in research. Although most often the person will be the parent(s), others are also called upon to act *in loco parentis* (Freedman, Fuks, & Weijer, 1993). Much of medical ethics can be divided into two general types of questions: "Who makes a particular decision?" and "What decision should be made?" This distinction between the procedural and substantive type of question has major ramifications for pediatric research ethics. The former generally results in looking to parents as decision makers. Often, this appeal to the procedural question deflects attention from important substantive questions raised by difficult cases. At best, this procedural approach allows for a more individualized assessment of various factors, with an effort to make a decision that reflects the authentic values of the child if this were possible to ascertain. This concept, defined as *substituted judgment* on behalf of the child, has limited relevance in pediatric ethics. The ethical foundation for use of the *substituted judgment* approach in pediatric ethics would be that because parents are best positioned to anticipate the values their children will develop as adults, they are given the prerogative to make decisions on their behalf. Such efforts at predicting the future and making current decisions based on those predictions are fraught with subjectivity.

In contrast, the concept of *best interests* promotes an effort to be more objective, weighing the potential benefits and burdens for a particular child. Best interest is like the Rosetta stone of pediatric ethics, and decoding its meaning is a central goal both in general and as applied to specific cases.

Although many of the general principles of medical ethics relate to both children and adults, the order of priority and application to specific cases differ in critical ways. For competent adults, the principle of respect for persons requires that patient autonomy take precedence over considerations of beneficence, which have been criticized as overly paternalistic (Siegler, 1985). The resulting emphasis on the rights of adults to control their own medical decisions has appropriately been applied to decisions in both clinical care and research (Veatch, 1981).

In contrast, pediatric ethics generally gives priority to beneficence over autonomy. The foremost consideration in *clinical* decision making for young children is the best interest of the child. This standard relies on the principles of beneficence (and nonmaleficence) to guide decision making on behalf of the child. The concept of best interests is more complicated in the *research* context. Research is, by definition, designed primarily to advance knowledge for the benefit of future patients (Levine, 1986). A narrow definition of best interests therefore precludes all pediatric research except, perhaps, research that offers a likelihood of direct benefit to the subject. The best interests standard has often been criticized as being overly malleable. This characteristic allows some interpretations of the standard to allow research with children while other understandings of best interest may prohibit such research. The question of whether a best interests standard can be reconciled with any pediatric research agenda lingers and requires continuing analysis.

Practical questions also remain about how to determine the child's best interests. These questions are especially complex when considering research participation. If the research carries the prospect of direct benefit, a best interests determination will be part of a more complex set of variables. For research deemed "nonbeneficial," a narrow best interests approach would suggest complete prohibition of pediatric research. In reality, other factors such as altruism, compensation to parents and/or child, maintenance of hope, and confusion stemming from the "therapeutic misconception" may enter the moral calculus (Appelbaum, Roth, Lidz, Benson, & Winslade, 1987). In summary, the best interests standard, commonly accepted as the moral foundation of clinical pediatric ethics, can be difficult to apply in the context of research on children. For this reason, some have suggested that the avoidance of harm serve as a basis for research ethics (Miller and Brody, 2003) and that this concept has particular resonance as an alternative foundation of pediatric research ethics that may be superior to best interests (Miller, 2003, p. 118).

Risk, Harm, and Wrong

The linchpin of the current U.S. system for protection of children in research does not depend on best interests or informed consent. Rather, the system mandates that research protocols be judged first and foremost on the potential risks facing children who are enrolled. Although it may be responsible for having slowed the pace of progress in pediatric medicine, the current system has generally served to provide effective protection to children. The governing regulatory framework relies on two separate kinds of decision makers: institutional and individual. The former responsibilities are assumed by the investigator and the IRB, whereas the latter involve informed consent, parental permission, and assent (see below). IRBs charged with assessment of risk are instructed to consider two aspects: probability and magnitude of harm. A more sophisticated ethical analysis should also consider the possibility that a child (or his or her parents) participating in research may be wronged without actually being harmed. For example, if an older child is misled during the course of research but is not physically injured, he or she may come to mistrust the medical establishment or feel that he or she was treated in a disrespectful fashion (Bartholome, 1996). This could result in the child being wronged without suffering actual harm. The National Bioethics Advisory Commission (2001) report referred to these as psychological and dignitary harms. These more subtle considerations should also be part of the assessment IRBs make on the ethical acceptability of pediatric research protocols.

The federal regulations governing pediatric research allow IRBs to approve three categories of pediatric research. Although provision for parental permission and assent is included, the crux of the regulations involves determination of risk and potential benefit. Risk accrues to the child-subject of research, but potential beneficiaries of research may include the child-subject, others, or both. The "others" who may stand to benefit from the participation of the child in research can include parents, siblings, physicians, investigators, research nurses, pharmaceutical sponsors, other children as a class, and society at large. Policy depends on threshold concepts such as "minor increase over minimal risk," but ambiguity exists around the definition and understanding of both minimal risk and what constitutes minor increase.

In the Code of Federal Regulations (45 CFR 46.102), minimal risk is defined as meaning "that the probability and magnitude of harm or discomfort anticipated in the research are not greater in and of themselves than those ordinarily encountered in daily life or during the performance of routine physical or psychological examinations or tests." Minimal risk studies may be approved by IRBs under 45 CFR 46.404 regardless of whether the research offers the prospect of direct benefit to the child. A more limited category of nonbeneficial research involving a minor increase over minimal risk may also be approved by IRBs under 45 CFR 46.406 nonbeneficial. These two categories use the concept of anticipated risk (minimal and minor increase over minimal) to limit allowable research involving children.

For controversial and important studies that carry greater than minimal risk, such as early gene therapy research or phase I oncology trials, approval hinges on interpretation of "prospect of direct benefit" (Kodish, 2003b). Despite a genuine effort to provide regulatory guidance, this language seems to raise more questions than answers. Does a 1–3% chance of tumor shrinking in a terminally ill child with cancer constitute the prospect of direct benefit (Shah et al., 1998)? Simple definitions such as radiographic tumor measurements seem inadequate. How can IRBs and conscientious investigators weigh the possible benefit of keeping the child or parents' hope alive? What role should older child-subjects have in deciding whether a study offers them potential benefit? Should the child's or parent's desire to be altruistic be considered a possible benefit? Compelling questions such as these are a critical part of the rationale for this book.

The careful analysis that these complex questions demand will be found in the chapters that follow. Application of the currently approvable categories as they relate to actual cases will allow the reader to determine the strengths, weaknesses, and current relevance of the existing regulations.

Informed Consent, Parental Permission, and Assent

Informed Consent in Pediatrics = Parental Permission + Assent of Child

Informed consent provides a key moral foundation for the conduct of research with competent adults, symbolizing a partnership between investigator and participant in the research endeavor (Heymann, 1995). In fact, the consent document invokes the image of a legally binding contract between two parties, ending with the signature of subject and investigator. Because very young children cannot possibly be voluntary partners (or even sign the consent document), informed consent is of more limited relevance in the pediatric context. In pediatric research, parental permission often takes the place of informed consent (American Academy of Pediatrics Committee on Bioethics, 1995). However, the ethical distinctions between the informed consent of a competent adult and the decision made by parent(s) on behalf of a child are significant. Decisions that adults make on their own behalf may be morally robust, but decisions made for children by parents cannot have the same degree of authenticity (Kodish, 2003a). Questions about how parents make such decisions and the moral validity of pediatric research decisions abound. Factors such as risk to the child, potential for benefit (to the child and to others), significance of the research question, and compensation for participation must all be considered for each specific decision for each specific child.

Parents are usually, but not always, authorized to act as decision makers on behalf of their minor children. This presumption is rooted in a long-standing moral and legal tradition. However, courts have consistently ruled that society's commitment to protect the welfare of minors takes precedence over parental rights (Holder, 1983). Can research participation ever be so clearly in the best interests of a child that parents should be compelled to permit study entry? Although this seems an unlikely notion, the strong momentum toward clinical trials as the "standard of care" makes this scenario a real possibility in the not-too-distant future. Evidence for an "inclusion benefit" for clinical trial participation suggests a pressing need to examine this issue (Lantos, 1999).

Parental permission may be *necessary* but is not *sufficient* for the conduct of pediatric research. First, unlike previous times in history when children were considered chattel, parents are no longer considered owners of their children. Second, multiple other criteria must be satisfied for the ethical conduct of clinical research (Emanuel, Wendler, & Grady, 2000). These include a favorable risk: benefit ratio and respect for enrolled subjects.

A third requirement to consider is assent, a concept that allows for the participation of older children in the research decision. Defined in federal regulations as "a child's affirmative agreement to participate in research," assent is generally applicable to developmentally normal children between 8 and 14 years of age. Capacity to assent requires that the child have a reasonable degree of understanding about what to expect in research, and comprehension of his or her ability to decline participation. Among scholars in pediatric ethics, assent is a concept that has gained favor in recent literature (Baylis, Downie, & Kenny, 1999). Unfortunately, consensus on the role of assent in pediatric research ethics is still lacking (Bartholome, 1996). Should parents have "veto power" if an older child and pediatric researcher agree that the child should participate in research? What about cases where the child refuses (dissents) but parents and investigator agree that participating in the study would offer significant benefit to the child?

The triangular relationship among investigator, parent, and child depicted in Figure 1.1 makes analysis of ethical obligations in pediatric research more complex than analysis of studies involving competent adults. Children are not simply "little adults." There are critical differences between adults and children in the physical, intellectual, psychological, spiritual, political, and economic domains. These important differences between children and competent adults demand a different approach to pediatric ethics.

There is agreement that older children should participate in research decisions. However, major questions remain concerning the appropriate timing and extent of their participation. Children, by definition, are in a process of maturation

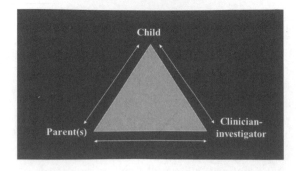

FIGURE 1.1.
The geometry of pediatric research ethics.

that requires pediatric ethics to utilize a developmental perspective. This continuum of development precludes a simple approach to the assent requirement. Any chronological age selected for a threshold above which children are expected to take part in decisions would be arbitrary and potentially counterproductive. A developmental assessment of a particular child's ability to participate in a particular decision represents a more defensible way to proceed.

Two specific, related issues of key importance for pediatric research ethics are decision-making capacity and developmental trajectory. Although newborns (or even fetuses) may be eligible to become research subjects, no rational claim for his or her own participation in the decision can be made. Capacity to participate in the decision about research is gradually acquired, without a bright line that divides capable from incapable. At the other end of the pediatric spectrum, a developmentally mature 17-year-old may not be legally permitted to sign an informed consent document. The moral justification for his or her participation in the research decision, though, is powerful. The ethical distance between the newborn and 17-year-old is immense and requires a strategy that recognizes this distance. A graduated approach provides a better fit to the reality of cognitive development than an artificial dichotomy between competent and incompetent.

The second, related domain of developmental trajectory also affects the child's participation in decisions about research. The maturation of children is not steady and linear; rather, it is subject to periods of acceleration and is influenced by life events. Some children with chronic illness may be developmentally advanced by virtue of their life experience with the illness, and this increases their ability to participate in research decisions. The developmental trajectory of children, however, is in the direction of full capacity. By contrast, geriatric research ethics has often grappled with the issue of declining competency in dementia patients. This mirror image, juxtaposing those with increasing ability to make research decisions (children) with subjects who may have diminishing capacity, provides for an interesting contrast. This is not to imply that dementia or even diminishing decisional capacity affects all who are elderly. When it does tragically take place, research decisions can sometimes be made in accordance with previously expressed wishes. For those children who have not yet attained decisional capacity, this is not an option.

The rights of children to participate in decisions about their own health care have been the focus of intense controversy. Despite this controversy, there is increasing consensus that older children should be empowered to make their own decisions. The concept of assent provides a framework for allowing such participation. In 1995, the American Academy of Pediatrics Committee on Bioethics issued a statement on "Informed Consent, Parental Permission, and Assent in Pediatric Practice." These helpful clinical guidelines do not address research participation decisions for children (American Academy of Pediatrics Committee on Bioethics, 1995).

A fundamental ethical difference between clinical and research decisions must be recognized, with major implications for pediatric ethics. In clinical pediatrics, decisions are determined by the best interests standard. If a 7-year-old refuses a vaccination that her parents and doctor agree must be administered, the dissent of the child must be acknowledged, and clinicians may owe the child an apology, but the vaccination will be given (Bartholome, 1995). Parents and pediatricians do have a moral obligation to address the child's concerns but must proceed with administration of the vaccine based on their commitment to the child's well-being. One such moving example is found in the classic short story by pediatrician and writer William Carlos Williams. In the Williams (1932) story, "The Use of Force" is justified to save the life of a young girl with diphtheria.

By contrast, research participation by children may never be morally obligatory. Because of the supererogatory nature of a decision to participate in research, parents, investigators, and IRBs should give more power to the voice of the child in research. As such, the U.S. Code of Federal Regulations defines assent as "[a] child's affirmative agreement to participate in research. Mere failure to object should not, absent affirmative agreement, be construed as assent" (CFR 46.402(b)). For children in research, silence does not imply acquiescence. To presume so risks basing pediatric research on the "violent and false presumption" that Ramsey feared (Ramsey, 1976).

Material presented in this book can help to make assent more meaningful and robust. Developing an enriched understanding of the assent concept will assist clinical investigators who conduct research with pediatric subjects, parents with children who are candidates for clinical trials, and older children faced with a decision about research participation. When research involves younger children, the very language of informed consent becomes problematic (Kodish, 2003a). The operative concept of parental permission more accurately characterizes the ethical transaction. Parental permission may be augmented by the concept of assent for older children, and assent may dominate permission in some cases. One helpful approach to the problem may be to separate the educational from the authorization components of assent. Although all children should be informed about research in which they may be asked to take part, the actual decision can still rest with parent(s). These two aspects relate to distinctive ethical domains and can be reasonably separated in cases where operationalizing the concept of assent are challenging.

Several chapters in this book analyze cases that point out important questions involving these concepts. Does informed consent by the competent adult provide a more firm moral foundation than does parental permission on behalf of a child? Do distinctions between the clinical and research contexts change the relevance of parental permission? Is adequate parental understanding of the research trial an ethically mandatory requirement for children to participate in research in which the child may benefit? Alternatively, is the combination of parental trust and the current system for the protection of children as vulnerable research subjects sufficient to justify research with the prospect of direct benefit to the child? What about nonbeneficial pediatric research? What might be the implications of policy designed to promote pediatric research with or without the prospect of direct benefit?

Subject Selection

Adult volunteers are routinely paid to participate in nontherapeutic research. Although questions persist about the amount of money that may make such research coercive or distort subject decision making, there is general agreement that competent adults should be allowed to make their own judgments on this issue (Dickert & Grady, 1999). Once again, pediatric research ethics are more complex; the practice of paying for the participation of children in research presents challenging questions (Gidding et al., 1993). Who should make the decision to participate, and who should receive payment? Can and should older children take part in the consent process, provide assent, or be allowed to supersede the decision of their parents? What systems might be established to assure that the monetary inducement to participate is just and equitable, and that children will not be exploited by parents, investigators, or the pharmaceutical industry? How can the altruistic motivation to take part in research coexist with economic incentives for subject recruitment? What messages do we send to children by paying them to take part in research?

In research without the prospect of direct benefit to the child, subject selection is a critical issue. One pivotal conceptual question is whether it is morally preferable to conduct "nonbeneficial" research in sick children or in healthy children (Ross, 2003; Wendler, Shah, Whittle, & Wilfond, 2003). Scientific and ethical issues intertwine to make this a difficult question to answer.

To determine the scientifically appropriate research subjects, investigators must assess the metabolic capabilities of healthy and of sick children who are candidates for research studies. For example, a child with sickle cell disease, admitted to the hospital for pain crisis, may be recruited to participate in a pharmacokinetic study of a new intravenous preparation of an anti-fungal drug. Because children with sickle cell disease are not at particularly high risk for fungal disease, an IRB might consider this study under the category of research without potential benefit to the subject. Children with sickle cell disease do, however, often have abnormal liver and kidney function. Based on these clinical scientific issues, healthy children may be scientifically better subjects for these early drug studies than are children with metabolic impairment from chronic illness. Subjects who have the closest physiological resemblance to those for whom a new drug is intended are likely to provide the most reliable knowledge during initial studies of a new drug.

The fact that healthy children would be scientifically preferable for such a study must be balanced against the practical consideration of subject availability. Children with sickle cell disease are hospitalized frequently for complications, whereas healthy children are not so accessible for research. Ultimately, the investigator must decide whether to enroll healthy children, sick children, or both in any particular study in this category.

Another critical consideration is the need for parsimony in research design. Good science and the principle of justice support studying those subjects who will provide data that can be generalized to a large number of patients. Sound research design also requires that a minimal number of subjects should be enrolled when the goal of research is clearly to help future patients rather than current subjects. This consideration of human subjects as valuable resources to be carefully allocated raises the troubling prospect of using children as a means to an end. If policy does allow for such research, subsequent questions about whether to use healthy children or sick children in early drug studies still remain. If it were anticipated that a new drug under study would eventually be targeted at a particular disease, parsimony would suggest that early, nonbeneficial studies be conducted in children with the target disease. Thus, scientific considerations yield conflicting guidance regarding the question of sick versus healthy children in research without the prospect of direct benefit to the subject.

Subject selection also raises practical issues related to geography and access. Because both pediatric investigators and sick children tend to inhabit academic children's hospitals, children with chronic or acute illness are often the most convenient sample. These children generally have baseline lab values that are readily available. Many children become familiar with and even comfortable in the hospital environment, making research participation less frightening for sick children than for healthy children. Another advantage is that for hospitalized children there is ready access to emergency medical services in the case of an untoward event or anaphylactic reaction.

These practical considerations favor the preferential use of sick children in research studies, but they are not determinative. It might be possible to recruit healthy children as subjects in studies conducted at a general clinical research center at a major children's hospital. One could also imagine the construction of free-standing pediatric research centers designed for the study of healthy children, providing many of the practical advantages mentioned above. This solution might be more costly but could be accomplished if the reasons were compelling. In fact, several major pediatric medical centers have recently established clinical trials offices to partner with the pharmaceutical industry in response to the recent call for increased pediatric research (Abzug & Esterl, 2001). Although this trend is likely to benefit children, it raises the possibility of exploitation in individual cases if caution is not exercised.

A second important practical issue relates to the need to acquire blood for testing in pediatric research. Frequent blood sampling is commonly required for drug research. Children with acute illness often have a peripheral intravenous line, and those with serious chronic disease may have a central venous access device. Peripheral intravenous lines are designed to allow for the infusion of fluids and medication but do not generally permit the removal of blood. By contrast, central venous access devices allow for both infusion and sampling of blood in a manner that does not hurt the child. Most children with central lines adjust quickly to the procedure of a simple blood draw, and even young children grow to appreciate the benefits of these devices. Compared with children who are not sick and therefore do not have a central line, the burden is relatively minimized in children for whom central access is already established. These practical issues, in general, suggest good reasons for preferentially enrolling children who are sick rather than those who are healthy in pediatric research.

But it is not enough to consider only the scientific and practical issues in subject selection. Investigators and IRBs must attend to the ethical issues. Contrary to many of the arguments reviewed above, an ethics analysis supports recruiting healthy children for nonbeneficial research. Patients participating in research often assume that the study is being conducted for their benefit (Lidz & Appelbaum, 2002). A very significant ethical advantage to conducting nonbeneficial research studies in healthy children is the fact that this would mitigate or prevent the therapeutic misconception. Children in good health and their parents are unlikely to mistake nonbeneficial research for medical treatment. The need to avoid the therapeutic misconception is one compelling argument for conducting such studies in healthy children.

A second ethical reason to favor healthy children as candidates for nonbeneficial research is the imperative to protect sick children. An argument from justice can be constructed to claim that a fair sharing of burdens and benefits points toward recruiting healthy children. Children with acute and chronic illness already experience a great deal of burden. Unlike many adult conditions related to alcohol, tobacco, or other lifestyle choices, children are almost never responsible for their illness. Ethical analysis would suggest that investigators and IRBs recognize the need for just distribution of the burdens of pediatric research. If the burden of illness is part of this calculation, policy that encourages research with healthy children may contribute to this goal. The contrary stance risks a subtle devaluing of sick children and should be discouraged (National Commission, 1977). However, protecting sick children from nontherapeutic research risk must be clearly distinguished from overly aggressive protection in the context of potentially beneficial clinical trials. A "one size fits all" approach to this complicated set of questions may unintentionally harm both healthy and sick children.

Equally dangerous, but even more seductive, is the notion that current participants in research will potentially derive some ultimate benefit by virtue of the knowledge gained from the current study. The nature of research is such that most studies do not produce "home runs" for very sick subjects; incremental progress against disease will likely come too late for their own personal benefit. Investigators must not delude themselves or their subjects into thinking that there will be ultimate benefit in exchange for participation. Those caring for and studying children may be at highest risk for this tendency, because the prospect of a child's death is so tragic and dedication to lifesaving efforts can be so powerful.

It is difficult to provide specific recommendations about the question of which children should be research subjects. Policy, IRB review, and study design should incorporate and reflect the scientific, practical, and ethical considerations discussed here and avoid blanket generalizations and categorical determinations. In the end, successful policy will likely produce a reasonable admixture of studies on children who are healthy and children who are sick, and a diverse portfolio of pediatric research. Getting there will require hard work and careful deliberation.

THE VALUE OF CASES

This book is subtitled "A Case-Based Approach" and formatted so that each chapter centers on a particular case, for several reasons. First, I am a doctor. By training and temperament, education for me has always been about cases. In clinical medical education, cases are the units through which knowledge is transmitted. Good teachers know how to use a case to make a point, and the format of this book emerges from my experience as a teacher on rounds. Second, for medical ethics to be practical, it must tell the stories of patients and subjects, of physicians and investigators. A theoretical book on pediatric research ethics might make for an excellent doctoral dissertation but would not fulfill the need for a hands-on resource to assist those who are grappling with the real issues. Finally, a format using cases paired with analysis allows for us to maximize the quality of work in this edited volume. The gifted and diverse contributors to this book had the freedom to select their own case in pediatric research ethics, giving them an opportunity to analyze issues that each finds most engaging. This strategy was designed to provide the reader with the best possible understanding of pediatric research ethics.

Narrative bioethics has recently emerged as a way to enrich the "principles"-based approach (Murray, 1997; Hunter, 1994). The foundation for this case-based approach to medical ethics is recounted in *The Abuse of Casuistry*, by Jonsen and Toulmin (1988), who provide arguments that support reasoning up from cases rather than down from principles. This book also traces the history, from popularity to decline and resurrection, of the case-based approach to ethics and moral reasoning. Of note, *The Abuse of Casuistry* had its genesis in the deliberations of the National Commission for the Protection of Human Subjects of Biomedical and Behavioral Research over the *Belmont Report*, upon which current U.S. federal regulations governing research ethics are based. Thus, it seems only appropriate to continue in this spirit with this book.

The perils of a case-based approach also deserve mention. Each chapter in this book analyzes hard questions that required answers in real time. Investigators, IRBs, parents, and children must make decisions prospectively and do not have the benefit of hindsight that the authors and readers of this book may sometimes possess. This limitation of a case-based approach must be acknowledged, but it does not mitigate the value of learning from cases. Revisiting difficult decisions that were made at a time the outcome was not known can be a very educational strategy indeed.

HOW TO USE THIS BOOK

A wide range of interested readers will find this book helpful. Students of medical ethics and those taking the NIH-required courses in research integrity may use this as a textbook or resource. Members of IRBs are charged with making many of the difficult decisions we describe in the chapters that follow. This book can serve as a guide and companion to those important deliberations. Pediatric investigators who have responsibilities for both scientific discovery and the protection of the children they study may find ideas in these cases that will illuminate the difficult challenges they may face. Similarly, pediatricians providing medical care for children are confronted with requests from older children and parents for advice about research participation. The cases and analyses in this book can be a resource for these clinicians. The book will also be a resource for pharmaceutical industry sponsors designing or conducting clinical trials involving children, and federal officials administering research policy. In summary, we hope that all individuals engaged in the delicate balancing of protecting children from research risk and assuring access to research for children will find the book useful.

Finally, we hope that this book will be of use to parents and children faced with a decision about whether to take part in research. Despite the current emphasis on risk–benefit analysis by IRBs, informed parental permission and assent represent an important aspiration for how things should be in pediatric research ethics. Although shaped by social and cultural factors, decisions such as these are ultimately personal and value driven. Children and their families respond in a wide variety of ways to questions about altruism, community, and risk. Through reading these cases and analyses, parents and older children may deepen their understanding and be empowered to make the decisions that are right for them.

This book is not intended to be a historical, legal, or regulatory document. We recognize that good ethics start with good facts. We have done our best to get the facts right and have cited sources when available. The point of this book, however, is the ethics that can be learned from the cases. This disclaimer, then, must be emphasized. Although the editor and contributors take full responsibility for the moral analysis presented here, the authenticity of the facts are only as good as the publicly available reference materials and cited scholarship we have been able to provide. Although we have done our best to get the facts right, the reader must understand both the limits we describe here and the priority given in this book to ethical analysis.

To assist students and teachers using this book in the classroom setting, each chapter includes a list of questions for discussion. These questions are found at the end of the ethical analysis at the conclusion of each chapter, prior to the references. The format for each of the following chapters, then, includes three sections: case description, ethical analysis and discussion, and questions for discussion. Some students and instructors may wish to review and discuss the questions prior to reading the ethical analysis and discussion, in order to stimulate independent thinking. Others may prefer to utilize the questions after having read the contributors' analysis of the case.

Many ethical dilemmas, almost by definition, have no "right" answer. On this basis, it is often said that doing ethics well means asking the right questions.

The questions for discussion that accompany each chapter have been developed in this spirit. The Socratic method provides a wonderful pedagogical tool for teaching medical ethics; we hope that the questions found here will engage readers and catalyze the magic of the educational process. We have provided this text, but that is only the beginning. The magic happens when you work with the text. If this book can help students to become independent askers of the right questions, it will have met this editor's definition of success.

CONCLUSION

The story never ends, but this chapter ends with Abby. When Abby looked at me and asked if she should be in the study, I did not have an easy answer. On further reflection, there are no easy answers to compelling questions like this. The best we can do is struggle to understand the question and offer the most thoughtful and compassionate best answer we can. We start to answer with words, but we must complete the response with action. Careful ethical analysis is sterile if not accompanied by moral action. Telling the story is the first step in active response, and telling the story begins to provide an answer to Abby's question.

The development of a pediatric ethics that is based on genuine respect for children and their best interests requires that the justification for pediatric research go beyond pure utilitarian motivation. The research imperative is founded on the commitment to progress, and research has become like a religion for many investigators and subjects. This may place children at risk for harm in clinical research; more important, the overwhelming power of the research imperative can quickly dominate respect for a particular child and family. Pediatric ethics depends on this respect, even if it requires that such respect come at the expense of progress against childhood diseases. Individual beneficence must take precedence over collective notions of beneficence, and the pediatric research community must remember that our responsibilities to individual children outweigh more speculative concerns about potential benefits to future generations of children. The balance shown in Figure 1.2 must never tip to favor science that benefits others over the best interests of the child-subject.

The American Academy of Pediatrics vision statement declares: "We believe in the inherent worth of all children. They are our most enduring and vulnerable legacy" (AAP, 2004). The conduct of research involving children challenges us

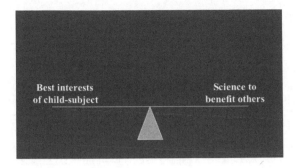

FIGURE 1.2.
Pediatric research ethics.

to confront this vision. Knowledge gained from research is part of our commitment to this legacy but must be acquired in a way that recognizes the vulnerability of children and respects their inherent worth. This book is one effort to produce work that is worthy of this vision. Ultimately, we hope this volume will provide the thoughtful guidance for pediatric research ethics that children deserve.

References

Abzug, M., & Esterl, E. (2001). Establishment of a clinical trials office at a children's hospital. *Pediatrics, 108*, 1129–1134.

Additional protections for children involved as subjects in research. (1983). *Federal Register, 48*, 114–117.

American Academy of Pediatrics Committee on Bioethics. (1995). Informed consent, parental permission, and assent in pediatric practice. *Pediatrics, 95*, 314–317.

American Academy of Pediatrics Core Vision Statement. (2004, July 27). Retrieved from http://www.aap.org/new/reachchild.pdf

Appelbaum, P. S., Roth, L. H., & Lidz, C. (1982). The therapeutic misconception: Informed consent in psychiatric research. *International Journal of Law and Psychiatry, 5*, 319–329.

Appelbaum, P. S., Roth, L. H., Lidz, C. W., Benson, P., & Winslade, W. (1987). False hopes and best data: Consent to research and the therapeutic misconception. *Hastings Center Report, 17*(2), 20–24.

Bartholome, W. G. (1995). Hearing children's voices. *Bioethics Forum, 11*(4), 3–6.

Bartholome, W. G. (1996). Ethical issues in pediatric research. In H. Y. Vanderpool (Ed.), *The ethics of research involving human subjects: Facing the 21st century* (pp. 339–370). Frederick, MD: University Publishing Group.

Baylis, F., Downie, J., & Kenny, N. (1999). Children and decisionmaking in health research. *IRB: Ethics and Human Research, 21*(4), 5–10.

Belmont Report: Ethical Principles and Guidelines for the Protection of Human Subjects of Research. (1978). Washington, DC: U.S. Government Printing Office.

Blumer, J. L. (1999). The therapeutic orphan—30 years later. *Pediatrics, 104*(3 Suppl.), 581–645.

Dickert, N., & Grady, C. (1999). What's the price of a research subject? *New England Journal of Medicine, 341*, 198–203.

Dresser, R. (2002). The ubiquity and utility of the therapeutic misconception. *Social Philosophy and Policy, 19,* 271–294.

Dresser, R. (2001). *When science offers salvation: Patient advocacy and research ethics.* New York: Oxford University Press.

Ellis, G. B., & Puglisi, J. T. (1998). *NIH policy guidance on the inclusion of children in research.* Rockville, MD: OPRR Reports, National Institutes of Health.

Emanuel, E. J., Wendler, D., & Grady, C. (2000). What makes clinical research ethical? *JAMA, 283,* 2701–2711.

Freedman, B., Fuks, A., & Weijer, C. (1993). In loco parentis: minimal risk as an ethical threshold for research upon children. *Hastings Center Report, 23*(2), 13–19.

Gidding, S. S., Camp, D., Flanagan, M. H., Kowalski, J. A., Lingl, L. L., Silverman, B. L., & Langman, C. B. (1993). A policy regarding research in healthy children. *The Journal of Pediatrics, 123,* 852–855.

Henney, J. (2000). Speech to the Annual Meeting of the Society for Pediatric Research, Boston, May 15.

Heymann, S. J. (1995). Patients in research: Not just subjects, but partners. *Science, 269,* 797–798.

Holder, A. R. (1983). Parents, courts, and refusal of treatment. *Journal of Pediatrics, 103,* 515–521.

Hunter, K. M. (1994). *Narrative and medical knowledge.* Baltimore, MD: Johns Hopkins University Press.

Ingelfinger, F. J. (1973). Ethics of experiments on children. *The New England Journal of Medicine, 288,* 791–792.

Jonsen, A. R. (1998). *The birth of bioethics.* New York: Oxford University Press.

Jonsen, A. R., & Toulmin, S. (1988). *The abuse of casuistry.* Berkeley: University of California Press.

Kodish, E. (2003a). Informed consent for pediatric research: is it really possible? *Journal of Pediatrics, 142*(2), 89–90.

Kodish, E. D. (2003b). Pediatric ethics and early-phase childhood cancer research: Conflicted goals and the prospect of benefit. *Accountability in Research, 10,* 17–25.

Lantos, J. (1999). The "inclusion benefit" in clinical trials. *Journal of Pediatrics, 134,* 130–131.

Lederer, S. E., & Grodin, M. A. (1994). Historical overview: Pediatric experimentation. In M. A. Grodin & L. H. Glantz (Eds.), *Children as research subjects: Science, ethics, and law* (pp. 3–28). New York: Oxford University Press.

Levine, R. J. (1986). *Ethics and regulation of clinical research* (2nd ed.). New Haven, CT: Yale University Press.

Lidz, C. W., & Appelbaum, P. S. (2002). The therapeutic misconception: Problems and solutions. *Medical Care, 40*(9 Suppl.), V55–V63.

McCormick, R. (1974). Proxy consent in the experimental situation. *Perspectives in Biology and Medicine, 18,* 2–20.

Miller, F. G., & Brody, H. (2003). A critique of clinical equipoise. Therapeutic misconception in the ethics of clinical trials. *Hastings Center Report, 33*(3), 19–28.

Miller, R. B. (2003). *Children, ethics, and modern medicine.* Bloomington: Indiana University Press.

Mozes-Kor, E. (1992). The Mengele twins and human experimentation: A personal account. In G. Annas and M. Grodin (Eds.), *The Nazi doctors and the Nuremberg Code* (pp. 53–60). New York: Oxford University Press.

Murray, T. H. (1997). What do we mean by "narrative ethics"? *Medical Humanities Review, 11*(2), 44–57.

National Bioethics Advisory Commission. (2001). *Ethical and policy issues in research involving human participants.* Bethesda MD: Author.

National Commission for the Protection of Human Subjects of Biomedical and Behavioral Research. (1977). *Research involving children: Report and recommendations*. DHEW Publication No. (OS) 77-0004, Appendix. DHEW Publ. No. (OS) 77-0005. Washington, DC: Author.

National Institutes of Health. (1998). *NIH policy and guidelines on the inclusion of children as participants in research involving human subjects*. Bethesda, MD : Author.

Olechnowicz, J., Eder, M., Simon, C., Zyzanski, S., & Kodish, E. (2002). Assent observed: Children's participation in leukemia treatment and research discussions. *Pediatrics, 109*(5), 806–814.

Ramsey, P. (1976). The enforcement of morals: Nontherapeutic research on children. *Hastings Center Report,* 21–30.

Ross, L. F. (2003). Do healthy children deserve greater protection in medical research? *Journal of Pediatrics, 142*, 108–112.

Shah, S., Weitman, S., Langevin, A.-M., Bernstein, M., Furman, W., & Pratt, C. (1998). Phase I therapy trials in children with cancer. *Journal of Pediatric Hematology/Oncology, 20*, 431–438.

Siegler, M. (1985). The progression of medicine. *Archives of Internal Medicine, 145*, 713–715.

U.S. Department of Health and Human Services. (1983, March 8). 45 Code of Federal Regulations 46. Subpart D—Additional protection for children involved as subjects in research. *Federal Register, 48*, 9818.

U.S. Department of Health and Human Services. (1997, August). FDA proposes to require pediatric data prior to drug and biologic product approvals. *HHS News,* pp. 1–3.

U.S. Food and Drug Administration. (2004, February 27). *One Hundred Seventh Congress: Best Pharmaceuticals for Children Act* Washington, D.C.: Author. Retrieved from http://www.fda.gov/cder/pediatric/#bpca July 27, 2004.

Veatch, R. M. (1981). *A theory of medical ethics*. New York: Basic Books.

Wendler, D., Shah, S., Whittle, A., & Wilfond, B. S. (2003). Nonbeneficial research with individuals who cannot consent: Is it ethically better to enroll healthy or affected individuals? *IRB: Ethics and Human Research, 25*(4), 1–4.

Williams, W. C. (1932). *The doctor stories*. New York: New Directions Books.

I

Research Involving Healthy Children

2

Evaluating Benefits and Harms in Research on Healthy Children

Paul B. Miller and Charles Weijer

This chapter provides a case-based illustration of institutional review board (IRB) evaluation of the benefits and harms of research involving healthy children. We commence with a case description of a controversial study of airway hypoxia in healthy infants. Then, in the ethical analysis and discussion that follows, we identify issues raised by this study and explain why the relevant federal regulations require a conceptual framework for IRB implementation. We then provide a brief overview of component analysis, a systematic conceptual framework for IRB evaluation of benefits and harms in research. Next, we appeal to the airway hypoxia study to explain the implementation of component analysis, and illustrate that it usefully directs and governs IRB evaluation of research. Finally, we reflect further on the limitations of component analysis and its important contribution to effective IRB review.

CASE DESCRIPTION

A controversial study of airway hypoxia in infants (Parkins, Poets, O'Brien, Stebbens, & Southall, 1998) serves well to illustrate the challenges that IRBs face when evaluating the benefits and harms of research involving healthy children. The researchers in the study sought to investigate physiological responses to airway hypoxia (low oxygen) in infants. The question was: What happens to infants who are exposed to oxygen levels lower than the normal 21% fraction of inspired oxygen that exists in room air? The study was conducted on the basis of evidence suggesting that airway hypoxia, brought on by such circumstances as intercontinental air travel, may be associated with severe respiratory distress and sudden death in infants. Stimulated by reports of two infant deaths from sudden infant death syndrome (SIDS) shortly after intercontinental air travel, researchers hoped that the study would provide further insight on "the physiological effects of airway hypoxia on respiratory function in infants" (Parkins et al., 1998, p. 887).

29

The study included 34 healthy infants whose mean age was 3.1 months. Twenty-one infants were recruited from an obstetrics unit run by family practitioners. Thirteen infants were recruited by approaching families who were receiving support in caring for an infant after a sibling had died of SIDS. All infants were born at term and without history of respiratory distress or congenital anomalies. No infant in the study had a history of an apparent life-threatening event.

Parents of potential study participants were sent a letter explaining the scientific interest, purpose, and methods of the study. Those who responded with interest were provided with further information verbally, either in person or by telephone. The researchers noted in particular that "information was presented to parents on the relation between the administration of 15% oxygen and airline flights, holidays at altitude, and sudden infant death syndrome" (Parkins et al., 1998, p. 888). Importantly, the researchers say that the parents "knew that [there was] a small risk of sudden death" (Southall, Poets, O'Brien, Stebbens, & Parkins, 1998, p. 893). Parents were also informed of their right to withdraw their child from the study at any time.

The study itself involved prechallenge, challenge, and postchallenge measurement of oxygenation levels and the frequency of apnea. During each of the three phases of the study, pulse and oxygen saturation were measured transcutaneously, and respirations were measured with a volume expansion capsule placed on the abdominal wall. During the challenge phase, the infant was placed in an oxygen tent and a mixture of oxygen (15%) and nitrogen (85%) was provided. During this phase, additional measurements were taken. Respired oxygen and carbon dioxide levels were measured with a cannula placed on the upper lip, and blood carbon dioxide levels were measured transcutaneously. More invasive measurements, such as electroencephalogram, electro-oculogram, and quantifying ventilation were decided against, in part, because they would interfere with normal sleep patterns of the infant.

The prechallenge, challenge, and postchallenge phases of the study took place over two nights. The infant's mother was present at all times. The prechallenge phase took place in the infant's home and lasted an average 7.7 hours. Baseline values for oxygen saturation and respiratory variables were collected. Infants with oxygen saturation levels less than 94% were removed from the study for safety reasons. The challenge and postchallenge phases took place one or more nights later in hospital and close to the intensive care unit. In the challenge phase, which lasted 6.3 hours on average, infants were placed in an oxygen tent in which the fraction of inspired oxygen was 15%. Infants and monitors were continuously observed by an experienced pediatrician. Infants were removed from the oxygen tent if their oxygen saturation fell to 80% or less for 1 minute or more. Immediately after the challenge session, the postchallenge recording session commenced, in which the response of infants to return to room air (21% FI O_2: Fraction of Inspired Oxygen) was measured. Postchallenge recordings lasted the duration of the night, on average, 4.5 hours.

Responses to airway hypoxia were variable and unpredictable. None of the 34 infants that met the study eligibility criteria were withdrawn during the prechallenge phase. Six of 34 infants had the challenge phase of the study terminated, four of whom had prolonged oxygen desaturation in response to hypoxia. However, no significant differences were observed between infants with and without a family history of SIDS. Parents of children who were withdrawn from the challenge phase were advised not to expose their infant to high altitude until the infant reached the age of 1 year. One infant died suddenly 3 weeks after the study, but its cause of death was ultimately determined to be homicide rather than SIDS.

ETHICAL ANALYSIS AND DISCUSSION

The Underdetermination of Research Regulation

Research on healthy children has been the subject of considerable controversy of late (Friedman Ross, 2002, 2003; Glantz, 2002; Kopelman, 2002; Mastroianni & Kahn, 2002), much of it stirred by the judgment of the Maryland Court of Appeals in *Grimes v. Kennedy Krieger Institute* (2001). Ostensibly, much of the concern has centered on the ethical and legal issues associated with the exposure of healthy children to risk solely for research purposes. The fundamental question, which many commentators propose to explore and, in some cases, answer is: to how much risk, if any, may healthy children be exposed in research that does not offer them the prospect of therapeutic benefit?

That said, the current debate reads in a disjointed and confusing way. This is because different subsets of questions arise depending on which of the fundamental *Belmont Report* principles (respect for persons, beneficence, or justice); (National Commission, 1979) one adopts as one's starting point, and from what perspective one investigates their application to the conduct of research (e.g., the perspective of children, parents, physician-researchers, institutions, or IRBs). Further confusion is generated by the fact that, on top of differences of moral principle and perspective, various legal and regulatory mechanisms and standards are applicable to the conduct of the various parties involved in research involving healthy children.

From a generally disjointed debate, certain core questions have emerged and received sustained attention. First and foremost are questions concerning the extent of parents' decision-making authority given the special moral and legal status of the parent–child relationship. Parents are widely understood to be morally and legally obliged to make decisions in their children's best interests. To what extent, if at all, consistent with these duties may they authorize their children's involvement in risky but socially beneficial activities, including research? Ought the child's best interests be understood broadly, to encompass the development of moral character, or narrowly, in terms of physical and psychological health and well-being?

Also subject of considerable attention have been a range of questions concerning the potential for injustice associated with the involvement of healthy children in research. Some are of the view that it is inherently exploitative to allow healthy children to shoulder the risks of an endeavor the benefits of which will largely accrue to others. Others argue that by enabling limited involvement of healthy children in research an injustice is mitigated to the extent that children who suffer illness are provided relief from risks associated with participation in research.

These questions all engage, on some level, the acceptability of imposing risk on healthy children without compensatory therapeutic benefit. Yet, distinct questions concerning standards of acceptable risk have been neglected in analyses primarily concerned with issues of justice and the limits of parental discretion. Key among these are questions concerning the process and standards according to which IRBs ought to assess the benefits and harms associated with research involving children.

IRBs are charged with a broad mandate of protecting the rights and welfare of human subjects of research. In fulfillment of this mandate, they ensure that researchers comply with the *Belmont Report* principles and derivative regulations, including special regulatory norms relating to research involving children. IRBs fail to meet their mandate if they do not confront and resolve outstanding issues relating to the scope of parental decision making, and the potential for exploitation of child research subjects. That said, the principle of beneficence requires that IRBs evaluate the acceptability of the benefits and harms of research. Our analysis focuses on how IRBs ought to conduct this evaluation.

In fairness, it should be noted that some commentators have subjected to extensive treatment questions concerning IRB evaluation of risks of research involving healthy children (Friedman Ross, 2002, 2003; Kopelman, 2002). However, almost invariably these accounts focus on studies involving healthy children as a means by which to highlight already well-known conceptual and practical difficulties faced by IRBs in assessing risk under existing federal regulation. These accounts leave open the question under what conditions IRBs may deem risks posed to healthy children in research acceptable.

The Common Rule instructs IRBs to ensure that (1) "risks to subjects are minimized" and (2) "risks to subjects are reasonable in relation to anticipated benefits, if any, to subjects, and the importance of the knowledge that may be reasonably expected to result" (45 CFR 46.111 (a)(1,2)). But how precisely are IRBs to do this? The answer is not obvious because regulations are not self-interpreting. In the absence of a conceptual framework for the ethical analysis of benefits and harms in research, IRBs fall back upon the vagaries of moral intuition in order to implement these rules. Predictably, reliance on intuition results in inconsistent decisions within and among IRBs (Shah, Whittle, Wilfond, Gensler, & Wendler, 2004). Further, intuition will tend to rupture when difficult cases, such as the case under discussion, are encountered. Indeed, in the absence of a conceptual framework, it is difficult to see how the IRB can effectively fulfill its mandate. The National Bioethics Advisory Commission (2002) came to the same conclusion:

> [An] IRB's assessment of the risks and potential benefits of research is central to determining whether a research study is ethically acceptable. Yet, this assessment can be a difficult one to make, as there are no clear criteria for IRBs to use in judging whether the risks of research are reasonable in terms of what might be gained by the individual or society. (p. 13)

If IRB decision making is to be principled, a conceptual framework for the ethical analysis of benefits and harms in research is required. A successful framework must answer questions that flow directly from the text of the Common Rule:

1. Which risks to subjects must be minimized?
2. To what extent must they be minimized?
3. Which risks and which benefits enter into the second requirement, that is, that "risks to subjects are reasonable in relation to anticipated bene-fits"?
4. How does one determine that risks are reasonable in relation to benefits to subjects?
5. How does one determine that risks are reasonable in relation to knowl-edge that may be reasonably expected to result?

Component Analysis

A conceptual framework for IRB evaluation of benefits and harms in research called component analysis has recently been proposed (Weijer, 2000). It answers the questions stemming from the Common Rule and to our knowledge is the only systematic framework for the ethical analysis of research benefits and harms con-sistent with federal regulation. It was endorsed by the U.S. National Bioethics Advisory Commission in its final report, *Ethical and Policy Issues in Research*

Involving Human Participants (2000), and by a variety of commentators (Burke, 2002; Clarke, 2002; Emanuel, Wendler, & Grady, 2000).

Component analysis relies upon the understanding of research benefit and harm of the National Commission for the Protection of Human Subjects of Biomedical and Behavioral Research. Benefit is defined as a favorable outcome, harm as an adverse outcome, and risk as the probability and magnitude of an adverse outcome. Importantly, benefits and harms are taken not merely to refer to physical outcomes. Rather, benefits and harms are appropriately understood as concepts broad in scope, encompassing physical, psychological, social, and economic outcomes (Levine, 1988).

The fundamental insight of component analysis is recognition of the fact that clinical research may contain a mixture of interventions administered with differing purposes and warrant.[1] Therapeutic procedures, such as drug, surgical, or behavioral interventions, are administered with therapeutic warrant, that is, on the basis of evidence that the intervention may benefit individual research participants. Nontherapeutic procedures, on the other hand, such as venipuncture for pharmacokinetic drug levels, imaging procedures or questionnaires not used in clinical practice, are administered without therapeutic warrant and solely to answer the scientific question at hand. As therapeutic procedures hold out the prospect of benefit for study participants and nontherapeutic procedures do not, separate moral calculi are required for IRB assessment of the legitimacy of each type of study procedure (Freedman, Fuks, & Weijer, 1992).

Therapeutic procedures are assessed according to the standard of clinical equipoise (Freedman, 1987a). Clinical equipoise is a research-friendly response to the question: when is a physician morally permitted to offer enrollment in a clinical trial to his or her patient? Clinical equipoise answers this question as follows: the physician may do so when the administration of the various therapeutic procedures in a clinical trial is consistent with competent medical care. Clinical equipoise formalizes this requirement as condition for IRB approval[2] as follows: the IRB must certify that at the outset of a trial there exists a state of honest, professional disagreement in the community of expert practitioners as to the preferred treatment (Freedman, 1987a). Procedurally, in making this determination, the IRB does not survey practitioners. Rather, the IRB scrutinizes the study justification, reviews relevant literature, and, where appropriate, consults with independent clinical experts.[3] Clinical equipoise is satisfied if the IRB concludes that the evidence supporting the various therapeutic procedures is sufficient that, were the evidence widely known, expert clinicians would disagree as to the preferred treatment for the condition.

Nontherapeutic procedures do not, by definition, offer the prospect of therapeutic benefit to study participants. When assessing risks associated with nontherapeutic procedures, the IRB must ensure that two standards are met: (1) nontherapeutic risks must be minimized consistent with sound scientific design and (2) such risks must be reasonable in relation to the knowledge that may be gained from the study. The IRB implements the first standard by eliminating unnecessary nontherapeutic procedures and by requiring, where feasible, the substitution of "procedures already being performed on the subjects for diagnostic and treatment purposes" (45 CFR 46.111 (a)(1)(ii)). The implementation of the second standard requires that the IRB judge the study's scientific value sufficient to justify risks to subjects (Weijer, 1998). Since this judgment involves an appraisal of scientific priorities in social context, IRB membership should include community representatives (Freedman, 1987b).

When research involves a vulnerable population such as children, an important additional protection is applied under component analysis. Risks associated with nontherapeutic procedures are limited to a "minor increase over minimal risk." This standard requires that IRBs ensure that nontherapeutic risks posed to children in research are no more than a minor increase over the risks "ordinarily encountered in daily life" (45 CFR 46.406(a), 102(i)). To determine whether this standard is met by a particular study, the IRB reasons by analogy (Freedman, Fuks, & Weijer 1993). It must determine that the nontherapeutic risks posed are in fact the same as those encountered in daily life, for instance, "during the performance of routine physical or psychological examinations or tests," or that they are sufficiently similar to such risks (45 CFR 102(i)). The risk threshold aims to protect the welfare interests of children in research through shielding them from atypical levels of risk, while allowing important research to proceed. It remains controversial whether the referent for minimal risk ought to be the daily lives of healthy or sick children (Kopelman, 1981; Miller & Weijer, 2000).

Applying Component Analysis

Returning to the airway hypoxia study, we are now in a position to ask whether study participation poses an acceptable balance of benefits to harms. Recall that the study involved exposing healthy infants to a variety of procedures:

- Exposure to 15% oxygen in an oxygen tent (challenge phase)
- Transcutaneous measurement of pulse and oxygen saturation (prechallenge, challenge, and postchallenge phases)
- Measurement of respirations with a volume expansion capsule placed on the abdominal wall (prechallenge, challenge, and postchallenge phases)
- Measurement of respired oxygen and carbon dioxide with a cannula placed on the upper lip (challenge phase)

• Transcutaneous measurement of blood carbon dioxide levels (challenge phase)

Under component analysis, the first stage of IRB evaluation of research benefits and harms involves demarcation of therapeutic and nontherapeutic study procedures. It seems clear that none of the procedures in this study are administered with therapeutic warrant. No claims of potential therapeutic benefit to study participants are made by the investigators (nor would such claims be accepted by the IRB due to lack of evidence to substantiate them). Further, the study involves healthy children and does not involve the administration of a preventative therapy, such as a vaccine. Since the study involves no therapeutic procedure, the study interventions listed above are all nontherapeutic procedures. Thus in this case, as is usually the case in research involving healthy children, the IRB's task of benefit-harm analysis is simplified. The IRB must ensure that risks of nontherapeutic procedures are (1) minimized consistent with sound scientific design, (2) reasonable in relation to knowledge to be gained, and (3) no more than a minor increase over minimal risk.

We take it as obvious that the contentious intervention in this study is exposure of infants to hypoxic conditions (15% oxygen in an oxygen tent). Are the risks associated with this procedure minimized consistent with sound scientific design? A variety of steps were taken in this study to minimize risk from airway hypoxia to subjects. As our analysis is limited to the final publication of the study, it is difficult to know whether these efforts were undertaken by the investigators of their own initiative or were required by the IRB. First, alternative study methods were considered with an eye to the risks posed to subjects. Recall that the study was prompted by an apparent association between airline travel and SIDS deaths. One might have expected the study to be carried out on infants on trans-Atlantic flights or in a hypobaric chamber. Only under these conditions is the reduction in alveolar oxygen pressure due to reduced barometric pressure. The former possibility was rejected on grounds of feasibility; the latter was rejected on grounds of safety. The possibility of carrying out the study in a hypobaric chamber was rejected because "this would cause difficulties in monitoring the infants, and might increase the risks to the infants because of difficulties in access" (Southall et al., 1998, p. 893). Thus, the study was carried out using an intervention to reduce the alveolar oxygen pressure through a different mechanism, namely, a reduced fraction of inspired oxygen. This step was consistent with sound scientific design since there is no "data to suggest that there is a difference between a reduction in alveolar oxygen pressure due to reduced barometric pressure or due to a reduced fraction of inspired oxygen during constant atmospheric pressure" (Parkins et al., 1998, p. 890). Thus, carrying out the study in an oxygen tent rather than a hypobaric chamber minimized risks to infants consistent with sound study design.

Second, infants who may have been at undue risk from study participation were excluded. Infants with a history of respiratory distress or congenital abnormalities were excluded from study participation as they may have been at increased risk of an adverse event from exposure to airway hypoxia. Infants with a history of an apparent life-threatening event were also excluded from study participation. Several infants with this history were screened and found to have abnormally low baseline values of blood oxygen saturation. It was concluded that it would not be safe to expose any infant with this history to airway hypoxia. Further, during the prechallenge phase all infants were screened to ensure that their baseline blood oxygen saturation levels were greater than or equal to 94%. Thus, risks to subjects were minimized by excluding subjects for whom exposure to airway hypoxia constituted an undue risk (Weijer & Fuks, 1994).

Third, steps were taken to ensure the early detection and effective treatment of adverse outcomes. The challenge phase of the study was carried out in hospital and close to the intensive care unit to ensure that infants could be rapidly and definitively treated for any adverse event. Further, infants were carefully monitored for the following variables: respiration, pulse, blood oxygen saturation, blood carbon dioxide, respired oxygen, and respired carbon dioxide. Infants were removed from the oxygen tent if oxygen saturation fell to 80% or less for at least 1 minute. Also, infants and monitors were constantly observed by an experienced pediatrician. Finally, parents of infants who were withdrawn from the study due to a prolonged desaturation were advised not to expose their child to air travel until at least one year of age. Thus, risks to subjects were minimized by taking steps to detect and treat adverse events.

Aside from these steps taken to minimize risks from airway hypoxia, steps were also taken to minimize risks from the various monitoring interventions. We are told that investigators decided against more invasive monitoring techniques, including electroencephalogram, electro-oculogram, and quantifying ventilation, so as not to interfere with normal sleep patterns of the infants. While this step reduced risk to infants, it also limited the ability of the study to determine the cause of observed hypoxemia and thereby limited the scientific value of the research. Such compromises are often necessary to balance the protection of children from research risk against the imperative to produce generalizable knowledge.

It is clear, therefore, that significant efforts were undertaken in this study to ensure that risks to research subjects were minimized consistent with sound scientific design. Alternative study interventions that posed less risk to subjects were considered and implemented. Also, subjects who were at undue risk of an adverse outcome were excluded from study participation. Further, steps were taken to ensure that adverse events could be detected early and treated effectively. Finally, respiratory and cardiac variables were monitored with noninvasive rather than invasive means. Thus, we believe that an IRB reviewing the study could reasonably conclude that risks to study subjects were minimized consistent with sound scientific design.

The next step is for the IRB to determine whether risks are reasonable in relation to knowledge to be gained. Even if risks to subjects are minimized, a study may be unacceptable if nontherapeutic risks to subjects are excessive, or the study question is without sufficient merit or significance. According to the information presented by the investigators, the risks associated with exposing infants to airway hypoxia are not fully understood. The investigators were aware of two children who died of SIDS between 14 and 41 hours after a transatlantic flight. British Airways further reported to the investigators the death of one infant on a flight between London and Hong Kong. Infants born at high altitude have higher than predicted levels of blood oxygen saturation due to genetic adaptation. Infants who are moved to high altitude have low levels of oxygen saturation and experience a disproportionately high rate of sudden death in the period immediately following the move. Nonetheless, as the investigators point out, "[m]any infants traveling on airplanes or to holidays at high altitude are exposed to similar or even more markedly reduced partial pressures of inspired oxygen. Yet this exposure is considered safe" (Parkins et al., 1998, p. 890). The risks of monitoring respiratory and cardiac variables transcutaneously and via a cannula on the upper lip are known to be very small. Nonetheless, the IRB will want to ensure that these devices are safe for use in young infants.

What of the knowledge likely to be gained as a result of the study? The questions motivating the airway hypoxia study are important. The investigators document considerable gaps in scientific evidence on the harms associated with airway hypoxia for healthy infants, and explain the partial, but significant extent to which the study would fill the existing evidentiary void. The relative social priority of this study is also high. Given that infants are commonly exposed to reduced oxygen levels through respiratory infections and air and ground travel at high altitude, it is a matter of no small importance that sound scientific evidence of the effect on infants of exposure to reduced oxygen levels be generated. The authors acknowledge that the study does not answer all significant outstanding scientific questions concerning airway hypoxia in healthy infants. In particular, further research in which the conditions of exposure to reduced oxygen on prolonged flights and vacations at high altitude are emulated is required. The researchers also note that the study was not designed in such a way as to identify the underlying mechanisms of observed physiologic responses of infants to reduced oxygen.

The determination of whether the study's risks are adequately counterbalanced by the importance of the knowledge to be gained is a matter for the IRB's judgment. As the determination relies on assessment of not only scientific but also the broader social value of the study, input from community members is especially important. In this case, the risks presented by study participation are nontrivial and include a small but unquantified risk of death. The study seems likely, however, to generate information of considerable scientific and social importance. We believe therefore that an IRB could reasonably conclude that this study poses risks that are reasonable in relation to the knowledge to be gained.

The final step in IRB analysis of the benefits and risks of the airway hypoxia study is to determine whether the risks are no more than a minor increase over minimal risk. To determine whether this criterion is satisfied the IRB reasons by analogy. It must determine that the risks posed by the study are the same as those encountered in daily life, for instance, "during the performance of routine physical or psychological examinations or tests," or that they are sufficiently similar to such risks. Risks of daily life for children vary from place to place and from time to time. So then the question is what are the risks of daily life for healthy children in the United Kingdom currently? These risks certainly include going to the shop with their mother, driving in a car, and a check up by the pediatrician. These are risks that every child or the great majority of children encounter routinely. As the study exposed infants to airway hypoxia comparable to that of trans-Atlantic air travel, is this a risk of daily life? While this is an empirical question, our suspicion is that only a minority of infants are ever taken on a trans-Atlantic flight. The risks of air travel for children are likely not much different than the risks of other forms of travel. So we might ask more broadly whether infants are commonly taken on any sort of long trip. A majority of infants likely are.

But long trips are surely not undertaken daily, does this rule them out as a risk of daily life? Not necessarily. The routine physical examinations carried out in a pediatrician's office would like occur only a few times in the first year of life, and yet these are considered a risk of daily life. A risk of daily life may be posed by an activity undertaken by all or a majority of infants on a daily basis, or by an activity undertaken by all or a majority of infants less frequently provided that the risks posed are roughly *interchangeable* with those of activities carried out more commonly. Risks of daily life may productively be thought of as referring to a fairly constant background level of risk accepted by responsible parents on behalf of their infants and accepted by society in general. It seems to us that reasonable people could disagree about whether lengthy trips, including air travel, fall within or outside of this "fairly constant background level of risk." But the moral standard here is not minimal risk, but a minor increase over minimal risk. This higher threshold seems designed to allow for new and slightly riskier experiences. Just as responsible parents are given latitude by society to allow their children to be exposed to new and slightly riskier experiences, so to the IRB ought to allow children to be exposed to risks of nontherapeutic procedures that are a minor increase over minimal risk. Intercontinental air travel, or in this study, carefully monitored airway hypoxia, seems to be just this kind of activity.

However, this point, while valid, is not in itself determinative. While the risks of daily life are normative in a very important sense, they ought not be viewed as setting an unimpeachable standard. Uncommonly, activities may be undertaken routinely in daily life despite the existence of convincing evidence that such activities in fact pose undue risk. This possibility highlights the importance of the IRB assuming the perspective of the reasonable parent informed of the material facts. The IRB may therefore agree that a risk is commonly undertaken but reject its conformity with the minimal risk standard because of evidence that it *ought not* be commonly undertaken. In the case of the airway hypoxia study, as discussed in detail above, the evidence on the risks posed by airway hypoxia are inconclusive. Prior to the study, there was no evidence to rebut the presumption, acted upon in daily life, that exposing infants to reduced oxygen levels for significant but temporary intervals is relatively harmless. Thus, an IRB reviewing the hypoxia study under component analysis would appropriately find the challenge and monitoring procedures to pose less than a minor increase over minimal risk.

Under component analysis, the question whether a study involving healthy children poses an acceptable balance of benefits to harms breaks down into three questions. Have risks associated with nontherapeutic procedures been minimized consistent with sound scientific design? Are these risks reasonable in relation to the knowledge to be gained? And are the risks no more than a minor increase over minimal risk? We have shown that an IRB might reasonably answer in the affirmative to each of these questions. Thus, we conclude that the airway hypoxia study poses an acceptable balance of benefits to harms to subjects.

Further Reflection

The airway hypoxia study is an apt choice for demonstrating the use of component analysis for IRB analysis of the benefits and harms of research involving healthy children. As it involves the imposition of an intervention (airway hypoxia) with a small but unquantified risk of death on a vulnerable population (infants), it is precisely the sort of case in which moral intuition will tend to rupture. One might predict that in this sort of case strong feelings about the ethics of the study will conflict. Some motivated by a desire to protect infants from research which poses a risk of death will believe the study unethical. Others moved by the prospect of important scientific findings will deem the study ethical. In the absence of a conceptual framework for the ethical analysis of benefits and harms in research we are at an impasse. Intuitions about this case collide, and we have no way to move forward.

The ethical principle of beneficence is understood as requiring that we do no harm and maximize potential benefit while minimizing risk. Component analysis provides the procedure necessary to apply this moral principle to research on healthy children and other populations. As research on healthy children that does not involve a preventive intervention generally does not involve therapeutic interventions, the relevant moral standards are those that apply to nontherapeutic procedures. Thus, the question as to whether the study poses potential benefits that outweigh the risks is broken down into three discrete subquestions. First, have risks to subjects been minimized consistent with sound scientific design? Second, are study risks reasonable in relation to the knowledge to be gained? Third, are the risks posed no more than a minor increase over minimal risk? Only if all three questions are answered in the affirmative may we conclude that study benefits outweigh harms.

In our assessment of the airway hypoxia study, despite the strong intuitions of some to the contrary, each of the standards set by component analysis is met. One might ask: What is the relationship between moral principles and moral intuitions? We view them as having a reflexive relationship. Moral principles help refine our intuitions; while moral intuitions point out where principles require change. Of course, the difficulty in any particular case of conflict between the two is to know which is correct and which is in need of change. Generally, sound principles accord with intuition across a broad range of cases, and discord is limited to a small number of cases acknowledged a priori to be difficult. In our experience, component analysis functions very well across a diverse range of cases encountered in research ethics. Thus, we believe that the proper response for those whose intuitions differ with our analysis is to see that their intuitions have led them astray and are in need of change.

Having said this, some limitations of component analysis must be acknowledged. First, satisfaction of component analysis does not mean that a study as a whole is approvable. IRBs are charged with the social oversight of research. This task is guided by three ethical principles: respect for persons, beneficence, and justice. As component analysis only guides the IRB's implementation of the principle of beneficence, other aspects of the study may raise moral problems. Thus, a study with an acceptable benefit to harm ratio may pose problems with respect to consent, confidentiality, or selection of subjects. On the basis of these concerns, the IRB may determine that the study is to be rejected for its failure to fulfill the requirements of the principles of respect for persons or justice.

Second, component analysis involves the analysis of benefits and harms for defined groups, not individual research subjects. In conducting risk evaluation under component analysis, IRBs assess research harms and benefits in light of available scientific evidence, and what is known about the study population as defined by eligibility criteria. IRBs thus make differentiated, but still rather general risk judgments. If they conclude that a given procedure is acceptable for a defined population of healthy children, this does not mean it is so for each child who may be approached for participation. Thus, even though an IRB may conclude that the airway hypoxia study poses an acceptable balance of benefit to harms in general, a particular infant may be excluded because study participation poses undue risk to that infant. For example, the researcher and parents may deem participation inadvisable because the infant has done more intercontinental air travel than is considered routine.

Third, component analysis sets standards only for the IRB and does not set independent moral standards for parents or researchers. Indeed, a range of other parties are involved in the conduct of research and they operate under distinct moral and legal duties.[4] Researchers must conduct research in conformity with applicable federal regulations including the Common Rule. They must also act within bounds established by law, including tort and criminal prohibitions against negligent conduct, fraud, and nonconsensual physical interference. Researchers must also abide by professional codes of ethical conduct. Researchers are bound by trust-based obligations to investigate fully the circumstances of individual subjects approached for participation in approved research, and provide full and frank disclosure of all material information to parents to assist them in discharging their own obligations with respect to decision making on behalf of their children. In the case of the airway hypoxia study, for example, a researcher may decide to decline enrollment of a child, despite IRB approval and parental consent, out of concern for the motivation of the infant's parents to enroll the child.

Parents also have well-established moral and legal obligations, specifically obligations to care for their children. They must exercise discretion and act only in the best interests of their children. In its review of research on healthy children, the IRB adopts the perspective of the responsible parent informed of materials risks. It remains the case, however, that within bounds of the law parents have ultimate authority and responsibility for making decisions on behalf of their children. This is true for research participation as for other organized activities of social life. IRB approval suggests only that participation in a particular study represents a reasonable choice given what is known about the study population. It is for parents to decide, through consultation with researchers, whether participation is in their own child's best interests given their value system, the particular medical history of the child, their present psychological state, stage of development, and so on. In the case of the airway hypoxia study, some parents may decide that while risks posed are no more than a minor increase over minimal risk, they are unacceptable for their child.

Acknowledging these limitations, we feel that component analysis fills an important gap in research ethics literature and policy. Despite the considerable strides made in other areas of research ethics, the ethical analysis of study benefits and harms has long been underdeveloped. This situation has left IRBs with little or no guidance in the application of key aspects of federal regulation. Led only by intuition, IRBs have been beleaguered by inconsistency and the rupture of intuition when faced with difficult cases. Component analysis promises to remedy this situation. It provides IRBs with a principled approach to the ethical analysis of study benefits and harms that systematizes a central aspect of research review. As demonstrated by our analysis of the airway hypoxia study, it provides the IRB with a workable framework that illuminates the review of difficult and contentious studies.

Questions for Discussion

1. Is risky nontherapeutic research involving infants ever justified? If so, how can you defend against the argument that such research constitutes child abuse?

2. Is it proper to weigh the scientific value and knowledge to be gained from a study against risks that accrue to individual subjects? Does the fact that adults can make this assessment for themselves but parents must decide on behalf of young children change your answer to this question? What are some ways to assure that subject selection is equitable?

3. Were the infants who had a sibling that died of SIDS more or less appropriate as research subjects for this study? Explain your answer.

4. If you served on an IRB presented with this protocol, how would the inclusion of $200 as compensation per enrolled infant (to parents or physicians) affect your judgment about the study?

5. Given the facts of the study as presented in the chapter, do you think the study should have been approved?

6. If you were a parent approached to permit your child to be enrolled, what considerations would influence your decision?

7. How does component analysis facilitate clear thinking about the ethics of human subject research? What are the potential flaws in this kind of analysis?

Notes

1. The ethical analysis of risk.
2. Note that clinical equipoise is an essential, but only preliminary and partial answer to this question. IRBs are charged with ensuring only the satisfaction of ethical and regulatory standards for the protection of defined populations (the population from whom subjects may be drawn, as defined by inclusion and exclusion criteria). Clinical equipoise is an appropriate standard for IRB evaluation of the acceptability of therapeutic procedures, to the extent that it directs the attention of the IRB to evidence as to relative therapeutic merit for proposed and available therapeutic procedures, given the characteristics of a defined group. Yet satisfaction of clinical equipoise is not sufficient if it is understood as a condition justifying individual physicians' offer of trial enrollment to particular patients. It is insufficient to the extent that patients entrust physicians to make treatment recommendations on the basis of their appraisal of available scientific evidence and patient-specific evidence, including patient histories, contraindications, complicating conditions, and ongoing observation of side effects. Individual physicians may offer initial and ongoing trial enrollment to individual subjects only where they are in *patient-specific equipoise*, that is, genuinely uncertain as to the relative merit of therapeutic procedures under study, in light of clinically significant evidence as to their patient's treatment needs. See Miller and Weijer (2003).
3. The ethical analysis of risk.
4. For a more detailed review of the different responsibilities of various parties involved in research involving children, see Miller and Kenny (2002).

References

Burke, R. (2002). Minimal risk: The debate goes on. *Critical Care Medicine, 30,* 1180–1181.

Clarke, P. A. (2002). Placebo surgery for Parkinson's disease: Do the benefits outweigh the risks? *Journal of Law, Medicine & Ethics, 30,* 58.

Emanuel, E. J., Wendler, D., & Grady, C. (2000). What makes clinical research ethical? *JAMA, 283,* 2701–2711.

Freedman, B. (1987a). Equipoise and the ethics of clinical research. *New England Journal of Medicine, 317,* 141–145.

Freedman, B. (1987b). Scientific value and validity as ethical requirements for research. *IRB: A Review of Human Subjects Research, 9,* 7–10.

Freedman, B., Fuks, A., & Weijer, C. (1992). Demarcating research and treatment: A systematic approach for the analysis of the ethics of clinical research. *Clinical Research, 40,* 653–660.

Freedman, B., Fuks, A., & Weijer, C. (1993). *In loco parentis:* Minimal risk as an ethical threshold for research upon children. *Hastings Center Report, 23*(2), 13–19.

Friedman Ross, L. (2002). In defense of the Hopkins Lead Abatement Studies. *Journal of Law, Medicine & Ethics, 30,* 50–57.

Friedman Ross, L. (2003). Do healthy children deserve greater protection in medical research? *Journal of Pediatrics, 142,*108–112.

Glantz, L. H. (2002). Nontherapeutic research with children: Grimes v. Kennedy Krieger Institute. *American Journal of Public Health, 92,* 1070–1073.

Grimes v. Kennedy Krieger Institute Inc. 782 A.2d 807 (Md. 2001).

Kopelman, L. (1981). Estimating risk in human research. *Clinical Research, 29,* 1–8.

Kopelman, L. (2002). Pediatric research regulations: *Grimes* narrows their interpretation. *Journal of Law, Medicine & Ethics, 30,* 38–49.

Levine, R. J. (1988). *Ethics and regulation of clinical research* (2nd ed.). New Haven, CT: Yale University Press.

Mastroianni, A. C., & Kahn, J. P. (2002). Risk and responsibility: Ethics, Grimes v. Kennedy Krieger, and public health research involving children. *American Journal of Public Health, 92,* 1073–1076.

Miller, P. B., & Kenny, N. P. (2002). Walking the moral tightrope: Respecting and protecting children in health-related research. *Cambridge Quarterly of Healthcare Ethics, 11,* 217–229.

Miller, P. B., & Weijer, C. (2000). Moral solutions in assessing research risk. *IRB: A Review of Human Subjects Research, 22*(5), 6–10.

Miller, P. B., & Weijer, C. (2003). Rehabilitating equipoise. *Kennedy Institute of Ethics Journal, 13,* 93–118.

National Commission for the Protection of Human Subjects of Biomedical and Behavioral Research. (1979, April 18). The Belmont report: Ethical principles and guidelines for the protection of human subjects of research. *OPRR Reports,* pp. 1–8.

Parkins, K. J., et al. (1998.) Effect of exposure to 15% oxygen on breathing patterns and oxygen saturation in infants: Interventional study. *British Medical Journal, 316,* 887–890.

Shah, S., Whittle, A., Wilfond, B., Gensler, G., & Wendler, D. (2004). How do institutional review boards apply the federal risk and benefit standards for pediatric research? *JAMA, 291,* 494–496.

Southall, D., Poets, C. F., O'Brien, L. M., Stebbens, V.A., & Parkins, K. J. (1998). Authors' reply. *British Medical Journal, 316,* 893–894.

National Bioethics Advisory Commission. (2000, June 11). *Ethical and policy issues in research involving human participants.* Retrieved from http://bioethics.Georgetown.edu/nbac/human/overvol1.html.

Weijer, C. (1998). The IRB's role in assessing the generalizability of non-NIH-funded clinical trials. *IRB: A Review of Human Subjects Research, 20*(2–3), 1–5.

Weijer, C. (2000). The ethical analysis of risk. *Journal of Law, Medicine & Ethics, 28,* 344–361.

Weijer, C., & Fuks, A. (1994). The duty to exclude: Excluding people at undue risk from research. *Clinical and Investigative Medicine, 17,* 115–122.

3

Optimizing Risks and Benefits:
The Case of Rotavirus Vaccine

Susan E. Coffin and Robert M. Nelson

In August 1998, the U.S. Food and Drug Administration (FDA) licensed a new vaccine to prevent rotavirus, the most common and serious cause of gastroenteritis among children living in either developed or developing nations (CDC, 1999a). Fourteen months later, the vaccine was withdrawn from the U.S. market due to concerns about a rare gastrointestinal side effect known as intussusception (CDC, 1999b, 1999c). The estimates of the attributable risk of the vaccine have varied in several well-designed case–control studies (Chang, Smithe, Ackelsberg, Morse, & Glass, 2001; Kramarz, France, & Destefano, 2001; Murphy, 2001; Simonsen et al., 2001); thus, the debate about the significance of the association between rotavirus vaccine and intussusception continues. Some researchers and public health officials have questioned the wisdom of revoking the original recommendation to vaccinate U.S. infants (Murphy, 2003). In addition, international public health agencies continue to weigh the risks and benefits of this vaccine for children who live in developing nations (Schael-Perez, 2001; Walker, Akaramuzzaman, & Lanata, 2001; Weijer, 2000).

In this chapter, we examine the events surrounding the development, licensure, and discontinuation of this rotavirus vaccine. We explore ethical issues that are raised by this case and that have dominated the growing debates over national and international vaccine research: how the risks and benefits of vaccines are measured, what is considered an acceptable balance between vaccine-related risk and benefit, and what happens when U.S. vaccine policy clashes with international public health concerns.

CASE DESCRIPTION

The Disease

Worldwide, rotavirus is the most common cause of serious gastroenteritis. In both developed and developing countries, virtually all children are infected with rotavirus by 3 years of age (Prashar, Breese, Gentsch, & Glass, 1998a). In the United States, one out of seven infected infants requires medical care, resulting in approximately 500,000 office visits and 50,000 hospitalizations each year (Prashar, Holman, Clarke, Breese, & Glass, 1998b; Tucker et al., 1998). In addition, between 20 and 40 children die in the United States each year due to complications of rotavirus infection (Glass et al., 1996).

Although rotavirus is a cause of significant childhood morbidity in the United States, the burden of disease is much greater in the developing world. Each year, approximately 640,000 children die of rotavirus gastroenteritis (Clark, Glass, & Offit, 1999); approximately 85% of these deaths occur in children who live in low-income countries (Miller & McCann, 2000).

The Vaccine

On August 31, 1998, the FDA licensed the first rotavirus vaccine for use in children (CDC, 2003); 1 month later, vaccine distribution began (CDC, 1999a). This vaccine (RotaShield) was an oral, live attenuated, tetravalent vaccine. Phase III clinical trials demonstrated that the vaccine had 70–90% efficacy against severe diarrhea and 100% efficacy against hospitalization (Clark et al., 1999). The manufacturer (Wyeth-Lederle Vaccines and Pediatrics, Radnor, PA) and vaccine advisory committees recommended that infants receive three doses at ages 2, 4, and 6 months (American Academy of Pediatrics, 1998; CDC, 1999a).

During the course of four prelicensure studies, more than 10,000 infants received the tetravalent reassortant rhesus rotavirus vaccine (Rennels et al., 1998). Fever was the only adverse event that was consistently and significantly associated with vaccine administration; when compared to placebo, the vaccine was associated with a 3.5-fold increased incidence of fever $> 38.0°C$ after the first dose (CDC, 1999a). In placebo-controlled studies, there was no evidence that the vaccine was associated with vomiting. In a single trial, diarrhea was more common among vaccine recipients than among placebo recipients (2.8% vs. 1.4%; Joensuu, Koskenniemi, & Vesikari, 1998).

Upon review of all prelicensure studies, researchers observed that intussusception occurred in 5 of 10,054 recipients of any vaccine formulation (Rennels et al., 1998). In contrast, one case of intussusception was diagnosed in the 4,633 infants who received placebo vaccine. Although this difference was not statistically significant and the incidence of intussusception among vaccine recipients was similar to that previously reported for U.S. children, intussusception was listed on the package insert as a possible vaccine-related adverse event (CDC, 2003). In addition, the manufacturer funded a phase IV study of vaccine efficacy and safety.

Sounding the Alarm

By May 1999, nine cases of intussusception were reported to the Vaccine Adverse Events Reporting System (VAERS), a nationwide passive surveillance system that is jointly administered by the Centers for Diseases Control and Prevention (CDC) and the FDA. Preliminary review revealed that six of these cases had developed between 3 and 6 days after the first dose of rotavirus vaccine. During the prior 8 years, only four cases of intussusception had been reported to VAERS. Initial analysis suggested that as many as 16 cases of intussusception might be expected within 1 week of vaccine administration based upon prior rates of intussusception, estimates of the number of vaccine doses administered, and 100% reporting of all cases. Data from the ongoing postlicensure study were rapidly analyzed, systematic case finding was undertaken, and a multistate case–control study was initiated. Within 6 weeks of initial recognition, the CDC's Advisory Committee on Immunization Practices recommended temporary suspension of all rotavirus vaccination pending further study (CDC, 1999c).

The Early Evidence

As cases were sought, the number of reports to VAERS of intussusception after rotavirus vaccine rose rapidly (CDC, 2003). By October 1999, 101 presumed or confirmed cases had been reported. More than half of the identified cases had the onset of intussusception within 7 days of vaccination. Many of these affected children had undergone surgery to reduce the intussusception, and 10% had required bowel resection. One fatal case of intussusception was reported in a 5-month-old infant (CDC, 1999b).

Initial case–control analysis revealed an association between rotavirus vaccination and intussusception (relative risk = 2.37; 95% confidence interval, 1.31–4.30; CDC, 1999c). A subsequent case-series analysis revealed that cases of intussusception were not evenly distributed over time after vaccination; when compared to other time intervals, the risk of intussusception was greatest between 3 and 14 days after the first dose of vaccine. In October 1999, the manufacturer voluntarily withdrew its product and the CDC revoked its recommendation for vaccination (CDC, 1999b).

ETHICAL ANALYSIS AND DISCUSSION

Assessing the Risks of Vaccines

Vaccines are not inert; they are intended to engage the recipient's immune system and thus induce immunologic protection. Therefore, all vaccines have side effects associated with their administration. Fever, pain, and erythema at the site of vaccine administration are evidence that a vaccine is inducing an immune response. Live viral vaccines, such as the measles vaccine, are composed of an attenuated virus designed to undergo several cycles of replication in order to stimulate an immune response that closely mirrors that triggered by a natural infection. Because vaccine viruses have been modified, both the duration of viral replication and the expression of virulence factors are dramatically less than that which occurs after infection with wild-type viruses. In this way, viral immunogenicity and pathogenicity are dissociated in live viral vaccines. Nonetheless, some individuals who receive a live viral vaccine may develop mild symptoms associated with the transient replication of the vaccine virus. For example, approximately 6% of children who received the varicella vaccine will develop vesicles near the site of vaccine administration (Krause & Klinman, 1995).

The incidence and profile of vaccine-related side effects are determined during clinical trials prior to vaccine licensure. Common side effects, such as fever and erythema at the inoculation site, are typically first recognized during small phase I trials and their incidence determined more precisely during the course of larger phase II and III trials. During phase III clinical trials, when thousands of doses of a candidate vaccine are administered to child-subjects, adverse events that occur uncommonly are recognized. This step in the development of a vaccine provides an opportunity to identify vaccine-related adverse events that may affect as few as 1% of vaccine recipients. Recognizing rare vaccine-related adverse events remains a serious challenge for vaccine research. Although several rare adverse events might occur during the development of a vaccine, phase III trials typically lack the power to determine whether the observed event is related to the vaccine administration. This challenge is heightened when an adverse event is not exclusively associated with vaccine administration, but is also a spontaneously occurring medical condition. The development of the rotavirus vaccine illustrates this difficulty.

As described above, six cases of intussusception occurred during prelicensure testing of rhesus rotavirus vaccine, affecting five individuals who received vaccine and one individual who received placebo (Rennels et al., 1998). Analysis of these data revealed that cases of intussusception (1) did not occur significantly more frequently in vaccine compared to placebo recipients, (2) were not temporally clustered in the time window immediately after vaccine administration, and (3) occurred at a rate similar to that observed in the general population. Therefore, vaccine developers and the FDA concluded that intussusception was unlikely to be a vaccine-related adverse event and RotaShield was licensed for general use in infants. Intussusception was, however, listed on the package insert as a possible adverse event (Halpern, Karlawish, & Berlin, 2002). In addition, postlicensure studies were designed to monitor vaccine recipients for intussusception. By May

27, 1999, when an estimated 900,000 doses of vaccine had been administered, vaccine safety experts recognized the first signal that the risk of intussusception might differ among vaccinated and unvaccinated infants. Within 1 month, postlicensure data was reviewed and vaccine use was suspended (CDC, 1999c). Subsequent studies have suggested that with full implementation of a national rotavirus vaccine program, one case of intussusception would occur for every 4,670 to 9,474 vaccinated infants (Murphy, 2001).

The case of RotaShield provoked a debate among the private and governmental groups responsible for the development and licensure of new vaccines. Pharmaceutical companies and regulatory agencies wrestle with questions such as how safe is safe enough and what evidence is needed to identify and quantify the risks associated with a candidate vaccine (Cohen, 2001; Jacobson, Adegbenro, Pankratz, & Poland, 2001; Murphy, 2003). Vaccine researchers consider whether phase III clinical trials—traditionally considered efficacy trials—should be designed with sufficient power to examine potential rare vaccine-related adverse events (Halpern et al., 2002; Jacobson et al., 2001; McPhillips, Davis, Marcuse, & Taylor, 2001). Finally, experts are divided on whether postlicensure studies are an acceptable strategy to identify rare but serious adverse events (Danovaro-Holliday, Wood, & LeBaron, 2002; Jacobson et al., 2001; McPhillips et al., 2001) and if novel strategies are necessary to enhance the early detection of adverse events (Niu, Erwin, & Braun, 2001; Verstraeten et al., 2001; Weiss & Davis, 2002).

The logistic and financial challenges of identifying rare vaccine-related adverse events and accurately determining their incidence could be significant. Statisticians have calculated that prelicensure studies would have had to include more than 250,000 infants to determine (with 90% power) if vaccination was associated with a doubling of the risk of intussusception (Jacobson et al., 2001). Representatives from public health agencies, regulatory bodies, and industry debate who should pay for this additional expense (Murphy, 2003). Leaders from pharmaceutical companies have complained that revenues from vaccine sales represent a small component of their profits although vaccine development currently consumes a large fraction of their research budget (Lang & Wood, 1999). Although a phase III trial of this magnitude would undoubtedly enhance public confidence in the efficacy and safety of a newly licensed vaccine, public health and government officials worry that pharmaceutical companies will be unwilling to shoulder this additional expense for a product that has a low profit margin. Finally, the increased time to conduct such large phase III trials would further delay the licensure of a potentially live-saving vaccine.

Measuring the Benefits of Vaccines: Who Are the Beneficiaries

As one of the greatest public health achievements of the past 100 years, the benefits of vaccination seem obvious (CDC, 1999d). Vaccines have led to the eradication of one organism (variola virus), the global control of others (measles and polio), and the significant reduction of common disease in some countries (varicella). However, as vaccine-preventable diseases become rare, the benefits individual children derive from vaccination become less apparent.

Direct Benefits of Vaccination Ironically, the successes of childhood vaccines have led to recent skepticism about their necessity (Allen, 2002; Gellin, Maibach, & Marcuse, 2000; Wolfe, Sharp, & Lipsky, 2002). Recent outbreaks of vaccine-preventable diseases in the United States, England, and Ireland, however, have demonstrated that immunization remains a vital component of disease control in developed countries (CDC, 1985; Salmon et al., 1999). In the United States, endemic transmission of measles had been virtually eradicated by the early 1980's; however, measles outbreaks occurred in cities throughout the United States from 1989 through 1991. These outbreaks, which affected both unvaccinated and previously vaccinated children, were associated with a modest drop in immunization rates among preschool children. In 1990 alone, an estimated 26,672 children were infected and 89 children died as a result of these outbreaks (CDC, 1991). Subsequent analysis revealed that the risk of developing measles was 35-fold greater among children who had not been vaccinated (Salmon et al., 1999). Fortunately, by the mid-1990s measles was again controlled through the expanded use of measles vaccine.

The individual benefits of vaccination are modified by characteristics that are unique to each child, vary over time, and are often difficult to measure. Factors such as the likelihood of being exposed to a given organism, the risk of developing clinically apparent disease (which may be associated with the virulence of a specific organism and the immunocompetence of the host), and the ability to access medical care help to determine the benefits of vaccination. For example, although rotavirus is endemic in the United States and has a high clinical attack rate, the *severity* of rotavirus infections is greater among children living in poverty (Glass et al., 1996). Therefore, the benefits of rotavirus vaccination might be greater for a child living in poverty. This may be due to his or her limited access to health care. In contrast, the risk of hepatitis B exposure is not uniform throughout the U.S. population (Alter, 2003). Nonetheless, hepatitis B vaccine is recommended for universal administration at birth. Because the perceived risk of exposure is low among newborns born in the United States, some parents have challenged the recommendation that all neonates received hepatitis B vaccine (Marwick & Mitka, 1999). Public health authorities contend that all immunized children benefit from hepatitis B vaccine because no one can identify a priori infants who in the future will adopt high-risk activities associated with hepatitis B exposure, and because of the potentially lethal severity of the disease. Thus, a tension exists between individual parents who feel confident in predicting their child's future behavior and public health authorities charged with the responsibility of developing a strategy to protect all children from vaccine-preventable diseases.

Indirect Benefits of Vaccination   Immunizations provide benefits to specific individuals other than the vaccinated child. For diseases that are transmitted person to person, rising rates of vaccine coverage are often associated with reductions in the incidence of disease in nonimmunized as well as immunized children ("herd immunity"). Givon-Lavi, Fraser, and Dagan (2003) recently demonstrated that pneumococcal vaccination of children who attend daycare reduces the risk of colonization among their nonimmunized siblings. Similarly, pertussis vaccination of older siblings affords indirect protection to a new family member; thus, babies younger than 8 weeks, who are too young to receive pertussis vaccine but at highest risk of experiencing a serious infection, benefit from the pertussis vaccination received by other members of their family.

Community Benefits of Vaccination
Finally, vaccinations also provide benefit to an entire community. The benefits of herd immunity often reach beyond the level of an individual household. As discussed above, as the rates of vaccination rise, the risk of pathogen exposure falls. Thus, the benefits afforded by immunization may shift from the individual vaccine recipient to the community in which he or she lives (Fine & Clarkson, 1986). In areas where vaccine penetration is high and vaccine-preventable diseases are uncommon, vaccinated individuals help to sustain disease control that was initially achieved by prior high rates of vaccination. Within an individual community, high levels of vaccine coverage have been associated with reduced rates of numerous diseases in *unvaccinated* individuals, such as pertussis, measles, and influenza. This umbrella effect provides indirect immunologic protection for individuals who cannot or have not received vaccinations. Thus, a community can protect its most vulnerable members—the young and the immunocompromised—from endemic diseases by sustaining high levels of vaccine coverage.

To ensure control of vaccine-preventable diseases, the community relies upon broad participation in childhood vaccination programs. Although virtually all states offer medical and religious waivers of vaccine requirements upon school entry, relatively few parents seek these exemptions. Recent skepticism about the need for and safety of vaccines has been associated with a rapid rise in the number of states offering parents a "philosophic" exemption to vaccination (Orenstein & Hinman, 1999). At present, little data exist about the numbers of parents seeking these exemptions. In addition, few states track the percentage of philosophic exemptions granted. Although little is known about the individual beliefs of parents seeking philosophic exemptions from vaccinations, public health officials have speculated that this growing trend reflects a perception that the individual risks of vaccines outweigh their benefits (Rota et al., 2001). In fact, parents who elect to not vaccinate their children succeed in avoiding the risk of vaccine-associated adverse events. However, such families continue to reap the indirect benefits of vaccination if they live in a community where vaccine coverage remains high. This individual parental decision violates the principle of justice which requires the fair distribution of *both* risks and benefits, and raises the ethical issue known as the "free rider" problem (Arneson, 1982; Cullity, 1995). As the percentage of unvaccinated individuals in a community rises, the risk of disease increases (Fair, Murphy, Golaz, & Wharton, 2002; Gangarosa et al., 1998; Salmon et al., 1999). Thus, continued control of vaccine-preventable diseases relies upon the beneficence of individuals—the willingness of individuals to accept the individual risk of a vaccine-associated adverse event—so that they, and their community, may realize the full benefits of immunization.

Measuring the Benefits of Vaccine: Interpreting Efficacy Studies

Serotype Diversity Influences Vaccine Efficacy:

Vaccines are rarely 100% effective. Phase III clinical studies demonstrated that RotaShield was 40–60% effective in preventing all rotavirus infections; however, the vaccine was 70–80% effective in preventing severe infections (Coffin, 2000). In addition, prelicensure studies suggested that vaccination would prevent virtually all rotavirus-related hospitalizations (Tucker, 1998).

The benefits of a vaccine are dictated, in part, by characteristics of the targeted organism. The number of clinically distinct serotypes influences the actual and perceived benefits of vaccination. For example, the vaccines against two of the most common causes of bacterial meningitis, *Haemophilus influenzae* type B (HIB) and *Streptococcus pneumoniae*, were designed using virtually identical technology; however, one vaccine might be perceived to be more effective than the other. Typically, only one serotype of *H. influenzae* causes meningitis (type B). Thus, the HIB vaccine is designed to induce protection against virtually all cases of *H. influenzae* meningitis. In contrast, there are more than 90 serotypes of *S. pneumoniae*. The current formulation of the protein-conjugated *S. pneumoniae* vaccine contains antigens from the seven most prevalent serotypes. In the United States, however, approximately 15% of invasive *S. pneumoniae* infections are caused by serotypes that are not included in the vaccine. Thus, although both vaccines confer greater than 95% protection against vaccine-related serotypes, the efficacy of the HIB vaccine might be perceived to be greater than the *S. pneumoniae* vaccine.

RotaShield was a tetravalent vaccine that contained the four serotypes of rotavirus that were responsible for the majority of infections in the United States. Recently, novel serotypes of rotavirus have emerged in the United States (Cunliffe, Bresee, Gentsch, Glass, & Hart, 2002; Griffin et al., 2002). If these new viral strains become more prevalent in the U.S. population, future rotavirus vaccines might be less effective (in preventing all rotavirus infections) than was RotaShield. Similarly, the seroepidemiology of rotavirus differs in developed compared to developing countries (Adah, Wade, & Taniguchi, 2001; Kang, Green, Gallimore, & Brown, 2002). Therefore, geography may influence the ideal composition of a rotavirus vaccine. Consequently, international public health officials have emphasized the need for the vaccines that are developed for and evaluated in developing countries (Breese et al., 2001; Shann & Steinhoff, 1999).

Cost–Efficacy Studies: Quantifying Economic and Human Benefits of Vaccines
Recognizing finite resources, public health officials often rely upon cost–benefit and cost–efficacy analyses when they consider recommending a new vaccine for general use (Beutels et al., 2002; Nalin, 2002). Because the federally funded Vaccines for Children program purchases vaccines for use in public health clinics, an economic evaluation of the impact of a vaccine is a critical component of establishing national vaccine priorities. Vaccines are considered cost effective if their costs are lower than the costs associated with disease. Typically, factors such as the costs of medical care (direct costs) and the lost wages associated with parental absence from work (indirect costs) are included in these calculations. However, health economists have struggled to assign an economic value to the relief of suffering that is the natural consequence of disease prevention. Thus, virtually all cost efficacy analyses fail to take into account one of the most important goals of vaccination—the alleviation of children's suffering.

Balancing the Risks and Benefits of Vaccines

Unlike most other medical interventions, vaccines are usually administered to prevent, not treat, a disease. Thus, a healthy individual must accept a risk of illness or disability (i.e., a vaccine-related adverse event) to incur a somewhat intangible benefit—the prevention of possible disease. Because vaccines are typically given to healthy young children unable to make their own decision, establishing the appropriate balance between acceptable risk and anticipated benefit is critical. A federal advisory group, the National Vaccine Advisory Committee, is responsible for the oversight of public health policy so that the "optimal prevention of human infectious diseases through immunization and . . . the optimal prevention against adverse reactions to vaccination" is achieved (Peter et al., 1999). This charge is complicated by several major challenges. As illustrated by the case of RotaShield, adverse reactions to vaccines can sometimes be difficult to detect. Additionally, the benefits of vaccination are not fixed but rather a function of who are the designated beneficiaries and what is the local epidemiology of the targeted microorganism.

What Is Optimal Risk? What Is Optimal Benefit? Vaccine safety has become an issue of great concern to many parents in the United States. Although all medical interventions carry some associated risk, surveys suggest that the public may be less tolerant of risk associated with preventive, as compared to therapeutic, medical care (Kataoka-Yahiro & Munet-Vilaro, 2002). However, by accepting a small risk associated with a preventive intervention, an individual may dramatically reduce the future risk associated with a disease or its treatment. Thus, the balance between risk associated with prevention and the risk associated with treatment is strongly influenced by the incidence of disease. For example, each year in the United States the oral polio vaccine (OPV) led to four to eight cases of vaccine-induced paralytic poliomyelitis (Plotkin, 1991). This rare complication of vaccine was only recognized after wild-type polio had been eradicated in the Americas. Because the risk of infection in the United States was low, in 1998 public health officials recommended that vaccination with OPV be discontinued and that only the inactivated polio vaccine be given to infants in this country. However, in developing countries where polio remains endemic, vaccination with OPV continues; the benefits of immunization with OPV (induction of broad herd immunity) outweigh the risk of this rare vaccine-associated adverse event. Similarly, some experts have argued that the risks associated with preventing rotavirus disease (intussusception and mild vaccine-associated side effects) are far less than the risk of developing a serious rotavirus infection (Murphy, 2003). Recent studies suggest that the RotaShield vaccine induced one case of intussusception per 10,000 vaccine recipients. Unlike other more common vaccine-related side effects, intussusception is associated with greater morbidity. Although some cases of intussusception resolve spontaneously, most require medical attention to prevent complications such as peritonitis or intestinal perforation; approximately 50% of cases may require surgical intervention (Wylie, 2004). In contrast, studies have demonstrated that each year approximately 1 out of every 80 infants in the United States will require hospitalization due to rotavirus each year (Parashar et al., 1999; Parashar, Holman, Clarke, Breese, & Glass, 1997).

Thus, widespread vaccination might prevent 120 rotavirus-related hospitalizations for every vaccine-attributable case of intussusception (Glass et al., 1996).

National and International Vaccine Policy: Social Equity and Vaccine Safety

Geographic and economic factors may influence both the magnitude of and relative balance between vaccine-associated risks and benefits. The incidence and severity of some infectious diseases are strongly determined by geographic location, economic development, and political stability. Therefore, the benefits of vaccine use might be greater in developing compared to developed countries. Alternatively, reduced access to appropriate medical care for vaccine-related adverse events might increase the risks associated with vaccination in less developed countries. Thoughtful analysis of the ethical requirement for justice can guide policy in this area, as the fair distribution and balance of the risks and benefits of vaccination will likely differ between populations.

International public health officials have questioned whether the benefits of rotavirus vaccine might outweigh the risks in some developing countries (Breese et al., 2001; Hall, 2001; Linhares & Breese, 2000; Miller & McCann, 2000; Weijer, 2000). Each year, approximately 640,000 children are estimated to die from the complications associated with rotavirus infections. Most of these children live in developing countries. Factors such as unsanitary water supplies, poor access to health care, and crowding contribute to the dramatic mortality due to rotavirus. Because the burden of rotavirus disease is greatest in the developing world, an effective rotavirus vaccine might dramatically reduce childhood mortality. However, little is known about the risks associated with the use of RotaShield in developing countries since most clinical trials were conducted in North America and Europe. Thus, few data exist about the risk of vaccine-related intussusception among children who arguably have the most to gain from the introduction of a rotavirus vaccine (Breese et al., 2001).

In, 2000, officials from the World Health Organization (WHO) met to discuss the consequences of the U.S. decision to revoke licensure of the rotavirus vaccine (World Health Organization, 2000). Experts debated the risks and benefits of vaccine use in the developing countries. In addition, they wrestled with the logistical issues such as the production of a vaccine that was no longer being made by its original manufacturer. Data are scarce to define the risk of intussusception among children living in the developing world (Perez-Schael et al. 2003). Because access to advanced medical and surgical care is limited, the mortality associated with intussusception may be greater for children who live in the developing compared to developed world. Nonetheless, most international health experts believe that in the developing world the recognized burden of rotavirus-related disease far exceeds that which may be attributed to intussusception (Weijer, 2000). Similarly, experts wrestle with knowledge that a child who lives in the developing world has a much greater risk of death due to rotavirus infection than due to vaccine-related intussusception (Breese et al., 2001; Kang et al., 2002; Murphy, 2003; World Health Organization, 2000).

CONCLUSION

Rotavirus infections remain a serious threat to global child health. Although the point at which the benefits outweigh the risks associated with vaccinations differs for children living in developing compared to developed countries, all children must wait for a second-generation rotavirus vaccine. As second-generation rotavirus vaccines undergo phase III evaluation, national and international vaccine experts and public health officials must determine if any serious vaccine-associated adverse events are acceptable given the potential life savings associated with prevention of this infectious disease. In addition, vaccine researchers must address the role of postlicensure monitoring for vaccine safety and examine whether future phase III clinical trials should be designed with sufficient power to detect relatively rare vaccine-associated adverse events.

In the 21st century, vaccines remain one of our most important strategies to improve child health. The future success of vaccines will rely upon the preservation of public trust in the mechanisms used to assess vaccine safety and the development of vaccines that are effective for the most vulnerable children.

___

Questions for Discussion

1. Do you think the risks of vaccination research (probability and severity) should be weighed *only* against the benefits of vaccination that accrue to the child-subject, or that a more permissive analysis is warranted?
2. Phase III clinical trials in the development of a vaccine provide an opportunity to identify vaccine-related adverse events that may affect as few as 1% of vaccine recipients, but they may not detect events that occur with less frequency. What are the ethical implications of this challenge?
3. Had you been policy maker what would be the threshold, both in terms of probability and severity of side effects, at which you would stop the postlicensure clinical trials for safety reasons? What, if anything, is the ethical difference between pre- and postlicensure studies with regard to this question?

4. Discuss the logistic and financial challenges that are involved in identifying and accurately determining the incidence of rare vaccine-related adverse events. What ethical issues do these challenges raise?

5. What are the factors involved in the determination of the individual benefits of vaccination for children? Why is it so difficult to assess the individual child benefit?

6. Why is there a tension between some individual parents and public health authorities in determining policy regarding administration of vaccination to children for vaccine-preventable diseases? How would you suggest that this tension be resolved?

7. In light of the indirect benefits of vaccination ("herd immunity") and the umbrella effect associated with community benefits of vaccination, what is your response to the new trend of "philosophic" exemption to vaccination? Relate your answer to the problem of the "free rider." Do you find this exemption ethically problematic?

8. How would you measure the value that should be associated with the relief of suffering that is the natural consequence of disease prevention, as part of the economic cost efficacy analysis? What are the ethical implications of the ambiguity of existing measurement models?

9. Why is the establishment of the appropriate balance between acceptable risk and anticipated benefit so critical when dealing with universal childhood vaccination?

10. What is the role of geographic and economic factors in both the magnitude of and relative balance between vaccine-associated risks and benefits? What are the ethical and social implications of the difference in vaccine-associated risks and benefits balance between populations?

11. How would you apply the principle of justice with a commitment to fair distribution to the case of rotavirus vaccination discussed in this chapter?

—

References

Adah, M. I., Wade, A., & Taniguchi, K. (2001). Molecular epidemiology of rotaviruses in Nigeria: Detection of unusual strains with G2p[6] and G8p[1] specificities. *Journal of Clinical Microbiology, 39,* 3969–3975.

Allen, A. (2002, September). Bucking the herd. *The Atlantic Monthly,* pp. 40–41.

Alter, M. J. (2003). Epidemiology and prevention of hepatitis B. Seminars in liver disease. *Seminars in Liver Disease, 23,* 39–46.

American Academy of Pediatrics, Committee on Infectious Diseases. (1998). Prevention of rotavirus disease: Guidelines for use of rotavirus vaccine. *Pediatrics, 102,* 1483–1491.

Arneson, R. J. (1982). The principle of fairness and free-rider problems. *Ethics, 92,* 616–633.

Beutels, P., Edmunds, W. J., Antonanzas, F., De Wit, G. A., Evans, D., Feilden, R., et al. (2002).

Viral hepatitis prevention board. Economic evaluation of vaccination programmes: A consensus statement focusing on viral hepatitis. *Pharmacoeconomics, 20,* 1–7.

Breese, J. S., El Arifeen, S., Azim, T., Chakraborty, J., Mounts, A. W., Podder, G., et al. (2001). Safety and immunogenicity of tetravalent rhesus-based rotavirus vaccine in Bangladesh. *Pediatric Infectious Disease Journal, 20,* 1136–1143.

Centers for Disease Control and Prevention. 1985. Measles in a population with religious exemption to vaccination—Colorado. *Morbidity and Mortality Weekly Report, 25,* 3411–3415.

Centers for Disease Control and Prevention. (1991). Measles—United States, 1990. *Morbidity and Mortality Weekly Report, 40,* 369–372.

Centers for Disease Control and Prevention. (1999a). Rotavirus vaccine for the prevention of rotavirus gastroenteritis among children. *Morbidity and Mortality Weekly Report, 48,* 1–20.

Centers for Disease Control and Prevention. (1999b, October 22). ACIP Revokes Recommendation for Rotavirus Vaccine Use [Press Release]. Atlanta: Centers for Disease Control and Prevention.

Centers for Disease Control and Prevention. (1999c). Intussusception among recipients of rotavirus vaccine—United States (1998–1999). *Morbidity and Mortality Weekly Report, 48,* 577–581.

Centers for Disease Control and Prevention. (1999d). Achievements in public health (1900–1999). *Morbidity and Mortality Weekly Report, 48,* 243–248.

Centers for Disease Control and Prevention. (2003). Surveillance for safety after immunization: Vaccine adverse event reporting system (VAERS)—United States, (1991–2001). *Morbidity and Mortality Weekly Report, 52,* 5–7.

Chang, H. G., Smithe, P. F., Ackelsberg, J., Morse, D. L., & Glass, R. I. (2001). Intussusception, rotavirus diarrhea, and rotavirus vaccine use among children in New York state. *Pediatrics, 108,* 54.

Clark, H. F., Glass, R. I., & Offit, P. A. (1999). Rotavirus vaccines. In S. A. Plotkin & W. A. Orenstein (Eds.), *Vaccines* (pp. 987–1005). Philadelphia: W.B. Saunders.

Coffin, S. E. (2000). Rotavirus vaccines: Current controversies and future directions. *Current Infectious Disease Reports, 2,* 68–72.

Cohen, J. (2001). Rethinking a vaccine's risk. *Science, 293,* 1576–1577.

Cullity, G. (1995). Moral free riding. *Philosophy and Public Affairs, 24,* 3–34.

Cunliffe, N. A., Bresee, J. S., Gentsch, J. R., Glass, R. I., & Hart, C. A. (2002). The expanding diversity of rotaviruses. *Lancet, 359,* 640–642.

Danovaro-Holliday, M. C., Wood, A. L., & LeBaron, C. W. (2002). Rotavirus vaccine and the news media, (1987–2001). *Journal of the American Medical Association, 287,* 1455–1462.

Fair, E., Murphy, T. V., Golaz, A., & Wharton, M. (2002). Philosophic objection to vaccination as a risk for tetanus among children younger than 15 years. *Pediatrics, 109,* e2.

Fine, P. E. M., & Clarkson, J. A. (1986). Individual versus public priorities in the determination of optimal vaccination policies. *American Journal of Epidemiology, 124,* 1012–1020.

Gangarosa, E. J., Galazka, A. M., Wolfe, C. R. Phillips, L., Gangarosa, R. E., Miller, E., & Chen, R. T. (1998). Impact of antivaccine movements on pertussis control: The untold story. *Lancet, 351,* 356–361.

Gellin, B. G., Maibach, E. W., & Marcuse, E. K. (2000). Do parents understand immunizations? A national telephone survey. *Pediatrics, 106,* 1097–1102.

Givon-Lavi, N., Fraser, D., & Dagan, R. (2003). Vaccination of day-care center attendees reduces carriage of *Streptococcus pneumoniae* among their younger siblings. *Pediatric Infectious Disease Journal, 22,* 524–531.

Glass, R. I., Kilgore, P. E., Holman, R. C., Jin, S., Smith, J. C., Woods, P. A., et al. (1996). The epidemiology of rotavirus diarrhea in the United States: Surveillance and estimates of disease burden. *Journal of Infectious Diseases, 174*(Suppl. 1), s5–s11.

Griffin, D. D., Nakagomi, T., Hoshino, Y., Nakagomi, O., Kirkwood, C. D., Parashar, U. D., et al., and National Rotavirus Surveillance System. (2002). Characterization of nontypeable rotavirus strains from the United States: Identification of a new rotavirus reassortant (P2a[6], G12) and rare P3[9] strains related to bovine rotaviruses. *Virology, 294,* 256–269.

Hall, A. J. (2001). Ecological studies and debate on rotavirus vaccine and intussusception [Commentary]. *Lancet, 358,* 1197–1198.

Halpern, S. D., Karlawish, J. H. T., & Berlin, J. A. (2002). The continuing unethical conduct of underpowered clinical trials. *Journal of the American Medical Association, 288,* 358–362.

Jacobson, R. M., Adegbenro, A., Pankratz, V. S., & Poland, G. A. (2001). Adverse events and vaccination—the lack of power and predictability of infrequent events in pre-licensure study. *Vaccine, 19,* 2428–2433.

Joensuu, J., Koskenniemi, E., & Vesikari, T. (1998). Symptoms associated with rhesus-human reassortant rotavirus vaccine in infants. *Pediatric Infectious Disease Journal, 17,* 334–340.

Kang, G., Green, J., Gallimore, C. I., & Brown, D. W. (2002). Molecular epidemiology of rotaviral infection in South Indian children with acute diarrhea from (1995–1996) to (1998–1999). *Journal of Medical Virology, 67,* 101–105.

Kataoka-Yahiro, M. R., & Munet-Vilaro, F. (2002). Barriers to preventive health care for young children. *Journal of the American Academy of Nurse Practitioners, 14,* 66–72.

Kramarz, P., France, E. K., & Destefano, F. (2001). Population-Based study of rotavirus vaccination and intussusception. *Pediatric Infectious Disease Journal, 20,* 410–416.

Krause, P. R., & Klinman, D. M. (1995). Efficacy, immunogenicity, safety, and use of live attenuated chickenpox vaccine. *Journal of Pediatrics, 127,* 518–524.

Lang, J., & Wood, S. C. (1999). Development of orphan vaccines: An industry perspective. *Emerging Infectious Diseases, 5,* 749–756.

Linhares, A. C., & Breese, J. S. (2000). Rotavirus vaccines and vaccination in Latin America. *Pan American Journal of Public Health, 8,* 305–331.

Marwick, C., & Mitka, M. (1999). Debate revived on hepatitis B vaccine value. *Journal of the American Medical Association, 282,* 15–17.

McPhillips, H. A., Davis, R. L., Marcuse, E. K., & Taylor, J. A. (2001). The rotavirus vaccine's withdrawal and physicians' trust in vaccine safety mechanisms. *Archives of Pediatric and Adolescent Medicine, 155,* 1051–1056.

Miller, M. A., & McCann, L. (2000). Policy analysis of the use of hepatitis B, *Haemophilus Influenzae* type B, *Streptococcus Pneumoniae*-conjugate, and rotavirus vaccines. *Health Economics, 9,* 19–35.

Murphy, B. R., Morens, D. M., Simonsen, L., Chanock, R. M., LaMontagne, J. R., & Kapikian, A. Z. (2003). Reappraisal of the association of intussusception with the licensed live rotavirus vaccine challenges initial conclusion. *Journal of Infectious Diseases, 187,* 1301–1308.

Murphy, T. V., Gargiullo, P. M., Massoudi, M. S., Nelson, D. B., Jumaan, A. O., Okoro, C. A., et al. (2001). Intussusception among infants given an oral rotavirus vaccine. *New England Journal of Medicine, 344*(8), 564–572.

Nalin, D. R. (2002). Evidence based vaccinology. *Vaccine, 20,* 1624–1630.

Niu, M. T., Erwin, D. E., & Braun, M. M. (2001). Data mining in the U.S. vaccine adverse event reporting system (Vaers): Early detection of intussusception and other events after rotavirus vaccination. *Vaccine, 19,* 4627–4634.

Orenstein, W. A., & Hinman, A. R. (1999). The immunization system in the United States—the role of school immunization laws. *Vaccine, 17,* S19–S24.

Parashar, U. D., Chung, M. A., Holman, R. C., Ryder, R. W., Hadler, J. L., & Glass, R. I. (1999). Use of state hospital discharge data to assess the morbidity from rotavirus diarrhea and to monitor the impact of a rotavirus immunization program: A pilot study in Connecticut. *Pediatrics, 104*, 489–494.

Parashar, U. D., Holman, R. C., Clarke, M. J., Breese, J. S., & Glass, R. I. (1997). Hospitalizations associated with rotavirus diarrhea in the United States, 1993 through 1995; Surveillance based on the new *ICD-9-Cm* rotavirus-specific diagnostic code. *Journal of Infectious Diseases, 177*, 13–17.

Perez-Schael, I., Escalona, M., Salinas, B., Meteran, M., E.Perez, M., & Gonzalez, G. (1998). Intussusception-associated hospitalization among Venezuelan infants during 1998 through 2001: Anticipating rotavirus vaccines. *Pediatric Infectious Disease Journal, 22*, 234–239.

Peter, G., des Vignes-Kendrick, M., Eickhoff, T. C., Fine, A., Galvin, V., Levine, M. M., et al. (1999). Lessons learned from a review of the development of selected vaccines. National vaccine advisory committee. *Pediatrics, 104*, 942–950.

Plotkin, S. A., (1991). Current issues in evaluating the efficacy of oral poliovirus vaccine and inactivated poliovirus vaccine immunization. *Pediatric Infectious Disease Journal, 10*, 979–981.

Prashar, U. D., Breese, J. S., Gentsch, J. R., & Glass, R.I. (1998). Rotavirus. *Emerging Infectious Diseases, 4*, 561–570.

Prashar, U. D., Holman, R. C., Clarke, M. J., Breese, J. S., & Glass, R. I. (1998b). Hospitalizations associated with rotavirus diarrhea in the United States, 1993 through 1995. *Journal of Infectious Diseases, 177*, 13–17.

Rennels, M. B., Parashar, U. D., Holman, R. C., Le, C. T., Chang, H. G., & Glass, R. I. (1998. Lack of an apparent association between intussusception and wild or vaccine rotavirus infection. *Pediatric Infectious Disease Journal, 17*, 924–925.

Rota, J. S., Salmon, D. A., Rodewald, L. E., Chen, R. T., Hibbs, B. F., & Gangarosa, E. J. (2001). Processes for obtaining nonmedical exemptions to state immunization laws. *American Journal of Public Health, 91*, 645–648.

Salmon, D. A., Haber, M., Gangarosa, E. J., Phillips, L., Smith, N. J., & Chen, R. T. (1999). Health consequences of religious and philosophic exemptions from immunization laws: Individual and societal risk of measles. *Journal of the American Medical Association, 281*, 47–53.

Schael-Perez, I. (2001). Future of research into rotavirus vaccine. *British Medical Journal, 322*, 106–107.

Shann, F., & Steinhoff, M. C. (1999). Vaccines for children in rich and poor countries. *Lancet, 354*, SII7–SII11.

Simonsen, L., Morens, D. M., Elixhouser, A., Gerber, M., Van Raden, M., & Blackwelder, W. C. (2001). Effect of rotavirus vaccination programme on trends in admission of infants to hosptial for intussusception. *Lancet, 358*, 1224–1229.

Tucker, A. W., Haddix, A. C., Bresee, J. S., Holman, R. C., Parashar, U. D., & Glass, R. I. (1998). Cost-effectiveness analysis of a rotavirus immunization program for the United States. *Journal of the American Medical Association, 279*, 1371–1376.

Verstraeten, T., Baughman, A. L., Caldwell, B., Zanardi, L., Haber, P., & Chen, R. T. (2001). Enhancing vaccine safety surveillance: A capture-recapture analysis of intussusception after rotavirus vaccination. *American Journal of Epidemiology, 154*, 1006–1012.

Walker, D., Akaramuzzaman, S. M., & Lanata, C. F. (2001). Future of research into rotavirus vaccine: Cost-effective of vaccine is being assessed. *British Medical Journal, 322*, 106a.

Weijer, C. (2000). The future of research into rotavirus vaccine. *British Medical Journal, 321*, 525–526.

Weiss, N. S., & Davis, R. L. (2002). In nonrandomized studies, can we use a person's preimmuni-zation experience to help gauge the safety and efficacy of immunization? *American Journal of Epidemiology, 156,* 395–396.

Wolfe, R. M., Sharp, L. K., & Lipsky, M. S. (2002). Content and design attributes of antivaccination web sites. *Journal of the American Medical Association, 287,* 3245–3248.

World Health Organization. (2000). Report of the Meeting on Future Directions for Rotavirus in Developing Countries. Geneva: Author.

Wyllie, R. (2004). Ileus, adhesions, intussusceptions, and closed loop obstructions. In R. E. Behrman (Ed.), *Nelson's Textbook of Pediatrics* (17th ed.). Philadelphia: W. B. Saunders & Company.

4

Bioethics Meets the Barrio: Community-Based Research Involving Children

Molly Martin and John Lantos

The last two decades have been marked by an effort to move research out of the ivory tower of academic medical centers and into the community. This move has been positive for three reasons. First, it provides a research setting that more closely mimics the real world. Second, it allows the identification of research projects that have a tangible benefit to research subjects and creates a mechanism for "closing the loop" and allowing the results of studies to get back to the people who participated in those studies. Finally, it empowers mediating institutions, such as community organizations, religious groups, or other citizens' groups, to scrutinize and revise research protocols according to their own moral priorities. In this way, protocols become more culturally appropriate and may ultimately lead to better information yields since the material is understandable and relevant to subjects.

These positive aspects of community-based participatory research have also created some controversies and challenges for research ethics. To the extent that the research setting more closely mimics the real world, it has also been messy in ways that the real world is messy. It is more difficult to conduct the sort of well-controlled clinical trials that are the hallmark of scientific validity in the community than it is on the wards of teaching hospitals. The demand that research have tangible results limits the sorts of projects that are allowable. Some projects are of scientific interest but have no direct or even indirect benefits to the participants. The acceptance of community-based alternative moral considerations raises questions about the generalizability or universality of moral principles. What if a community would allow or even encourage a research project that the IRB or the U.S. government would not? Is it ever acceptable to bend our rules to accommodate the rules of others? Can they be right and we wrong? These issues were illustrated nicely, recently, by a controversy that arose over a proposal that we submitted to our IRB describing a project that involved collaboration with community organizations.

CASE DESCRIPTION

The following protocol was submitted to an institutional review board (IRB):

Title: An evaluation of a community health worker asthma intervention program in a Latino community in Chicago.

The background of the proposal was the recognition that a half million Latino children in the United States have asthma (Flores et al. 2002). In Chicago, the asthma mortality rate for Latinos doubled in the last decade (Thomas & Whitman, 1999). This rate has increased more rapidly than that for African Americans or whites, even after adjustment for increases in the population (Thomas & Whitman, 1999). The reasons for the disproportionate increase in asthma mortality among Latinos and their children are not clear. The asthma prevalence within the Latino community subgroups also has unexplained significant differences. A recent study from 1999 in Brooklyn in a predominantly Puerto Rican/Dominican neighborhood found the prevalence of asthma to be 12% (97% confirmed by a physician). Unexpectedly, Puerto Ricans had a 13.2% prevalence of asthma while Dominicans and other Latinos had only a 5.3% prevalence (Ledogar, Penchaszadeh, Garden, & Garden, 2000).

The current medical structure is failing to understand and provide service to these high-risk populations, and perhaps more community-based approaches are needed to identify, involve, and educate families on asthma and asthma management. Several previous studies have concluded that the community health worker (CHW) model is useful in helping the medical community to identify Latino communities at risk for asthma and in gaining access to difficult-to-reach minority populations (Butz et al. 1994; Ledogar et al. 2000; Stout et al. 1998). This suggests the CHW model may also be able to improve asthma management and outcomes. To determine this, we proposed the evaluation of a Latino CHW program in Chicago to test the effectiveness in improving knowledge and outcomes of pediatric asthma.

CHWs are local inhabitants who are trained to provide specific basic health and nutrition services to the members of their surrounding communities (Berman, Gwatkin, & Burger, 1987) or community members who educate and assist individuals and groups in gaining control over their health and their lives (Center for Policy Alternatives, 1998). They live in the home village or neighborhood, have limited health care training, usually work part-time as CHWs, may be volunteers or receive salaries, and usually are not civil servants or professional employees of any government agency. They have many names, including community health advisors, lay health workers, health auxiliaries, barefoot doctors, health promoters (prometoras), family welfare educators, health volunteers, village health workers, and community health aids. Their duties are just as varied: serving as outreach worker, advocate, translator, educator, mentor, role model, counselor, cultural mediator, and community organizer; dispensing first aid, medicines, and family planning services; making health care referrals; maintaining records; and giving health advice.

In the field of asthma, the evaluation of CHWs is very limited. A study in Baltimore used CHWs to gather information on asthma using home visits and schools, but they did not use this information for further evaluation (Butz et al. 1994). CHWs in New York participated in a similar study where they went door to door in their community to identify people of different Latino backgrounds with asthma. No comments were made on interventions or follow-up done after the people with asthma were identified (Ledogar et al. 2000). In Chicago, Rush Medical School and the members of the Henry Horner Homes worked together to train several CHWs in asthma education. They measured graduation from their program, but they did not measure any changes in asthma or behavior (Baier, Grant, Daugherty, & Eckenfels, 1999). A recent pilot study from Seattle was able to show slight decreases in hospital admissions and emergency department visits using a CHW, but this study population consisted only of 23 families.

In the Chicago Latino community, CHWs have worked to improve and unify their communities. Centro Comunitario Juan Diego (CCJD) is a grassroots organization founded in 1994 by Latina women to work for social change in the low-income, problem-plagued neighborhood of South Chicago. They focus their community organizing efforts in the areas of violence prevention, local school council elections, literacy, human rights, and environmental health and creating opportunities for youth and women in organizing, HIV education, diabetes education, asthma education, and fostering alliances between Latino and African American organizations in South Chicago. After extensive interaction with CCJD, the investigators and the CHWs developed a study protocol that included the following sections as "purpose" and "protocol."

Purpose
This study will attempt to evaluate the current asthma intervention at Centro Comunitario Juan Diego in order to understand the efficacy of the CHW model in asthma management in an underserved Latino neighborhood. Showing improvements in asthma knowledge and outcomes would add much needed validity to the CHW model. The model could then be more extensively used to improve access to care in Latino and other underserved populations.

Study Questions
1. Do CHWs improve asthma outcomes in Latino children and adults?
2. Do CHWs improve asthma knowledge in Latino children and adults?
3. Do CHWs facilitate behavior changes in Latino families with children or adults with asthma?
4. Do CHWs increase access to medical care in Latino children and adults?

CHW Training
CHWs undergo extensive training in asthma pathophysiology and treatment.

They take two classes from the American Lung Association: Asthma 101 and Asthma for Children. These classes are offered in English and Spanish; they last 1 day each for 6 hours a day for a total of 12 hours of training. CHWs receive continuing education sessions for physicians and others at CCJD three or four times a year.

They evaluate each other every several months by attending each other's sessions and critiquing their performance. Before the start of this program, the CHWs will be given a test that has been developed to standardize their knowledge. The CHWs will receive an in-service on how to use the pulmonary function machine.

Recruitment
Recruitment for the asthma programs occurs simultaneously with recruitment for all programs at CCJD. They encourage people to sign up for a general home evaluation at their food pantry, churches, HIV program, and other programs and community centers.

When a person signs up for a home evaluation, they are called by telephone by a CHW to set up a visit time. If they have no telephone, the CHW attempts to find them at their house or through letters.

The CHW goes to the home for an initial evaluation where they ask screening questions about asthma, diabetes, HIV, finances, immigration status, domestic violence, drug use, and others to identify areas in which the family will need assistance. If the family identifies an adult or child with asthma, they are asked to allow a second visit for asthma education. The screening questions used for asthma will be based on the recommendations in the Guidelines for the Diagnosis and Management of Asthma by the National Institutes of Health (NIH, 2004).

The Intervention
The CHW returns with asthma education materials after a household has been identified with a member with asthma. First, the CHWs will obtain consent

for the evaluation from participating family members. Then they will help the participants to complete an asthma form that contains questions on demographics, asthma knowledge, asthma history and symptoms, and access to the medical system. They will measure the pulmonary functions of the family member with asthma. They will then begin the teaching intervention using whatever materials they feel are appropriate. The materials include education brochures, videos, flipcharts, practice inhalers, and peak flow meters. The house will be evaluated for exacerbating factors. An asthma action plan will be filled out and explained to the family. Appropriate referrals will be made to local health clinics or social service agencies if needed. If the full education cannot be completed in one visit, the CHW will make a second home visit. The CHW will then call or visit the family every several weeks until they feel the family understands their medicine and triggers, has tried to change their home, and has access to medical care.

The CHW will revisit the family at 6 months and 1 year from the original visit. At this time, they will repeat the pulmonary function tests. They will also complete the follow up form that includes questions on asthma knowledge, asthma history and symptoms, and access to the medical system.

ETHICAL ANALYSIS AND DISCUSSION

The central moral dilemma of clinical research is that it requires research subjects to take risks in order to seek knowledge that might benefit others. The research subjects, then, are inevitably a means to an end rather than an end in themselves. To the extent that this is not so, that is, to the extent that a research protocol offers tangible benefits to the actual subjects of the protocol, the moral dilemmas of research disappear. (That is not to say the regulatory dilemmas disappear, but that is another matter entirely.)

This dilemma is explored and analyzed best in relation to individual participants in research. For individuals, the "solution" to the dilemma has been threefold. First, we require institutional oversight of clinical research through the mechanism of IRBs. Second, we require the voluntary and informed consent of the research subject. Finally, we allow a variety of post hoc remedies for those injured as a result of research, ranging from free emergency medical care to tort liability for researchers who, in spite of IRB approval and informed consent, can still be shown to have deviated from the appropriate standards.

One of the problems with the creation of academic–community partnerships derives from different ideas about the proper regulation of research. There is a phenomenon that occurs in the regulation of any human endeavor by which the regulation is directed not at those who have the most to gain or lose but instead at those who are most likely to comply with the burdens of regulation. In research regulation, this leads to a system wherein the research subjects, who have the most to lose, are not the main targets of regulation. Instead, the researchers, who arguably have the most to gain and little to lose, become the focus of the regulatory apparatus. This is, perhaps, as it must be, but it leads to distorting effects. The punishments for those who are regulated must be tied to distinct and particular rules. The rules are devised in order to create certain behaviors, but following the rules does not necessarily mean that those behaviors are, in fact, being followed, only that they are being documented. Documentation becomes the surrogate behavior that can be observed, measured, and evaluated.

The best example of this paradoxical effect is in the development of the practice of obtaining informed consent from subjects for standard medical treatment. The movement to require such consent developed out of subjects' desire for more information and protection from researchers. They attempted to operationalize this desire this through legal means—they sued doctors for harms that resulted from innovative therapies. Thus, regulation was imposed on researchers from outside the profession through a series of malpractice cases. In one of the earliest cases, the physicians caring for Martin Salgo, a 55-year-old man with cramping leg pains, recommended that Mr. Salgo undergo an aortogram. When Mr. Salgo awoke after the procedure, he could not move his legs. He sued the doctors for failing to warn him of the risks of paralysis inherent in the procedure. Mr. Salgo's claim was poignant because the doctors, although apparently not negligent in performing the procedure, made the patient worse than he was before he sought their help. In such situations, the judges ruled that it was not justifiable to withhold information about toxicity (*Salgo v. Leland Stanford University Board of Trustees,* 1957).

Similarly, in *Natanson v. Kline* (1960), a patient suffered damage from radiation therapy that was given to her after a mastectomy in order to prevent recurrence of her breast cancer. She later sued her doctor for not warning her about the effects that radiation therapy would have on her. Again, this was a situation in which a patient suffered a foreseeable side effect of a therapy that had not been negligently delivered.

These cases were buttressed by moral arguments that asserted that patients, like all citizens, had a right to make autonomous decisions and that they needed information that only doctors could provide in order to make those decisions. Doctors initially howled in protest at the new, legally imposed standard for communication and truth-telling. Even doctors engaged in clinical research felt that discussing procedures in detail with patients was inappropriate. As recently as 1965, Donald Fredrickson, Director of the National Heart Institute, could oppose disclosure because it might "unduly alarm the patient and hinder his reasonable evaluation of procedures important to his welfare" (Rothman, 1991).

More recently, doctors have embraced the concept of informed consent. Unfortunately, this has not always been for reasons initially imagined by judges and philosophers. The requirement that patients give informed consent was initially thought to be a fundamental change in the moral basis of the doctor–patient relationship. In particular, it was seen as a way of allowing patients and doctors to share responsibility for decision making, of reducing the silence that Katz (1984) abhorred, and of equalizing the power balance between doctors and patients. In reality today, it more often disempowers patients. In his recent novel *Operation Wandering Soul*, Powers (1994) describes a girl from Laos trying to explain an informed consent form to her father who speaks no English: "If you want them to treat me, you must agree not to ask for lots of money if they make a mistake and something bad happens." Informed consent is like the disclaimer on the back of a ski lift ticket: "Surgery is a dangerous sport. . . ." If we tell patients about bad outcomes, and they consent, then they are responsible, not us. Rather than a way of sharing power, truth-telling and the process of seeking consent have become a way of evading accountability.

The goals of law and the goals of ethics are not the same. The law is better at defining minimally acceptable behavior and leads to the development of standards that represent the lowest common denominator of social acceptability. Fine distinctions are drawn between what is minimally acceptable and what is impermissible, rather than between what is good and what is excellent. This self-protective legal approach, rather than the more idealistic ethical approach, has shaped truth-telling and informed consent in American medicine. This is not to blame the lawyers. Instead, responsibility lies with the doctors who often do not heed *moral* critiques but will quickly change their behavior in response to punishments meted out to their colleagues by judges or juries and, even then, tend to do what they must rather than what they ought.

With regard to research, as opposed to clinical care, the system of IRB oversight limits researchers' discretion even more. If they refuse to follow the IRB, their entire institutions' research operations will be shut down. If the IRBs were better at protecting the interests of the research subjects than the investigators were, this would be acceptable. However, IRBs today often focus less on protecting research subjects and more on protecting the institutions that they serve. In many cases, they seem to have lost sight of the central purpose of the central concept of informed consent.

This can be seen, in our case, by looking at the IRBs response to our protocol to use CHWs to improve asthma care.

The IRB Response

The response of the IRB to this proposal was interesting. The first response was to insist on a Memorandum of Agreement (MOA) between the community agency and the University of Chicago to ensure that the "ethical guidelines for research" were followed. The IRB insisted the community agency sign the following text:

MEMORANDUM OF AGREEMENT

Whereas Centro Comunitario Juan Diego, for whom the Director is Olivia Hernández, wishes to cooperate with The University of Chicago in the conduct of the project entitled "An Evaluation of a Community Health Worker Asthma Intervention" directed by Dr. John Lantos (primary investigator) and Dr. Molly Martin (contact),

The Parties agree as follows:

A. Protection for the Use of Human Subjects in Research

Centro Comunitario Juan Diego hereby gives assurance that they will comply with the requirements of The University of Chicago Multiple Project Assurance for the Protection of Human Subjects during their participation in the above referenced project and specifically agree as follows:

1. Centro Comunitario Juan Diego agrees to be guided by the ethical principles regarding research involving humans as subjects as set forth in the report of the National Commission for the Protection of Human Subjects of Biomedical and Behavioral Research entitled, Ethical Principles and Guidelines for the Protection of Human Subjects of Research (The Belmont Report) and agrees to satisfy the intent and procedures specified in 45 CFR Part 46 and other Federal, state or local laws or regulations that may apply.
2. Centro Comunitario Juan Diego acknowledges and accepts their responsibility for protecting the rights and welfare of human research subjects involved in research under this Agreement and for complying with all applicable provisions of the UC IRB and UC MPA under which this Agreement is implemented.
3. Centro Comunitario Juan Diego assures that before human subjects are involved research covered by the Memorandum of Agreement, proper consideration will be given to:
   a. the risks to the subject (being possible breech of confidentiality),
   b. the anticipated benefits to the subjects and others (such as subjects learning more about asthma and how to control it and Centro Comunitario Juan Diego making better programs for the community),
   c. the importance of the knowledge that may reasonably be expected to

result (an improvement in the understanding of asthma in Latinos and the roles community health workers can play),

d. the informed consent process to be employed (written), and

e. the need for additional safeguards if the human subjects are especially vulnerable.

4. Centro Comunitario Juan Diego will abide by determinations of the UC IRB and will accept the final authority and decisions of that IRB.

5. Centro Comunitario Juan Diego has reviewed the protocol as approved by the UC IRB and agrees to follow said protocol as described in Attachment A without deviation. [Note: Attachment A should be a summary of the protocol indicating in clear and precise language the steps to be followed by the physician.]

6. In the event that Centro Comunitario Juan Diego determines that a modification of the protocol is programmatically, scientifically, or clinically mandated, they will notify Dr. Molly Martin, who will be responsible for proposing an amendment to the approved Protocol. In no event will Centro Comunitario Juan Diego initiate the change until approved by the UC IRB.

7. Centro Comunitario Juan Diego will secure subject informed consent as described in the protocol and will use the consent form as approved by the UC IRB. A Centro Comunitario Juan Diego representative should sign the consent form to indicate that protocol procedures were followed. Original consent forms should be forwarded to Dr. Molly Martin who is responsible for maintaining project files. Centro Comunitario Juan Diego will retain copies of consent form in their files.

8. Completed case reports should be forwarded to Dr. Molly Martin in the form and format specified by Dr. Molly Martin.

9. Any adverse reactions must be reported immediately to Dr. Molly Martin (by a letter, which includes client's initials, description of adverse event, outcome).

10. Annually, Centro Comunitario Juan Diego will supply Dr. Molly Martin with appropriate information (e.g., progress to date, number of subjects, results, etc.) to allow the protocol to be renewed.

This MOA was interesting for two reasons. The first was that it challenged the relationship that had developed between the University of Chicago researcher and CCJD. CCJD was concerned about collaborating with University of Chicago because they saw themselves as the protectors of the rights of their clients and saw the academic medical center as traditionally the locus of exploitation. The MOA assumed just the opposite—that the university was the ultimate protector of the rights of research subjects, and that, in that role, the university had to make sure that CCJD was upholding all of the safeguards for research subjects that are guaranteed by federal law. This is, in itself, and on its face, admirable. The university should be doing that. The subjects do need to be protected. At the same time, there is something ironic or ludicrous about the implication that the university will do a better job in that role by following the federal guidelines for IRBs than CCJD, which is a community run center that has long defended the rights and needs of its community.

The second interesting thing about this MOA was that it was written in English. There was no discussion of or option for translation. The director of CCJD spoke very poor English and probably could not read or fully understand this document even though she is a well-educated and intelligent woman, any more than the University of Chicago's legal counsel could have understood the document if it had been written in Spanish. This sort of heedlessness signaled the sort of cluelessness that would be in evidence in all that followed.

Take the matter of informed consent. In collaboration with the folks at CCJD, we developed a consent form, written in simple Spanish, that explained the purpose of the project. We suggested that this be administered orally, rather than in written form, since many of the research subjects had low literacy. We explained the role of CHWs and the seriousness of asthma. We asked potential subjects if they would be willing to participate. The script was straightforward, easy to read, and included all of the essential elements of informed consent.

The IRB insisted that, instead, we include their "boilerplate" language that essentially insulates the university from liability for the project. The result was a four-page consent form in complicated English with multiple legal terms and references. The Spanish translation was required to have a certification that all content and terms were equal to those in the English version, which meant we could not alter the Spanish to be more understandable and to incorporate the slang of the target community. The CHWs at CCJD assured us that most potential subjects would not be able to understand it, but that they would sign it anyway, because they trusted the CHWs.

Some examples of the required text:

I agree to permit Dr. John Lantos and Dr. Molly Martin at the University of Chicago Hospitals and the Division of Biological Sciences to use and disclose my Protected Health Information (PHI) for the purposes described below. Protected Health Information includes any identifiable health information that is collected about me which would include my medical history and new information collected as a result of this study. Disclosure means that my Protected Health Information may be given to individuals outside the University of Chicago. I also agree to permit my doctors or other health care providers to disclose PHI to this Principal Investigator and research staff for the purposes described.

Yo estoy acuerdo en permitir a Dr. John Lantos y Dra. Molly Martin de la Universidad de los Hospitales de Chicago (University of Chicago Hospitals) y a la División de Ciencias Biológicas (Division of Biological Sciences) que usen y divulguen mi Información Médica Protegida (PHI, por sus siglas en inglés) para los propósitos descritos a seguir. La Información Médica Protegida incluye toda información médica identificable que haya sido recolectada sobre mi persona, que podría incluir mi historial médico y toda información nueva que se obtuviese como resultado de este estudio. Divulgación significa que mi Información Médica Protegida podría ser revelada a personas afuera de la Universidad de Chicago. Además, yo también autorizo a mis médicos y a otros proveedores de cuidados de salud para que revelen esta PHI a este Investigador Principal y al personal de investigación, para los propósitos descritos.

And:

The research study and the treatment procedures associated with it have been explained to me. The experimental procedures have been identified and no guarantee has been given about the possible results. I have had the opportunity to ask questions concerning any and all aspects of the study and any procedures involved. I am aware that I have the right to choose not to sign this form. However, if I decide not to sign, I cannot participate in this research. I understand that I may withdraw my consent at any time, but if I withdraw I will no longer be allowed to participate in this research and the protected health information collected prior to my written request may still be used. If I want to withdraw, I must write to: Dr. Molly Martin, 5841 S. Maryland Ave, MC2007, Chicago, IL 60637. I am aware that my decision not to participate or to withdraw will not restrict my access to health care services normally available at the University of Chicago Hospitals or Centro Comunitario Juan Diego. Confidentiality of records concerning my involvement in this study will be maintained in an appropriate manner. When required by law, the records of this research may be reviewed by applicable government agencies including the Federal Food and Drug Administration (FDA) and Office of Human Research Protections (OHRP). In addition, representatives of the University of Chicago, including the Institutional Review Board, a committee that oversees the research at the University of Chicago, may also view the records of the research.

El estudio de investigación y los procedimientos para el tratamiento asociados con el estudio se me han explicado. Los procedimientos experimentales han sido identificados y no se me ha dado garantía alguna acerca de sus resultados posibles. He tenido la oportunidad de hacer preguntas sobre cualquier aspecto del estudio y sobre cualquier procedimiento asociado con él. Yo tengo el derecho de elegir no firmar este formulario. Asimismo, si decido no firmarlo, no puedo participar de este estudio de investigación. Yo puedo cambiar de opinión y puedo anular esta Consentimiento en cualquier momento. Para anular esta Consentimiento yo debo escribir a: Dra. Molly Martin, 5841 S. Maryland Ave, MC2007, Chicago, IL 60637. No obstante, si anulo esta Consentimiento no podré continuar participando en este estudió de investigación. Además, el Investigador Principal aun así puede continuar usando mi Información Médica Protegida obtenida antes de mi pedido escrito, si esta información fuese necesaria para el estudio.

Estoy consciente de que si mi decisión es la de no participar, esta decisión no se interpondrá con mi acceso al cuidado médico en el Centro Comunitario Juan Diego ni con el acceso al cuidado médico normalmente disponible en los Hospitales de la Universidad de Chicago. La confidencialidad de todos mis datos respecto a este estudio será mantenida de la manera apropiada. Si fuera requerido por la ley, los datos de esta investigación pueden ser revisados por agencias del gobierno relevantes, incluyendo la Administración Federal de Drogas y Alimentos (FDA, por su sigla en inglés) y la Oficina de Protección de Sujetos Humanos Participantes de Estudios de Investigación (OHRP, por su sigla in inglés). Además, los registros de la investigación también pueden ser inspeccionados por representantes de la Universidad de Chicago, incluyendo la Junta de Revisión Institucional (Institutional Review Board), un comité que supervisa los estudios de investigación en la Universidad de Chicago.

As predicted, most potential subjects signed the form. It did not appear to have been any indication of their truly informed consent. But it met the letter of the IRB regulations, and so protected the University of Chicago from federal sanctions.

SUMMARY AND CONCLUSIONS

The university's approach to collaboration with community partners is essentially paternalistic. The university, operating under federal mandates, assumes that it alone knows what is "ethical" and that it alone can insure the protection of human subjects. The university's behavior in this regard is a massive overreaction to past abuses of vulnerable populations with a negative impact on the potential benefits of partnering with community-based collaborators. The dilemmas that it raises mirror the dilemmas of doing research in other countries. In particular, we must ask how much we should impose our standards of subject protection upon those who come from different traditions. In this case, however, the issues are somewhat more mundane than those that arise in, for example, trials of antiretroviral agents in developing countries. Nevertheless, the fundamental issues that they raise are similar. The central question is whether our mechanisms for protecting human subjects are better than those of other communities or whether, by contrast, our methods in fact function primarily to protect the institutions conducting the research from accusations that they have deviated from federal law. In some cases, overscrupulous adherence to federal guidelines may decrease, rather than increase, the empowerment of the most vulnerable participants in research.

▬

Questions for Discussion

1. What is the shift that most characterizes the field of research ethics in the last two decades? What are the implications of the shift?
2. Generally speaking, which framework protects the rights of subjects more extensively, community-based research or an academic institution research? Explain your answer, and discuss the importance of the question.
3. What are the primary ethical and legal challenges for physicians in American medicine at this time? How are these challenges generally approached?
4. Whose interests are weighed against each other within the CHW's MOA? According to the memorandum, who receives stronger protection?
5. Do you agree with the author's conclusion regarding the paternalism of the University of Chicago as it is reflected in the MOA?
6. Do you think that there is a need to create balance to the university's power in community-based research? How would you construct the right balance?

▬

References

Baier, C., Grant, E. N., Daugherty, S. R., & Eckenfels, E. J. (1999). The Henry Horner Pediatric Asthma Program. *Chest, 116*(4 Suppl. 1), 204S–206S.

Berman, P. A., Gwatkin, D. R., & Burger, S. E. (1987). Community-based health workers: Head start or false start towards health for all? *Social Science and Medicine, 25*(5), 443–459.

Butz, A. M., Malveaux, F. J., Eggleston, P., Thompson, L., Schneider, S., Weeks, K., et al. (1994). Use of community health workers with inner-city children who have asthma. *Clinical Pediatrics (Philadelphia), 33*(3), 135–141.

Center for Policy Alternatives. (1998). Community health workers: A leadership brief on preventive health programs. Washington DC.

Flores, G., Fuentes-Afflick, E., Barbot, O., Carter-Pokras, O., Claudio, L., Lara, M., et al. (2002). The health of Latino children: Urgent priorities, unanswered questions, and a research agenda. *Journal of the American Medical Association, 288*(1), 82–90.

Katz, J. (1984). *The silent world of doctor and patient.* New York: Free Press.

Ledogar, R. J., Penchaszadeh, A., Garden, C. C., & Garden, I. (2000). Asthma and Latino cultures: Different prevalence reported among groups sharing the same environment. *American Journal of Public Health, 90*(6), 929–935.

Natanson v. Kline, 186 Kansas 393, 406407, 350 P.2d 1093 (1960).

National Institutes of Health. (2004). National Asthma Education and Prevention Program Expert Panel Report 2: Guidelines for the Diagnosis and Management of Asthma. Bethesda, MD: author.

Powers, R.. (1994). *Operation wandering soul.* New York: Harper Perennial.

Rothman, D. J. (1991). *Strangers at the bedside.* New York: Basic Books.

Salgo v. Leland Stanford University Board of Trustees, 154 Cal.App.2d 560, 317 P.2d 170 (1957).

Stout, J. W, White, L. C., Rogers, L. T., McRorie, T., Morray, B., Miller-Ratcliffe, M., & Redding, G. J. (1998). The asthma outreach project: A promising approach to comprehensive asthma management. *Journal of Asthma, 35*(1), 119–127.

Thomas, S., & Whitman, S. (1999). Asthma hospitalizations and mortality in Chicago: An epidemiological overview. *Chest, 116*(4), 135S–141S.

University of Arizona. (1998). *The Final Report of the National Community Health Advisors Study: A Policy Research Project of the University of Arizona.* Baltimore, MD: Annie E. Casey Foundation.

5

Adolescent Research and Parental Permission

Lauren K. Collogan and Alan R. Fleischman

CASE DESCRIPTION

An investigator proposes to conduct structured interviews of adolescents to examine the relationship between sexual and drug use practices, as well as social and psychological background and human immunodeficiency virus (HIV) status. The results of the study will be used to further understanding of social determinants of HIV prevalence in adolescents and to generate hypotheses about prevention programs. The study is not designed to benefit participants, but rather to increase general knowledge.

The participants in the study will be patients at a general adolescent clinic in a large urban medical center. All patients will be recruited to become research participants at the time of enrollment for care in the clinic, and those who agree to participate in the study will complete a structured interview and will be tested for HIV using discarded blood drawn for other routine tests. The results of the HIV test will be linked only to the anonymous interview surveys so that associations with HIV status can be identified for research purposes. Participants will not be informed of their HIV status from the study test results, and the seroprevalence results will be anonymous and will not be linked to patient identifiers. However, all patients will be referred for voluntary HIV testing and counseling as is routine practice in this clinic.

Some of the topics that the interview will address include sexual behavior, partner history, contraceptive and barrier protection use, treatment for sexually transmitted diseases, and specifically whether or not the participant has engaged in anal, survival, unprotected, man to man, or oral sex. Participants will also be asked to discuss drug use and habits as well as any history of physical and sexual abuse.

In her application for institutional review board (IRB) approval, the investigator contends that the study does not place the participants at more than a minimal risk of harm, given the anonymous nature of the interview and the blinding of the HIV testing. She argues that she should not be required to obtain the permission of parents in order for adolescents to enroll in the study, and she claims that the sensitive nature of the questions might make some adolescents uncomfortable by involving parents in obtaining permission to take part in the study. The investigator feels that study participation will be limited if parental consent is required. Accordingly, the investigator requests that adolescents between 13 and 17 years of age be permitted to consent for enrollment in the study without parental permission.

ETHICAL ANALYSIS AND DISCUSSION

This chapter explores the ethical issues involved in consent for research involving adolescents and the use of waivers of parental permission for participation. We discuss the legal standing of adolescents and their capacity to make complex decisions about clinical care and research participation. Next, we review existing federal regulations governing research with children and adolescents in order to focus on the role of waiver of parental permission in adolescent research. The chapter ends with a review of the case example and considerations for IRBs faced with requests to forgo parental involvement in consent for research involving adolescents.

Adolescents

The adolescent population consists of individuals who are approximately 10–21 years of age, characterized by a state of dynamic physiological and psychological development (English, 1990; Fleming, Towey, & Jarosik, 2001). This rapid and continual state of physical and mental growth distinguishes adolescents from children and adults and defines a group of individuals with unique health needs and risks (Santelli et al., 2003). Pubertal development results in physical changes to members of this group, including fluctuation of hormone levels and progressive maturation of reproductive systems, in ways that set them apart from younger children and fully developed adults. Furthermore, the onset of puberty and maturation also changes adolescent decisional capacity and influences the health behaviors of members of this group (Santelli et al., 2003). Adolescents face distinct social pressures that combine with developing cognitive skills to place this group at risk for beginning a number of high-risk behaviors with potential long-term negative health consequences, such as violence, sexual activity, substance abuse, and poor nutritional health (Santelli et al., 2003). Consequently, adolescents face an increased risk of physical injury, sexually transmitted diseases (including HIV

infection), unplanned pregnancy, illness or injury due to substance abuse, and conditions such as obesity and diabetes. Many medical professionals, educators, public health officials, and others have called for interventions to educate adolescents, reduce risky behaviors, and prevent poor health outcomes (Fleming et al., 2001).

Research is an important tool in developing interventions to address the health needs of adolescents, particularly in distinguishing the characteristics of this group from those of other populations (Santelli et al., 2003). The physical and mental characteristics of this age group cause this population to respond differently than do adults or children to therapeutic drug treatment, educational interventions, counseling efforts, and other responses designed to alleviate medical conditions and decrease health risks to individuals (English, 1995). Clinical investigation allows those working to improve adolescent health to tailor their efforts and make them more responsive to the specific problems faced by this population. For example, investigational studies with adolescent populations found that sexually transmitted *Chlamydia* infection is widespread in this group, particularly among females, and more so than levels indicated in adults (Gaydos et al., 1998). Consequently, efforts have begun to educate adolescents specifically about this condition to help reduce its spread (Fleming et al., 2001). *Chlamydia* infection is just one preventable condition in adolescents identified by clinical research. Accordingly, research with adolescents generates benefits specific to this group in ways that similar research in adult or child populations cannot (Levine, 1995).

Definition of Minors in the Legal Context

Most adolescents are considered to be minors. Minors, or children, are those individuals under the legal age of majority, or the age at which individuals are presumed to be legally competent (Santelli et al., 2003). Competence as it is used here is not necessarily an indication of mental ability or decisional capacity, but a legal term that enfranchises individuals and gives them the status of "adults" (Gaylin, 1982). Competent adults are individuals who are assumed to possess a certain level of decisional capacity and are thus granted decisional and economic autonomy. Some of the rights granted to competent adults (and denied to minors) include the right to vote, the right to purchase alcohol and cigarettes, and the right to enter into legally binding contracts. It is possible for adults to be declared incompetent, thus losing some or all of these rights. However, adults are presumed to be competent, while individuals under the age of majority are presumed incompetent, without any proof of decisional capacity required (Gaylin, 1982).

Most state and federal laws define the age of majority as 18 years (Campbell, 2004). Individuals under 18 years of age are legally restricted from making many decisions. Often, minors are not legally authorized to make decisions in areas of their own lives, such as education and employment, without permission from or the consent of parents or guardians. Accordingly, until reaching the age of majority, most minors are legally dependent on their parents or guardians (English, 1990).

Definition of Minors in the Clinical Context

The clinical health care setting is another example of an area where minors have historically been legally restricted from making binding decisions. In general, when providing treatment for medical conditions, physicians are legally and ethically bound to obtain informed consent from patients before proceeding with that treatment. Informed consent here stems from a desire to respect individual autonomy and consists of informing the patient of his/her condition, the treatment options available to him/her, the risks and benefits of each option, and then allowing the patient to make a free and uncoerced choice (National Commission, 1978b; *American Academy of Pediatrics,* 1995). In the case of minor patients, however, most state and federal laws presume that minors lack the decisional capacity necessary to make appropriate decisions regarding medical treatment (Buchanan & Brock, 1989). These laws allow physicians to forgo patient informed consent and instead charge parents or guardians with making treatment decisions on behalf of minors (Buchanan & Brock, 1989; English, 1995). Parents or legal guardians, who in most cases are above the age of majority, are presumed to possess adequate decisional capacity and are therefore able to provide legally binding, informed permission for their minor children to receive treatment. This concept of informed permission has the same requirements as informed consent, except permission comes from the parent, not the patient (American Academy of Pediatrics, 1995).

In many cases, parental consent is all that is required for a minor to receive medical treatment, especially in cases of very young children. However, as children grow older and their decisional capabilities improve, many physicians feel ethically bound to obtain the assent of minor patients as well as the permission of their parents or guardians (American Academy of Pediatrics, 1995). Obtaining assent consists of informing the minor patient of his/her condition and of the test or treatment proposed, then asking the minor whether or not he/she is willing to undergo that test or treatment (American Academy of Pediatrics, 1995). A minor gives assent when he or she says that he or she is willing to undergo the test or treatment. Assent differs from consent in that while the willingness of a minor to accept treatment may be an important consideration, treatment may often proceed against the wishes of the minor if his or her parent or guardian consents. Thus, it is the permission of the parents or guardians, not the assent of the child, that is considered legally binding in these cases.

Changing Role of Adolescents in the Clinical Setting

Despite the precedent of considering minors incapable of providing informed consent in the clinical setting, the decisional role of older minors, or adolescents, in this context has changed (English, 1990). Although state laws still require parental permission for most forms of treatment for minors, exceptions to these laws now allow some adolescents to receive treatment without the permission or knowledge of their parents or guardians. Two categories of minors, emancipated minors and mature minors, have been outlined in common law, and a third exception exists in state statutes concerning specific medical categories.

Emancipated Minors   Common law has long since allowed for minors to be considered as adults, with all of the attendant rights and responsibilities, under certain conditions. These emancipated minors are treated under the law as though they had reached the age of majority and are no longer under the control of parents or guardians (Campbell, 2004; English, 1990). Historically, minors only became emancipated when they married or enrolled in the military, and usually with some form of tacit or explicit consent on the part of their parents or guardians (Capron, 1982). However, the courts have also found that minors may be considered emancipated if they live apart from their parents and are financially independent, and if the parents do not continue to care for them (Campbell, 2004; English, 1990). Many states currently have statutes outlining conditions that must be met before a minor may be considered emancipated. These conditions include marriage, active duty in the military, living independently (physically and economically) of parents or guardians, or the presence of a court order, though the conditions differ from state to state. Once they have been emancipated, minors may consent to their own medical treatment, though this ability to make medical decisions is not explicitly stated in all state laws (Campbell, 2004).

Mature Minors   The mature minor doctrine has evolved in the courts as a means for minors with adequate decisional capacity and understanding of their medical situation to be allowed to consent to treatment. Under this doctrine, minors who are not emancipated from their families and show the ability to comprehend the risks and benefits of treatment may provide consent to that treatment, thus eliminating the need for parental or guardian consent (English, 1990). As opposed to emancipation laws, which grant minors adult status for all decisions, the mature minor doctrine applies only to specific medical decisions. While many states have explicitly outlined mature minor exception statutes, some states have not (Campbell, 2004; Capron, 1982; English, 1990). In many states, the standards for allowing a minor to be considered a mature minor and able to make medical decisions involve marriage, pregnancy, or status as a minor parent (Campbell, 2004). In states where emancipation does not explicitly allow for medical decision making, emancipation is one means of being declared a mature minor (Campbell, 2004). However, beyond these explicit standards, courts have shown a willingness to invoke the doctrine in cases of treatment without parental permission if the minor patient seemed capable of providing informed consent (English, 1990). Many professional organizations, including the American Medical Association, recognize the importance of the mature minor doctrine and urge health care professionals to treat mature minors without parental consent, even in the absence of a specific state statute addressing mature minors (American Medical Association, 1992).

Medically Emancipated Minors   In addition to the emancipated and mature minor exceptions, all states have statutes that allow physicians to treat minors for certain medical conditions without the involvement of parents or guardians (English & Kenney, 2003). These conditions and the restrictions on treatment vary from state to state but generally permit adolescents to consent to treatment for conditions for which they might be reluctant to seek needed care if parental involvement was required, such as sexually transmitted diseases, mental illness, and substance abuse, as well as treatment pertaining to pregnancy and birth control.

Beyond these three categories of decision making by minors in the clinical context, health care providers have begun to give more weight to the decisions of minors, particularly older adolescents, even when their choices conflict with the decisions of parents or guardians. Particularly for children who are chronically ill or at the end of life, providers have begun to make attempts to involve minors in the decision making process with the goals of respecting patient autonomy and increasing parent and patient satisfaction with treatment (McCabe, 1996). Since the 1970s, both medical and legal professionals have begun to call for increased patient involvement in the treatment of minors, even in cases where the patients and their parents disagree (Derish & Heuvel, 2000; Weir & Peters, 1997). Such disagreements are especially common in cases involving parental decisions to commit minors to psychiatric facilities and care at the end of life. There is legal precedent for allowing minor adolescents to leave mental institutions or avoid commitment against the wishes of their parents (Holder, 1985; *Melville v. Sabbatino*, 1973). There is also precedent to reject the substituted judgment of parents and providers if the minor involved has adequate decisional capacity (*In re Swan*, 1990).

Decisional Capacity

Although numerous studies have attempted to assess and define decisional capacity, there exists no universally accepted standard definition (Appelbaum & Roth, 1982; Rosenstein, 2003; Roth, Meisel, & Lidz, 1977). However, there are several standards used to determine decisional capacity for competency evaluations in the legal setting, as laid out in Appelbaum and Grisso (1988). These standards include evidencing a choice, understanding the factual issues involved in the choice, manipulation of information, and appreciating the nature of the information and applying it to one's own situation (Appelbaum & Roth, 1982; Grisso & Appelbaum, 1995; McCabe et al., 1996; Roth et al., 1977). McCabe (1996) also cites a standard of "voluntariness or freedom from coercion," which is a key element of any informed consent to treatment or research participation (Beauchamp & Childress, 1994). These standards are not applied in the same ways to different decisional contexts; indeed, an individual may be capable of meeting standards of competency in one situation, but unable to in another (Rosenstein, 2004; Roth et al, 1977). Whether or not an individual possesses decisional capacity depends on the type of decision and the risks and benefits involved.

Testing decisional capacity using the above standards can be accomplished using interviews or tests in which various elements of capacity are examined. These examinations may include testing of intelligence (IQ), language skills, attention, orientation, and recall and recent memory (Appelbaum & Roth, 1982). Another measurement may involve presentations to individuals who are then asked to recount information given to them in their own words, which ensures a retention and understanding of information about the decision they are to make (Grisso & Appelbaum, 1995). Conversations including the use of example problems or "vignettes" to which individuals must respond may also measure whether or not an individual understands information and is able to weigh consequences of different decisions (Appelbaum & Roth, 1982; Grisso & Appelbaum, 1995). Dialogue with individuals can be used to measure their understanding and insight into a situation as well as the presence of any condition (denial, depression, psychosis, etc.) that may prevent decision making (Appelbaum & Roth, 1982; Grisso & Appelbaum, 1995). Although some of these criteria require formal psychiatric evaluation, many of these standards are measurable in the form of a simple discussion with or written test of an individual (Derish & Heuvel, 2000).

Children and adolescents develop decisional capacity in stages, and children of different ages have differing abilities to process information and manipulate it in order to make decisions. Jean Piaget defined several stages through which children progress in the development of mental capacity. The first stages involve young children from birth until approximately 7–8 years of age. In these stages, children learn to use language and representational skills, but they have a limited perspective of the world. Piaget classified children from age 7 or 8 to age 12 to be in the stage of concrete operations, in which children have multiple perspectives and can manipulate information (Piaget, 1962). However, they are not able to understand problems in the abstract. Piaget called the final and most important stage of development the formal operations stage (Buchanan & Brock, 1989). It is in this stage that children and adolescents develop the means to think abstractly and hypothetically, as would be required for choosing between options and consenting to treatment (Grisso & Vierling, 1978). Piaget observed that elements of formal operations appeared between the ages of 11 and 13, but many children do not enter this stage until later. Some individuals never reach this stage of development, even in adulthood (Grisso & Vierling, 1978). It follows that, despite this general understanding of cognitive development, there is no one age at which all individuals can uniformly be said to possess the decisional capacity to consent to treatment or research participation. Currently, 18 years of age serves as the brightline standard for presuming competency, but this standard does not take into account individuals between the ages of 13 and 18 who may have reached the formal operations stage and thus have reached the cognitive development of decisional capacity necessary to provide consent.

Findings from several studies indicate that many individuals younger than 18 years do possess elements of decision making necessary for providing consent to treatment and research participation. The most frequently cited of these studies tested the developmental differences in competency to make decisions regarding treatment (Weithorn & Campbell, 1982). The study took children, adolescents, and adults of four ages (9, 14, 18, and 21 years of age) and attempted to determine their ability to meet the four standards of competency discussed by Appelbaum and Roth (1982): evidencing a choice, making a reasonable choice given the predicted outcome, providing rational reasons for the choice, and understanding the risks, benefits, and alternatives to that treatment. The study presented participants with four hypothetical health-related decisions with two or more possible treatment options. The study rated the participants based on their responses to the hypothetical situations and indications that they met the four competency standards. The results of the study supported the study's hypothesis, based on Piaget's observations, that minors 14 years of age do not differ from adults in their level of competency in making treatment decisions. Even the 9-year-old participants were able to evidence a choice and give reasonable support for their choices. The study concluded that "the ages of 18 or 21 as the 'cutoffs' below which individuals are presumed to be incompetent to make determinations about their own welfare do not reflect the psychological capacities of most adolescents" (Weithorn & Campbell, 1982).

Other studies have also provided evidence that many minors possess elements of decisional capacity adequate for consent to treatment and research participation. A study involving interviews of children as young as 6 years old about participation in a flu vaccine trial found that even young children can understand information about clinical investigations and can evidence reasoned choices regarding participation in research (Lewis, Lewis, & Ifekwunigue, 1978). Another study involved patients 7–20 years of age who were receiving treatment for cancer or obesity (Susman, Dorn, & Fletcher, 1992). Each of these children, adolescents, and adults were enrolled in research protocols and were later interviewed about the research and the consent process to determine the participant's understanding of the research using 12 elements of informed consent. These elements consisted of knowing the purpose of the research, that participation was voluntary, the potential risks and benefits, and alternative treatments. The study found that the participants had a good understanding of the concrete elements of the research, such as the duration of the research and the potential benefits, but were less likely to understand the scientific purpose of the research. Only 15% of the participants could discuss the potential risks of participation. While these results indicate that children and adolescents vary greatly in their ability to meet all of the standards of informed consent, the results did not differ from similar studies with adult participants. That is, while children and adolescents vary in their abilities to understand research participation, these variations are no different than the variations in the adult population. This same study also found that knowledge about research participation was related to the psychological state of the participants, rather than developmental factors such as chronological age or cognitive development (Dorn, Susman, & Fletcher, 1995). These results lend support to the argument that age should not be the determining factor in an individual's ability to comprehend research participation.

With respect to the voluntariness element of informed consent, evidence indicates that minors are more likely than adults to perceive of pressure while making decisions concerning treatment or research participation, but not that they are incapable of making free choices in the proper environment. One study found that children 10–12 years of age were capable of understanding elements of research and possessed the capacity to consent to participation, but that these children did not understand or believe that their participation was voluntary or confidential (Abramovitch, Freedman, Thoden, & Nikolich, 1991). However, the study involved children who knew that their parents had consented to the research, a situation that prevents children from acting as "free agents," given their dependence on their parents. Another study indicated that although children and adolescents may not always be aware of their rights and therefore able to invoke them, this absence of knowledge is not necessarily related to lack of cognitive development as much as lack of experience (Ruck, Keating, Abramovitch, & Koegl, 1998). More research is needed, but there is no evidence to suggest that adolescents are not capable of reasoning about their rights once they know them.

Given existing research, psychologists have argued that normal adolescents 14 or more years of age possess the elements of decisional capacity necessary to provide informed consent for treatment and research participation (Grisso & Vierling, 1978; Weithorn, 1983). However, even for children and adolescents with cognitive development similar to that of adults, adolescents do possess characteristics that distinguish them from adults and may adversely affect their decisional abilities. Even children and adolescents who are able to weigh the risks and benefits of multiple options and manipulate hypothetical situations before making a decision may still not possess the life experience or perspective of an older individual. Research has indicated that many adolescents are still developing their decision making capabilities. Adolescents are more likely than adults to act impulsively, and they are more likely to be focused on their current situation, rather than their situation in the future (Leikin, 1983; Levine, 1995). Given the importance of differentiating between short and long-term consequences in making decisions about treatment or research participation, many adolescents may not be able to provide full and knowing consent in this context (Grisso & Vierling, 1978). Adolescents are also more likely than adults to be focused on bodily appearance over other considerations (Leikin, 1983). Finally, adolescents may be more likely to defer to authority, medical, parental, or otherwise, in situations concerning research participation (Grisso & Vierling, 1978). Thus, even minors who have reached the formal operations stage of cognitive development may require additional protections to ensure their ability to provide voluntary, informed consent in the research context.

Clinical Context Versus Research Context

Although there are sometimes similarities between the clinical and research settings, receiving treatment in a clinical context differs markedly from participating in a nontherapeutic research protocol. The most important difference between the two settings is that of purpose. A health care provider treats a patient with the goal of improving the condition of that patient. Given this goal, clinicians only recommend treatment that they believe will be in the best interest of the patient, and the benefits of the treatment are presumed to outweigh the risks involved. Alternatively, the primary objective of clinical research is to produce generalizable knowledge using sound experimental methods. The interests of individual participants in the experiment are secondary to this overall goal. While investigators must protect research participants from harm, they are not obligated to consider whether or not participation in a study is in the best interest of each individual participant. Often, individuals take part in experiments that involve no prospect of direct benefit to participants. Studies may also involve substantial potential risks to participants, or they may result in some participants receiving no treatment, experimental or otherwise, if the investigation involves a placebo or observational control group. The distinction between the objectives of clinical treatment and clinical research leads to differences in the way informed consent is achieved in the two contexts. Given that the benefits of treatment generally outweigh the risks involved and that the motivation for treatment is the best interest of the patient, making a decision to consent to treatment generally requires less manipulation of risks and benefits and weighing of competing options than consenting to participation in research. Consequently, clinicians accept and abide by most decisions to consent to treatment, even when those decisions are made by persons of limited decisional capacity (McCabe, 1996; Rosenstein, 2003). Conversely, a person deciding whether or not to participate in research must seriously consider the potential risks and benefits of participation, including the possibility of no personal benefit, as well as the possible competing motivations of the researcher. Furthermore, the doctrine of informed consent requires that potential participants understand the primary purpose of the investigation and that it may not provide the prospect of direct benefit (Appelbaum et al., 1987). Accordingly, it may be argued that providing informed consent in the research context requires more sophisticated decisional capacity than consent to clinical treatment.

Regulating Research

The differences between consenting to treatment and consenting to research participation necessitate greater protections for those with limited decisional capacity in the research context than in the treatment setting. While regulation of clinical treatment has been left to state statutes, federal regulations were created to govern all human subject research funded or overseen by federal agencies. These regulations require institutional review for all research with human participants as well as the need for voluntary informed consent from subjects or their guardians. These regulations, known as the Common Rule, (DHHS, 1991) are based on part of the regulations adopted by the Department of Health and Human Services (DHHS) to govern research under their purview and have been incorporated into the policies of 17 federal agencies. The Common Rule is based on respect for the autonomy of individual participants in research as well as the obligation of investigators and IRBs to protect participants from harm.

In addition to the Common Rule, the DHHS Policy for Protection of Human

Research Subjects also includes a subpart D with specific regulations for research involving children. These additional regulations, which have also been adopted (with one notable exception) by the Food and Drug Administration (FDA), define children as "persons who have not attained the legal age for consent to treatments or procedures involved in the research, under the applicable law of the jurisdiction in which the research will be conducted" (45 CFR 46.402(a)). It is important to note that children are not categorized here as being under the local age of majority, but rather under the age at which they can legally consent to the treatments or procedures contained in the research. Given the number of states that allow legally defined minors to consent to specific treatments, this definition implies that the regulations governing children are only applicable to those minors who do not meet any of the exceptions allowing them to consent to the treatment being employed in the research protocol. Research involving minors who are legally able to provide consent to the treatment would be regulated by considering the adolescents as similar to adults with full authority to consent or refuse research participation with no parental involvement.

The DHHS and FDA regulations describe four categories of permissible research involving children, defined by the level of potential risk and benefit of participation (45 CFR 46, subpart D). These categories are (1) research not involving greater than minimal risk, (2) research involving greater than minimal risk but with the potential for direct benefit to individual participants, (3) research involving a minor increase over minimal risk with no prospect for direct benefit to individual participants but likely to yield generalizable knowledge of vital importance about the participant's disorder or condition, and (4) research not otherwise approvable but that presents an opportunity to understand, prevent, or alleviate a serious problem affecting the health or welfare of children.

"Minimal risk" is defined as "the probability and magnitude of harm or discomfort anticipated in the research are not greater in and of themselves than those ordinarily encountered in daily life or during the performance of routine physical or psychological examinations" (45 CFR 46.102(i)). While the regulations do not explicitly distinguish between children of different ages, risks encountered in daily life necessarily change as children grow older. The daily risks encountered in the life of a toddler who is rarely if ever left unattended by an adult differ dramatically from the risks encountered by a 16-year-old adolescent who attends school, might drive, plays sports, and engages in many independent activities. Thus, research that might be considered to pose greater than minimal risk for a younger child might pose minimal risk for an adolescent.

This definition of minimal risk is considered to be an "objective" standard indexed to daily lives of healthy, average children, not a "subjective" one relative to social situations or level of illness (National Human Research Protections Advisory Committee, 2002).

Parental Permission and Minor Assent to Research

Each category of permissible research carries protective requirements that must be met before research can be approved. All of the categories require researchers to obtain parental permission for children to participate in research, including permission from both parents for research that involves greater than minimal risk and does not hold the potential for direct benefit to participants (45 CFR 46.408(c)). The regulations also require investigators to obtain the assent of the participants themselves, if the IRB finds that the minor participants are capable of providing it.

The requirement for parental permission for research with minors is based in the desire to protect a population whose members may not be capable of protecting themselves. Minors, in addition to being presumed legally incapable of making decisions, have limited life experience and are more likely to be members of an emotionally, financially, and intellectually vulnerable population than someone who is older. Adolescents in particular underestimate long-term consequences of participation and are more likely to be influenced by peer groups and considerations of appearance than adults (McCabe, 1996). These influences and the socially vulnerable role of minors may inhibit a realistic accounting of the potential risks and benefits of research participation. Accordingly, parental judgment is often substituted for the judgment of minors.

The role of parents as protectors and decision makers for their children is a concept present in many cultures and social groups (National Commission, 1978a). It also has a strong legal history in the United States (English, 1990). For most children, it is presumed that their parents, who are usually over the age of majority and therefore presumed competent to make decisions, will make better decisions for their children than any other person (Buchanan and Brock, 1989). Generally, parents know their children, have a desire to protect their best interests, and possess greater life experience (Derish & Heuvel, 2000; McCabe et al., 1996). Accordingly, parents generally behave in a manner consistent with the best interests of their children.

For research with participants who possess adequate maturity, investigators are also required to solicit the assent of minor participants in addition to parental permission. The assent requirement stems from a desire to respect children as individuals. In its 1978 report, the National Commission for the Protection of Human Subjects of Biomedical and Behavioral Research emphasized the need to recognize and respect the wishes of children as they develop cognitively and mature (National Commission, 1978a). This mental development allows children an increasing ability to determine their own best interests, and thus, as children age, respect for evolving autonomy obligates investigators to take their decisions into greater consideration. The commission recommended that investigators solicit assent from all potential subjects older than 6 years; the current federal regulations state that an attempt to solicit assent from potential subjects is necessary when the IRB finds that the participants are of appropriate "age, maturity, and psychological state" (45 CFR 46.408(a)). However, despite this requirement, the regulations also state that IRBs may permit research without assent of subjects if the research holds out the prospect of "direct benefit that is important to the health or well-being of children and is available only in the context of research," as long as parental permission is obtained (45 CFR 46.408(a)).

Importance of Adolescent Research and Use of Waivers of Parental Permission

Despite the long-standing tradition of requiring parental permission for research with minors, there are exceptions to the requirement in some circumstances.

Section 46.408(c) of the federal guidelines states:

> [I]f the IRB determines that a research protocol is designed for conditions or for a subject population for which parental or guardian permission is not a reasonable requirement to protect the subjects (for example, neglected or abused children), it may waive the consent requirements . . . provided an appropriate mechanism for protecting the children who will participate as subjects in the research is substituted. (45 CFR 46.408(c))

This exception to the parental permission requirement was developed from a recommendation by the National Commission report on research with children. The National Commission recommended that IRBs be able to waive the requirement of parental permission, if that requirement were not reasonable to protect participants, provided that other protections for the minor participants be implemented (National Commission, 1978a). In particular, the National Commission emphasized the "special needs of adolescents," especially the need for improved treatment of conditions involving sexual and reproductive health and drug use. The National Commission argued that requiring parental permission for research participation would make it difficult for these types of research to take place and for treatment to advance, given the sensitive nature of the research and the presumed reluctance of adolescents to request parental permission. Accordingly, they argued that the "assent of such mature minors should be considered sufficient with respect to research about conditions for which they have legal authority to consent to their own treatment" (National Commission, 1978).

The regulations also allow for a waiver of parental permission for certain research that is of minimal risk to participants. In 45 CFR 46.408(c), the regulations allow IRBs to waive the requirement for parental permission in circumstances where ordinary informed consent may be waived. These circumstances include research that is of minimal risk and cannot be practicably performed without a waiver, and where the waiver will not adversely affect the rights and welfare of participants (45 CFR 46.116(d)).

In recent years, progress in certain areas of research has been inhibited due to the requirement of parental permission. Many adolescents are unwilling to take part in certain types of studies if doing so involves disclosing their illness, condition, or behaviors to their parents or guardians. Research indicates that many adolescents would stop seeking certain types of beneficial treatments if their parents would be informed (Ford & English, 2002; Reddy, Fleming, & Swain, 2002). Accordingly studies involving substance abuse, mental health, sexual activity, and pregnancy, areas in which research is needed to improve adolescent health, often lack participants because adolescents do not feel comfortable with the requirement for parental permission.

Even if adolescents are willing to disclose their conditions by telling their parents that they want to participate in particular types of research, parents may not allow their children to take part in studies discussing certain topics. Parents may fear that allowing such research will affirm or promote undesirable lifestyle choices, such as substance abuse or sexual activity (Petersen & Leffert, 1995). Studies have shown that there is no correlation between research participation and inducing undesired behavior (Santelli et al., 1995). However unfounded these parental concerns, they may result in effectively preventing adolescent research when parental permission is required.

Despite regulations that permit waiver of parental permission, IRBs rarely invoke this option in research involving adolescents. A survey study in, 1994 indicated that most IRBs are not likely to grant waivers of parental permission for any kind of research with minors (Mammel & Kaplan, 1995). There are several potential reasons for this reluctance on the part of IRBs. The study indicated that different IRBs had different interpretations of the appropriate uses for the waiver, and that some IRBs would waive parental permission for research while other boards would require permission for the same research. Furthermore, while over half the review boards surveyed supported changing the regulations to allow minors to provide full informed consent for many different types of research, few were willing to waive the permission requirement under the current regulations. The study concluded that given the variable interpretations of the current guidelines and the overall support for adolescent consent, the current regulations should be clarified.

Although the regulations include an example of a situation in which it might be appropriate for an IRB to waive parental permission (for an abused or neglected child), they do not include an explication of other situations in which it might be "reasonable" to waive parental permission. Unlike the National Commission report that specifically cited research with adolescents, the regulations do not discuss what types of research or what type of minor participants might fall under this exception. As a result, there exists little federal guidance for IRBs faced with requests from investigators to waive the parental permission requirement. Additionally, although the regulations call for IRBs to make determinations of the decisional capacity of minor participants, for purposes of considering assent, the regulations do not provide any guidance or methods for determining decisional capacity, maturity, and psychological state.

In, 1995, the Society for Adolescent Medicine released a set of guidelines encouraging IRBs to utilize waiver of parental permission in order to allow certain types of research involving adolescents to take place. However, a study in 1999 indicated that the guidelines did not greatly influence IRB decision making (Rogers, Schwartz, Weissman, & English, 1999). The study approached 11 IRBs with a common protocol, dealing with observation of HIV-positive adolescents, that the authors believed posed only minimal risk. Only four of the IRBs determined the study to be of minimal risk and accordingly waived the parental permission requirement. Other IRBs found study participation to carry minimal risk but were reluctant to waive parental permission. Furthermore, only one IRB of the 11 in the study had a method for taking into consideration the risks and benefits of the study and the maturity of the potential participants when making decisions about waiving the parental permission requirement, even though the regulations specify that IRBs should consider these factors. The study concluded that IRBs varied in their definitions of minimal risk and the uses of waivers of parental permission. Additionally, the authors found that IRBs were more likely to make decisions about waiver of parental permission based on their desire to avoid institutional risk rather than on the risks and benefits of the study and the decisional capacity of the participants.

The Society for Adolescent Medicine re-released their 1995 guidelines in 2003 and reemphasized the need for research with adolescents and the need to increase the use of parental permission waivers (Santelli et al., 2003). However, as the paper accompanying the guidelines reports, researchers and IRBs remain unclear as to the correct interpretation of the federal regulations and how to apply state laws that apply to adolescents. Accordingly, they argue that research continues to effectively exclude adolescent participants, negatively impacting the development of treatment options for this group (Santelli et al., 2003).

An additional factor that may work to complicate IRB decision making and limit utilizing waivers of parental permission is the absence of a parental permission waiver in the FDA regulations governing research with children. In April 2001, the FDA published an interim rule concerning 21 CFR, parts 50 and 56, entitled "Additional Safeguards for Children in Clinical Investigations of FDA-Regulated Products" (National Human Research Protections Advisory Committee,

2001). The rule was an attempt to bring the FDA regulations in line with DHHS regulations, as was mandated in the Children's Health Act of 2000. However, in adopting the DHHS regulations, the FDA did not adopt 45 CFR 46.408(c), the section of the regulations allowing IRBs to waive parental permission when "reasonable." The FDA stated that legal constraints do not allow for waivers of informed consent under any condition, and accordingly, IRBs are not permitted to waive the parental permission requirement for any studies involving drug trials. Some have argued that invoking a waiver of parental permission empowers the adolescents to consent to research participation, thus providing full informed consent as required by FDA law (National Human Research Protections Advisory Committee, 2001). As it stands, the FDA and DHHS regulations remain in conflict over this issue.

Given that some research holds potential benefits for individual adolescents and the adolescent population, and given that many adolescents possess decisional capacity similar to that of adults, there are certain cases where IRB use of the parental permission waiver is both ethically justified and legally permissible. These cases would involve only developmentally mature adolescents and research that could not reasonably proceed without the waiver. Such research might include low-risk studies where potential adolescent participants fear a negative reprisal were they to reveal participation in the research to their parents or guardian.

CONCLUSION

Standards for Waiving Parental Permission

The case study presented in this chapter examines at-risk adolescents and the correlation of behavior to HIV status. IRBs faced with reviewing a proposal like this need to create a systematic method to evaluate the protocol based on the characteristics of the research and the characteristics of the proposed participant population. Not all studies involving adolescents require waiver of parental permission. However, if the study protocol carries low potential risk and involves an area about which adolescents are likely to be reluctant to share information with their parents, and the adolescents themselves are generally mature, IRBs may determine that the research cannot practicably proceed without a waiver of parental permission. Such a determination fulfills the "reasonable" standard for parental permission waivers set out in 46.408(c). There are several key aspects of this protocol that must be considered.

This study involves discussion of substance use habits, sexual behavior, and other sensitive information that adolescents may be reluctant to discuss with parents or guardians. Accordingly, it is reasonable to argue that the protocol will not enroll a representative sample of participants to ensure generalizability unless adolescents are allowed to participate without the permission of their parents or guardians. A fundamental tenet of research ethics is that bad science is inherently unethical. If the generalizability of the data collected is severely compromised, the scientific quality of this study may be so seriously undermined as to make it unethical to proceed.

The concept of potential risk is another key aspect of the protocol that IRBs must consider. In this study, merely questioning adolescents about their behavior in an environment where treatment, counseling, and education are available constitutes minimal risk. Such questions are a standard part of clinical care in the routine office visit for adolescent health maintenance. The participants will not be informed of their HIV test results (although they may choose to be tested apart from the study), so the risk of being negatively affected as a result of learning one's HIV status is not a factor.

If an IRB determined that the research entails a level of risk that is a minor increase over minimal, the standards set forth for the waiver of parental permission could still be met. However, the fact that the research involves a risk that is more than minimal with no prospect of direct benefit would necessitate the use of increased procedural safeguards in place of parental permission in order to ensure the safety of minor participants. Given that the relative potential risk is still low, the availability of an objective third-party independent of the research team to answer any questions potential participants may have during the consent process would be a reasonable procedural safeguard to protect the interests of potential participants. Other procedural safeguards might include the ongoing availability of this counselor throughout the study and careful monitoring by the IRB.

The second key consideration for IRBs is the maturity of the potential participant population. In the HIV study, the investigator requests a waiver of parental permission for participants 13–17 years of age. Although members of this population may be viewed as being mature and possessing adequate decisional capacity, especially in light of their choice to seek treatment at the adolescent clinic, the younger members of this population may require greater protections than older adolescents. In this case, the IRB might require that an independent assessment of capacity to consent by a clinician independent of the research team be conducted for younger potential participants. For older participants (perhaps 16 or more years of age), a more informal general capacity assessment by the investigator may be sufficient.

Studies that have the prospect of direct benefit to individual participants but entail greater than a minor increase over minimal risk may also be considered for waiver of parental permission. IRBs can use the same considerations of protocol subject matter, risk, and population maturity to make such determinations, though increased procedural safeguards should be used to protect participants as the risk of the study increases. Such safeguards may include independent capacity assessments of participants and availability of third-party counseling throughout the study. Waiver of parental permission is particularly applicable when clinical trials are being performed on conditions for which minor adolescents are legally permitted to consent to treatment. In other cases, IRBs should consider whether trials will be inhibited by the reluctance of potential participants to discuss their behaviors or illnesses with parents. In these circumstances, waiver of parental permission may be a reasonable option. However, even with such protections, the parental permission waiver may not be granted for certain studies. IRBs are reminded that in reviewing drug trials under the purview of the FDA, parental permission is mandatory and may not be waived, even for mature adolescent participants. Based on the arguments set forth in this chapter, we call for the FDA to reconsider this position.

Adolescence is a unique state in human development that requires research to increase understanding of growth, development, and disease in order to develop interventions to enhance health and well-being. Adolescents, in general, have the capacity to provide informed consent for participation in a broad range of clinical and research endeavors. IRBs responsible for protection of human subjects should utilize extant regulations including the definition of children (46.402(a)), the waiver of informed consent (46.116(d)), and the waiver of the requirement for parental permission (46.408(c)) to facilitate important research while utilizing necessary procedural safeguards to protect the interests of adolescent participants. The ethical obligation to nurture the developing autonomy of these individuals is critical, and research participation can be viewed as an opportunity for moral education (Bartholome, 1976; McCormick, 1974).

Questions for Discussion

1. What are the characteristics of adolescents that distinguish them from other populations (i.e., children and full adults) in the medical setting? How should the distinct needs of adolescents be taken into account when a researcher tailors clinical trials aimed at this population?
2. What are the ethical standards for decision making for adolescents?
3. What are the differences in the concepts of consent, permission, and assent in the clinical setting? How, if at all, do they differ in the research context?
4. What role ought parents play in permitting research involving children and adolescents?

5. According to studies presented in this chapter, it is agreed upon that even minors who have reached the formal "operations stage" of cognitive development may require additional protections to ensure their ability to provide voluntary, informed consent in the research context. What kind of protection would you offer to guarantee voluntary informed consent of minors in research?

6. What are the main differences between receiving treatment in a clinical context and participating in a nontherapeutic research protocol in terms of the adolescent's risk-benefit? What is the application of the difference on the legal situation regarding informed consent, parental permission, and minor patient assent in the two contexts?

7. Do you agree with the current definition of minimal risk as an "objective" standard indexed to daily lives of healthy, average children, or do you favor a "subjective" standard indexed to social situations or level of illness? Explain your answer.

8. Considering the current social context of parent-child relationships in the United States, do you think that the role of parents as protectors and decision makers for their adolescent children is appropriate?

9. How much weight ought we to give an adolescent patients' assent when the adolescent's wishes conflict with those of his or her parents/legal guardian? Does the type of decision (i.e., clinical vs. research, serious vs. trivial) affect your answer?

10. The current federal regulations (46.408(c)) set out "reasonable" standard for parental permission waiver for adolescent's participation in research. Do you think this standard is fulfilled in the case described at the beginning of this chapter?

11. What standards or process of review can an IRB use when faced with a request to waive parental permission in research involving adolescents?

12. In the conclusion to this chapter, the authors propose a model to be used to analyze the case. The model emphasizes the need for procedural safeguards to protect the interests of potential participants. Those safeguards could be independent capacity assessments of participants and availability of third-party counseling throughout the study. Do you support this model?

13. According to the authors, IRBs are reminded that in reviewing drug trials under the purview of the FDA, parental permission is mandatory and may not be waived, even for mature adolescent participants. What could be the rationale behind these guidelines? Do you think this requirement should be reinforced, maintained, or abandoned?

References

Abramovitch, R., Freedman, J. L., Thoden, K., & Nikolich, C. (1991). Children's capacity to consent to participation in psychological research: Empirical findings. *Child Development, 62,* 1100–1109.

American Academy of Pediatrics, Committee on Bioethics. (1995). Informed consent, parental permission, and assent in pediatric practice. *Pediatrics, 95*(2), 314–317.

American Medical Association. (1992). *Confidential Care for Minors.* Report of the Council on Ethical and Judicial Affairs. Chicago: American Medical Association.

Appelbaum, P., & Roth, L. H. (1982). Competency to consent to research: A psychiatric overview. *Archives of General Psychiatry, 39*(8), 951–958.

Appelbaum, P., & Grisso, T. (1988). Assessing patients' capacities to consent to treatment. *New England Journal of Medicine,* 319(25): 1635–1638.

Appelbaum, P., Roth, L. H., Lidz, C. W., Benson, P., & Winslade, W. (1987). False hopes and best data: Consent to research and the therapeutic misconception. *Hastings Center Report, 17*(2), 20–24.

Bartholome, W. (1976). Parents, children, and the moral benefits of research. *Hastings Center Report, 6*(6), 44–45.

Beauchamp, T. L., & Childress, J. (1994). *Principles of biomedical ethics* (4th ed.). New York: Oxford University Press.

Buchanan, A. E., & Brock, D. W. (1989). *Deciding for others: The ethics of surrogate decision making.* Cambridge: Cambridge University Press.

Campbell, A. T. (2004). State regulation of medical research with children and adolescents: An overview and analysis. Appendix B in: Ethical Conduct of Clinical Research Involving Children. Institute of Medicine of the National Academies. Washington D.C.: National Academy Press pp. 320–387.

Capron, A. M. (1982). The competence of children as self-deciders in biomedical interventions. In W. Gaylin & R. Macklin (Eds.), *Who speaks for the child: The problems of proxy consent* (pp. 57–114). New York: Plenum Press.

Department of Health and Human Services. Protections of Human Subjects in Research. Washington D.C. U.S. Government Printing Office, 1991 (Codified at 45CFR Part 46).

Derish, M. T., & Heuvel, K. V. (2000). Mature minors should have the right to refuse life-sustaining medical treatment. *Journal of Law, Medicine & Ethics, 28*(2), 109–124.

Dorn, L. D., Susman, E. J., & Fletcher, J. C. (1995). Informed consent in children and adolescents: Age, maturation and psychological state. *Journal of Adolescent Health, 16*(3), 185–190.

English, A. (1990). Treating adolescents: Legal and ethics considerations. *Medical Clinics of North America, 74*(5), 1097–1112.

English, A. (1995). Guidelines for adolescent health research: Legal perspectives. *Journal of Adolescent Health, 17*(5), 277–286.

English, A. & Kenney, K. E. (2003). *State Minor Consent Laws: A Summary,* 2nd edition. Chapel Hill, NC: The Center for Adolescent Health & the Law.

Fleming, M., Towey, K., & Jarosik, J. (2001). *Healthy youth 2010: Supporting the 21 critical adolescent objectives.* Chicago: American Medical Association.

Ford, C.l A., & English, A. (2002). Limiting confidentiality of adolescent health services: What are the risks? *Journal of the American Medical Association, 288*(6), 752–753.

Gaydos, C. A., Howell, R., Pare, B., Clark, K. L., Gaydos, J. C., Ellis, D. A., et al. (1998). Chlamydia trachomatis infections in female military recruits. *New England Journal of Medicine, 339*(11), 739–744.

Gaylin, W. (1982). Competence: No longer all or none. In W. Gaylin & R. Macklin (Eds.), *Who speaks for the child: The problems of proxy consent* (pp. 27–54). New York: Plenum Press.

Grisso, T., & Appelbaum, P. (1995). Comparison of standards for assessing patients' capacities to make treatment decisions. *American Journal of Psychiatry, 152*(7), 1033–1037.

Grisso, T., & Vierling, L. (1978). Minors' consent to treatment: A developmental perspective. *Professional Psychology, 9*(3), 412–427.

Holder, A. R. (1985). *Legal issues in pediatrics and adolescent medicine* (2nd ed.). New Haven, CT: Yale University Press.

In re Swan. 569 A.2d 1202 (Me.1990).

Leikin, S. L. (1983). Minors' assent or dissent to medical treatment. *Journal of Pediatrics, 102*(2), 169–176.

Levine, R. (1995). Adolescents as research subjects without permission of their parents or guardians: Ethical considerations. *Journal of Adolescent Health, 17*(5), 287–297.

Lewis, C. E., Lewis, M. A., & Ifekwunigue, M. (1978). Informed consent by children and participation in an influenza vaccine trial. *American Journal of Public Health, 68*(11), 1079–1082.

Mammel, K. A., & Kaplan, D. W. (1995). Research consent by adolescent minors and the institutional review boards. *Journal of Adolescent Health, 17*(5), 323–330.

McCabe, M. A. (1996). Involving children and adolescents in medical decision making: Developmental and clinical considerations. *Journal of Pediatric Psychology, 21*(4), 505–516.

McCabe, M. A., Rushton, C. H., Glover, J., Murray, M. G., & Leikin, S. (1996). Implications of the Patient Self-Determination Act: Guidelines for involving adolescents in medical decision making. *Journal of Adolescent Health, 19*(5), 319–324.

McCormick, R. (1974). Proxy consent in the experimentation situation. *Perspectives in Biology and Medicine, 18*(1), 2–20.

Melville v. Sabbatino, 313 A.2d 886 (Conn. Sup. Ct. 1973).

National Commission for the Protection of Human Subjects of Biomedical and Behavioral Research. (1978a). Research involving children: Report and recommendations of the National Commission for Human Subjects of Biomedical and Behavioral Research. *Federal Registrar, 43*(9), 2084–2114.

National Commission for the Protection of Human Subjects of Biomedical and Behavioral Research. (1978b). The Belmont Report: Ethical Principles and Guidelines for the Protection of Human Subjects of Research. Washington, DC: U.S. Government Printing Office.

National Human Research Protections Advisory Committee. (2001). Specific comment on FDA's decision to adopt HHS 45 CFR 46 subpart D, excluding 46.408(c). Letter to the Food and Drug Administration. Retrieved from http://ohrp.osophs.dhhs.gov/nhrpac/documents/nhrpac16 .pdf March 11, 2004

National Human Research Protections Advisory Committee. (2002). Report from NHRPAC: Clarifying specific portion of 45 CFR 46 subpart D that governs children's research. Retrieved from http://ohrp.osophs.dhhs.gov/nhrpac/documents/nhrpac16.pdf March 11, 2004

Petersen, A. C., & Leffert, N. (1995). Developmental issues influencing guidelines for adolescent health research: A review. *Journal of Adolescent Health, 17,* 298–305.

Piaget, J. (1962). The stages of the intellectual development of the child. *Bulletin of the Menninger Clinic, 26,* 120–128.

Reddy, D. M., Fleming, R., & Swain, C. (2002). Effect of mandatory parental notification on adolescent girls' use of sexual health care services. *Journal of the American Medical Association, 288*(6), 710–714.

Rogers, A. S., Schwartz, D. F., Weissman, G., & English, A. (1999). A case study in adolescent participation in clinical research: Eleven clinical sites, one common protocol, and eleven IRBs. *IRB: A Review of Human Subjects Research, 21*(1), 6–10.

Rosenstein, D. (2004). Decision making capacity and disaster research. Journal of Traumatic Stress, in press.

Roth, L. H., Meisel, A., & Lidz, C. W. (1977). Tests of competency to consent to treatment. *American Journal of Psychiatry, 134*(3), 279–284.

Ruck, M. D., Keating, D. P., Abramovitch, R., & Koegl, C. K. (1998). Adolescents' and children's knowledge about rights: Some evidence for how young people view rights in their own lives. *Journal of Adolescence, 21,* 275–289.

Santelli, J. S., Rogers, A. S., Rosenfeld, W. D., DuRant, R. H., Dubler, N., Morreale, M., et al. (2003). Guidelines for adolescent health research (a position paper of the Society for Adolescent Medicine). *Journal of Adolescent Health, 33*(5), 396–409.

Santelli, J. S., Rosenfeld, W. D., DuRant, R. H., Dubler, N., Morreale, M., English, A., & Rogers, A. S. (1995). Guidelines for adolescent health research (a position paper of the Society for Adolescent Medicine). *Journal of Adolescent Health, 17*(5), 270–276.

Susman, E. J., Dorn, L. D., & Fletcher, J. C. (1992). Participation in biomedical research: The consent process as viewed by children, adolescents, young adults, and physicians. *Journal of Pediatrics, 121*(4), 547–552.

Weir, R. F., & Peters, C. (1997). Affirming the decisions adolescents make about life and death. *Hastings Center Report, 27*(6), 29–40.

Weithorn, L. (1983). Children's capacities to decide about participation in research. *IRB: A Review of Human Subjects Research, 5*(2), 1–5.

Weithorn, L., & Campbell, S. (1982). The competency of children and adolescents to make informed treatment decisions. *Child Development, 53*(6), 1589–1598.

6

Recruitment of Pregnant, Minor
Adolescents and Minor Adolescents at
Risk of Pregnancy into Longitudinal,
Observational Research:
The Case of the National
Children's Study

John Santelli, Gail Geller, Donna T. Chen, Marjorie A. Speers,
Jeffrey R. Botkin, and Stacy Laswell

CASE DESCRIPTION

The Pregnant Minor Adolescent

Maria, a 16-year-old Hispanic female, is making her first prenatal visit to a
university hospital clinic in California. At the first visit she receives a battery
of clinical screenings, including blood and urine samples and a gynecological
exam. She meets with a social worker, who asks her to complete a psychosocial
risk assessment. These several assessments reveal that she is 18 weeks pregnant
and in general good health. She has a history of a *Chlamydia* infection 1 year
ago and states that she uses condoms, "but not always." She reports that abortion is not an option for her because she could never "kill her baby." She has
recently stopped smoking. She is currently repeating 9th grade and getting Bs
and Ds in school. She is living with her parents in an inner-city neighborhood
with high rates of drug use and street violence. Her parents emigrated from
Mexico 10 years ago. Maria reports that her father is "very angry" with her
about getting pregnant. She initiated intercourse at age 14. She denies physical
abuse by her family or her boyfriend Ramon, who is 18. Ramon hopes to join
the Army and Maria hopes to finish school after the baby is born. During the
course of this first prenatal care visit, the social worker asks if Maria would be
interested in enrolling herself and her new baby in a longitudinal study of child
health called the National Children's Study.

The Minor Adolescent at Risk of Pregnancy

Estelle, a 16-year-old white female, is visiting a university hospital adolescent health clinic for acne. Per clinic routine she is offered a comprehensive bio-psychosocial health assessment, which was designed based on the American Medical Association's *Guidelines for Adolescent Preventive Services* (Elster & Kuznets, 1994). She has a history of asthma controlled with intermittent use of an inhaler; she is allergic to penicillin. Estelle is currently in 10th grade, is getting As and Cs, but doesn't like school sports or clubs. She began smoking at age 11, reached menarche at 12, and initiated sexual intercourse at 15. She states that she uses condoms "but not always." She has had several boyfriends; her current boyfriend is 18 and goes to her school. She likes to hang out with her friends on weekends at the lake and likes to drink wine coolers, but only on weekends. She admits blacking out a number of times while drinking. She denies drug use but admits that some of her friends smoke pot. She lives with her parents and says that they don't know much about her smoking and drinking; they think she is still a virgin. During the course of this visit, the nurse practitioner asks Estelle about her pregnancy plans and whether she would be interested in enrolling herself in a longitudinal study of child health called the National Children's Study.

Importance of the NCS Study

The National Children's Study (NCS) has been proposed as an observational, cohort study of the influence of physical and social environmental factors on children's health and development (National Children's Study, 2003). Because the NCS is currently in the development phase, many aspects of the study design had not been finalized when this chapter was written. Approximately 100,000 mother–infant dyads would be recruited before mothers give birth, and a subsample may be recruited before a woman becomes pregnant. Infants would be followed to age 21. The effects of environmental factors on pregnancy outcomes, and the growth and development of infants and children would be investigated using a life-stage approach, to determine if these exposures are harmful, harmless, or helpful. Health outcomes would include miscarriage, premature birth, low birth weight, birth defects, and long-term impacts such as impaired neurobehavioral development, developmental disabilities, psychiatric outcomes, childhood injury, asthma, obesity, altered physical development, diabetes, and altered puberty.

The NCS is expected to shed considerable light on the effects of physical and social environmental exposures on child health and development, particularly exposures occurring in utero. Annual costs for the study may exceed $100 million during peak years of data collection. Extensive data on physical environmental exposures, social influences, genetics, behaviors, and psychological states would be collected to allow a broad investigation of the interactions among factors that may affect child health and development. Research procedures in the NCS will involve serial physical examinations and collection of blood and other biologic specimens to allow for assessment of exposure, subclinical health effects, and genetic studies. Sample size will be sufficient to examine the reasons for health disparities among various subgroups. The NCS will also assess exposure to known environmental agents that adversely affect child health and development, such as lead and tobacco smoke. The sampling and recruitment strategy for the NCS will employ a national probability sample with clustered sampling to enhance the efficiency of sampling and to measure the social and physical environment of communities. Regional centers will be involved in data collection from study participants (children and families). Data from the NCS will form a scientific basis for future health promotion and health care practices.

The mother, fetus, and offspring are all research subjects, and one must assess the ethical risks and benefits to each. Many research procedures within the NCS would individually be considered minimal risk, defined in the federal regulations as "the probability and magnitude of harm or discomfort anticipated . . . are not greater . . . than those ordinarily encountered in daily life or during the performance of routine physical or psychological examinations or tests." (45 CFR 46.102(i)). However, data will be collected on multiple exposures and health outcomes. One such measure will be testing for genetic susceptibility to disease. This may also be minimal risk, but risk will depend upon the specific test, and such testing has special implications in childhood (Kodish, 1999). Genetic procedures that are greater than minimal risk may be excluded from the NCS or conducted as special substudies to keep the main study as minimal risk. These special implications for children and the overall burden of the study will need to be considered and monitored carefully. The NCS will need to be prepared to provide feedback of information to mothers and families about new associations that may be uncovered between past exposures, genetic traits, and health outcomes.

The extensive and intensive nature of the NCS raises important ethical issues. These issues include ethical oversight in a multisite study, how and when to involve communities, justice in the recruitment of study subjects, how best to obtain informed consent, privacy of family information, genetic testing, use of stored samples, returning results to participants, reporting of child abuse and imperiled child health conditions, and avoiding stigmatization of groups in reporting study results. The NCS is wrestling with the potential need for ongoing consent in a longitudinal study where new research procedures may be added over the course of the study. The NCS is also considering future needs for child assent, as the newborn subjects grow into childhood and adolescence during the course of the study.

———

ETHICAL ANALYSIS AND DISCUSSION

This case study deals with a specific issue identified by the Ethics Work Group of the NCS: the recruitment of teenagers who are pregnant or who are sexually active and therefore at risk of pregnancy. This ethical discussion raises questions that are important to involving adolescents in other longitudinal studies of pregnant women and their offspring. In this case study, we address background information on teen pregnancy, the rationale for inclusion of teenagers who are pregnant or at risk of pregnancy, the risks and potential benefits of the research to these two groups of teens, the legal status of adolescents who are pregnant or at risk of pregnancy, and the legal status of these teenagers under the federal regulations on research. Two critical sets of ethical questions are addressed, the inclusion or exclusion from research participation and the process for obtaining informed consent:

1. Inclusion or exclusion. Should the NCS recruit minor adolescents who are currently pregnant or at risk of pregnancy? Is it ethical to exclude these adolescents from the NCS? Are there unique risks or vulnerabilities for teenagers who are pregnant or at risk of pregnancy?
2. Informed consent. Who should consent for the teenager and her baby? Is the permission of the teenager's parents needed? Is the permission of the baby's father needed? What is the legal status of the teenager to provide informed consent for herself and her baby?

The answers to these questions depend upon a thorough understanding of the legal, ethical, social, and developmental status of adolescents and the realities of adolescent pregnancy.

Teen Pregnancy in the United States

Almost 900,000 adolescents in the United States become pregnant each year, most of these pregnancies are unplanned, and almost one-third end in abortion (Ventura, Mosher, Curtin, Abma, & Henshaw, 2001). Most teenage mothers are unmarried. Childbearing as a teenager is associated with adverse social and health consequences for the mother, including dropping out of school, unemployment, poverty, welfare dependency, and single parenthood (Alan Guttmacher Institute, 1994).

Teen childbearing is also associated with unfavorable outcomes for the offspring, including early effects such as prematurity and infant mortality and longer term effects on health, educational, and social well-being. Teenagers who become mothers are more likely to have grown up in poverty and to have experienced a variety of social deprivations. Disentangling the health and social effects of young age itself from these preexisting social deficits is difficult.

Teenagers at highest risk of pregnancy generally initiate sexual intercourse earlier in adolescence and use contraception ineffectively or not at all. Although estimates vary across national surveys, almost half of young women in the United States initiate sexual intercourse before age 18 (Santelli, Lindberg, Abma, McNeely, & Resnick, 2000). A variety of biopsychosocial factors influence early initiation of sexual intercourse and childbearing (Hofferth, 1987; Moore, Miller, Glei, & Morrison, 1995), including earlier age at pubertal maturation, poverty, lower parental educational achievement, growing up in a single parent family, lower parental monitoring, involvement in other health risk behaviors such as drug use and delinquency, and lower educational achievement. Connectedness to school and family act as protective factors against early initiation of sexual intercourse (Resnick et al., 1997). Early initiation of intercourse has also been associated with sexual abuse. Among females who were 13 or fewer years of age at first sexual intercourse, 24% reported the experience as nonvoluntary, compared with 10% whose first intercourse was between age 19 and 24 (Abma, Driscoll, & Moore, 1998). Early initiation of intercourse and pregnancy has also been associated with lower cognitive abilities (Shearer et al., 2002). Factors associated with the adolescent's failure to use contraception are similar to those associated with initiation of intercourse. These include involvement in other risk behaviors, negative attitudes about contraceptive methods, and lower perceived support from partners and peers (Moore et al., 1995). Residence in neighborhoods characterized by poor supervision of adolescent behavior, inadequate community resources for adolescents, and high levels of adolescent behavior that departs from a conventional lifestyle (i.e., dropping out of school) have also been linked to a failure to use contraceptives during intercourse (Brewster, 1994; Hogan, Astone, & Kitagawa, 1985).

Should Adolescents Who Are Pregnant or at Risk of Pregnancy Be Excluded From the NCS?

Individual children must be included as research subjects in order for children, as a class, to fully benefit from that research. Draft federal regulations addressing children in research were proposed in 1978, and final regulations were adopted in 1983. During the early 1990s, federal policies on inclusion of women and minorities in research were adopted (Levine, 1995; Mastrionni, Faden, & Federman, 1994). Such policies recognize that ethical and scientific criteria should determine the inclusion of specific groups within a research study; the regulations reject the convenience of the investigators as a rationale for exclusion. In, 1998, the National Institutes of Health (NIH) issued NIH *Policy and Guidelines on the Inclusion of Children as Participants in Research Involving Human Subjects* (National Institutes of Health, 1998). The policy states:

> Children (i.e., individuals under the age of 21) must be included in all human subjects research, conducted or supported by the NIH, unless there are scientific and ethical reasons not to include them.

This policy applies to adolescents who are pregnant or at risk of pregnancy who may be recruited into the NCS. Births to minor adolescents represent a small but important percentage of all births in the United States. In 1999, 4.4% of all births were to mothers younger than 18 years; an additional 3.4% of mothers were 18 at delivery (Ventura et al., 2001), and many 18-year-old mothers would be minors at the time of NCS recruitment (i.e., age 17 while pregnant but turning 18 before the delivery).

The NCS will examine physical and social environmental influences on child health and development. Minor adolescent mothers are more likely than older mothers to experience adverse social influences (Alan Guttmacher Institute, 1994). Given poverty and minority status, they may be more likely to experience adverse physical environmental exposures. The children of teen mothers are more likely to suffer poor health and delayed development, in part because of these adverse environmental exposures. Given maturation differences between teenage and older women, teenagers may be differentially vulnerable to these exposures. Thus, mothers younger than 18 years are important to the research questions of NCS.

The NIH policy lists seven exceptions to inclusion of children in specific studies. We reviewed each exception in considering the inclusion of pregnant adolescents and those at risk of pregnancy:

1. "The research topic to be studied is irrelevant to children."

Clearly the research questions of the NCS are relevant to teen mothers and their offspring.

2. "There are laws or regulations barring the inclusion of children in the research. For example, the regulations for protection of human subjects allow consenting adults to accept a higher level of risk than are permitted for children."

A variety of state laws address the age and circumstances under which adolescents legally become adults (i.e., laws addressing age at majority or emancipation statutes) or adolescent rights to independently access health care services for specific conditions such as pregnancy. Such state laws do not address inclusion or exclusion of adolescents in research. In the few states where statutes address adolescents and research, these statutes have generally focused on requirements for parental permission (Speers, Santelli, Rhoden, Reza, & Nieburg, 2001). We are not aware of any state laws or regulations that prohibit the inclusion of children or adolescents in research.

Subpart D limits the risk to which children in research studies may be subjected. Many of the procedures in the NCS would involve minimal risk and research involving minimal risk is approvable under section 46.404 of subpart D, which governs research with children. Subpart D also allows approval of a study that carries a minor increase over minimal risk, if it involves procedures that are commensurate with the child's prior experience. The NCS will likely be highly selective in requesting procedures in this category. Higher risk procedures involving children are approvable under exceptional circumstances and the NCS is unlikely to request institutional review board (IRB) approval for these.

3. "The knowledge being sought in the research is already available for children or will be obtained from another ongoing study, and an additional study will be redundant."

While many smaller and previous studies have examined environmental risk to child health, they have often not done so prospectively. As a prospective study, the NCS is specifically designed to find new risks and particularly, risks that might not be apparent in a smaller study. As such, the NCS will not be redundant, nor will the data be available elsewhere. By including adolescents, the NCS would be able to compare risks for children of teenage mothers with those risks to children of older mothers.

4. "A separate, age-specific study in children is warranted and preferable."

Examples in the policy included diseases which are rare or where a nationwide pediatric disease research network currently exists, or where issues of study design preclude direct applicability of hypotheses and/or interventions to both adults and children because of different cognitive, developmental, or disease stages or different age-related metabolic processes. We see no need for a separate study of teen mothers and their offspring.

5. "Insufficient data are available in adults to judge potential risk in children. . . ."

Procedures such as surveys, genetic testing, and the taking of biological specimens involving pregnant minors would be the same as those for adult women who are pregnant.

6. "Study designs aimed at collecting additional data on pre-enrolled adult study participants (e.g., longitudinal follow-up studies that did not include data on children)."

Not applicable.

7. "Other special cases justified by the investigator and found acceptable to the review group and the Institute Director."

See discussion of risks and benefits below.

In summary, a strong preliminary case can be made for the inclusion of teenagers who are pregnant or at risk of pregnancy in the NCS, based on the criteria in the NIH policy. Of course, this ethical justification would fail if one were unable to fully and properly address subject protection for this vulnerable group. Therefore, before reaching a decision about inclusion, one must consider the unique risks and ethical considerations regarding recruitment of either group of teenagers: those who are pregnant and those at risk of pregnancy.

Unique Risks and Ethical Considerations in Recruiting Teenagers Who Are Pregnant or at Risk of Pregnancy

The unique risks for teenagers who are pregnant or at risk of pregnancy lead one to different ethical conclusions about involvement of these two groups in the NCS.

The risks of study involvement to pregnant teenagers are similar to the risks to older pregnant women; as currently planned, most study risks would be minimal. However, the NCS will need to consider the unique vulnerabilities of teenage mothers. As outlined above, teenage mothers are more likely to have grown up in poverty, to have experienced family disruption, to be disconnected from family and other social institutions, and to have experienced sexual abuse (Alan Guttmacher Institute, 1994). They may also have lower cognitive abilities than older mothers (Shearer et al., 2002). These vulnerabilities should not exclude them from study involvement; pregnant teens are commonly recruited into other studies of pregnancy. However, they will demand special sensitivity and protections on the part of study investigators. For example, investigators will need to be knowledgeable about definitions of child sexual abuse and the reporting requirements when abuse is discovered.

Pregnancy in adolescence is frequently stigmatized by families and communities. Disclosure of a pregnancy may be the first acknowledgement that a young woman is having sex and involved in other risk behaviors. As such, many adolescents refuse to acknowledge pregnancy symptoms and delay disclosure to family and to sexual partners. Eventually however, the pregnancy, if not aborted, is difficult to hide and usually becomes known to the family. Pregnancy may cause family disruption and even expulsion from the family although such extreme consequences are relatively rare. Because pregnancy recognition or disclosure is often delayed, teenagers are more likely to delay initiation of prenatal care, compared to older mothers. Thus, they would likely be delayed in recruitment into the NCS. This would create significant operational challenges for the NCS. This methodological issue could then become an ethical issue if delayed recruitment of teenagers degraded the scientific value of data from teens. Sound scientific design is a primary ethical requirement for research.

Involvement in the NCS might, in some cases, result in earlier disclosure of a pregnancy to the teenager's family. This would be true if the study required parental permission that was not needed for clinical care. This is not likely to change the family's response to the pregnancy, but study investigators would need to be cognizant of the potential consequences of pregnancy disclosure to family.

Although the NCS is not an intervention trial with the potential for direct benefit, a variety of "inclusion" benefits (i.e., direct benefits incidental to research participation) may accrue to the pregnant teen who is recruited into NCS. The study will offer frequent and thorough medical monitoring and referral for needed care. Contact with adult professionals is also likely to be beneficial to the teenager, through informal social monitoring and education and parenting advice. In addition, being a volunteer in research may contribute to a young woman's sense of altruism and self worth (Society for Adolescent Medicine, 2003).

More difficult concerns would exist when recruiting teenagers who were sexually active but not yet pregnant. Operationally, it would be difficult to recruit a group of sexually active teenagers at risk of pregnancy who would plan to continue a pregnancy. Few teens plan pregnancy or motherhood. It should be acknowledged that recruitment of adult women prior to pregnancy will be difficult, as many adult women do not plan pregnancy (Santelli et al., 2003). Likewise, women who plan pregnancy are likely to be systematically different from women who do not. For example, women with intended pregnancies are less likely to smoke or drink and more likely to use folate supplements than women who have unintended pregnancies (Santelli et al., 2003).

Ethically, recruitment of teens at risk of pregnancy raises difficult dilemmas: What should be the responsibilities of the NCS to prevent pregnancy in such a group? Would recruitment of a cohort at risk of pregnancy provide subtle messages endorsing pregnancy? How do NCS investigators avoid influencing decisions about terminating a pregnancy?

Many teens would be reluctant to disclose their sexual behaviors, if parents would be informed of such behaviors (Reddy, Fleming, & Swain, 2002). In such circumstances, requiring parental permission would discourage adolescent enrollment and may conflict with state laws and clinical practice allowing sexually active teens independent and confidential access to health care. Conversely, waiving parental permission with the intention of enrolling a sexually active teenager may be problematic. Following a group of sexually active teens and waiting for them to become pregnant without educating and counseling them about the risks could be seen by parents, IRB members, and others as unethical. Investigators would be obligated to inform and counsel sexually active adolescents about the consequences of unprotected intercourse and measures to prevent these. Trying to prevent pregnancy would, of course, conflict with the study's needs to enroll subjects.

In summary, the inclusion of pregnant teenagers in the NCS seems ethically justifiable, if appropriate safeguards are put into place that address the teenagers' specific needs and vulnerabilities. In fact, it would seem unethical to exclude pregnant teens. This recommendation is based on the *Belmont Report*'s principles of justice and beneficence (National Commission, 1978). Conversely, the recruitment of teenagers at risk of pregnancy with the intention of following them through pregnancy and into parenthood would be more difficult to justify ethically. Here, the decision to exclude teens is based on the principle of beneficence or nonmaleficence, of avoiding harm to the adolescent.

Next we turn to appropriate research protections, particularly issues related to informed consent. Given the discussion above, we focus on the recruitment of teenagers who are already pregnant.

Informed Consent When Recruiting Adolescents Who Are Pregnant

In designing informed consent requirements for the NCS one must consider the ability of adolescents to provide informed consent, the informed consent requirements of the federal regulations, and the legal status of teenagers who are pregnant or parents in providing informed consent for themselves or their babies. Special considerations are the potential need for permission from the teenager's parents and the baby's father. Importantly, both motherhood and pregnancy may change the teenager's legal status with regard to health care decisions, emancipation from parents, and research decisions.

Adolescent Decision-Making Capacity

Adolescence is the transition from childhood to adult status; with it emerges increasing desire for autonomy and the increasing ability to make independent decisions. Parenthood is understood in many cultures as a primary marker of adult status. Understanding the emerging capacity of adolescents to provide informed consent is essential in considering their ethical participation in research, particularly where one contemplates waiving parental permission. The ethical principle of respect for persons demands attention to this emerging capacity. Growth into adolescence is marked by an increasing capacity to make independent and intelligent decisions. Developmental psychologists recognize emerging cognitive abilities (i.e., changes in the ability of the human organism to understand increasingly complex and abstract concepts); research ethicists have recognized a related concept—capacity—the ability to provide informed consent (i.e., to appreciate the risks and benefits of participation in research activities and to make reasoned choices; 1983; Weithorn, 1983). Capacity is linked to both developing cognition (Leikin, 1983) and previous life experiences. Lack of experience with decision making in real-world situations may reduce adolescent capacity. A potential beneficial effect of involvement in research is an expansion of the adolescent's experience base, which may lead to an increase in the capacity to provide informed consent (Weithorn & Scherer, 1994; Melton, 1983).

Research on cognition and capacity suggests that both adolescents and younger children show significant ability to provide informed consent (Weithorn, 1983; Susman, Dorn, & Fletcher, 1992). Among mid and late adolescents (>14 years), understanding of research and the cognitive ability to make decisions about research participation are similar to these abilities in adults. Weithorn (1983) found that 14-year-olds were as skilled as adults in understanding multiple viewpoints and in considering conflicting information. Formal operational thinking, the ability to understand and use abstract concepts, begins to appear in adolescents from age 11 (Petersen and Leffert, 1995), although many adults never attain the ability to engage in this kind of formal operational thinking.

The capacity of an individual adolescent (or adult) to provide informed consent is an empirical question. For adults we assume capacity unless we have evidence to the contrary; for children we assume the opposite. The Society for Adolescent Medicine has sponsored *Guidelines for Adolescent Health Research* (2003), which address this issue of capacity. These guidelines suggest that for research of low risk (i.e., confidential or anonymous survey research), capacity can be assumed based on the reasonable expectation of capacity for the group of adolescents to be studied. For research involving greater risk, the guidelines propose an individual assessment of capacity.

Adolescents display an emerging desire for autonomy and privacy and may be threatened by disclosure to parents of health information, including research data (Petersen and Leffert, 1995). In addition, adolescents may display a differential and even enhanced "vulnerability" to research in comparison with younger children (Thompson, 1980). For example, adolescents may have a heightened developmental sensitivity to particular issues (i.e., self-concept or body image). Their increasing cognitive abilities may lead to greater vulnerability when deception is used in research studies or when comparisons are made between their personal performance and the performance of others (Thompson, 1980).

Informed Consent Requirements of the Federal Regulations and the Legal Status of Adolescents

Most minor adolescents and the children of minor adolescents are covered by the children's regulations (subpart D) of the federal regulations on research (45 CFR 46), although the definition of "children" in subpart D may be interpreted as not applying to pregnant and parenting adolescents (Department of Health and Human Services, 2001). Pregnant minors and the fetus would also be covered by subpart B of the federal regulations, which addresses additional protections for pregnant women, human fetuses, and neonates involved in research.

Under subpart D, children are defined in the 402(a) as "persons who have not attained the legal age for consent to treatments or procedures involved in the research, under the applicable law of the jurisdiction in which the research will be conducted." This definition has critical implications for the recruitment of pregnant adolescents and adolescent mothers of children who are potential subjects in the NCS. Under this definition, not all adolescents who are under the legal age of majority are defined as children. In common practice, the applicable law of the jurisdiction is state law, but it could include federal statutes. Children are not defined by age, but by local laws governing medical treatment, age of majority, and emancipation status. In 48 states the age of majority is 18; it is 19 in Alabama and 21 in Mississippi. Several states establish an age for consent to general health care that is lower than the general age of majority (English & Kenney, 2003). All states recognize the concept of emancipated minors, either explicitly or implicitly as part of their law on age of majority. (Emancipated minors are legally adults for all purposes before the law.) Under the federal regulatory definition, emancipated minors and those who can consent for general medical care are not children. Moreover, all states authorize certain groups of minors to give their own consent for health care, such as for treatment of pregnancy or drug use (English & Kenney, 2003). Adolescents who are authorized to consent to health care under a minor consent statute are also not children under the definition of children in the research regulations. Pregnant minors in 28 states may consent for their own health care; in a similar number of states, minors who are mothers can consent for the care of the child. Thus, in many states no specific provision exists which addresses pregnant or parenting teens. A literal reading of the definition of children would find that in many but not all states, pregnant and parenting teens are not children under the federal regulations. As such, subpart D would apply in certain states but not in others.

It is worthwhile to consider the National Commission's thinking about these issues of adolescents and their transitional status (National Commission, 1977). The National Commission recognized that obtaining parental permission is not always a good way to protect children who are research subjects. The National Commission was also well aware of the changing capacities of adolescents, their evolving legal status, and the potential need to develop alternative mechanisms for human subjects protection. The National Commission suggested a number of circumstances in which parental permission was not a reasonable requirement:

> [R]esearch designed to identify factors related to the incidence or treatment of certain conditions in adolescents for which . . . they may legally receive treatment without parental consent; research in which the subjects are "mature minors" and the procedures involved entail essentially no more than minimal risk that such individuals might reasonably assume on their own; research designed to meet the needs of children designated by their parents as "in need of supervision," and research involving children whose parents are legally or functionally incompetent.

Thus, the National Commission recognized the reality of adolescents' independent access to care under state minor treatment laws and acknowledged the developing capacity of adolescents and the concept of the mature minor. This thinking of the National Commission is reflected in the final definition of children in the regulations and the section that allows a waiver of parental permission.

Under subpart D, children are considered to be a vulnerable population for which special protections must be provided. A hierarchy of risk and benefit is used in defining the specific protections required, relying on the concept of minimal risk as a threshold for certain allowable research activities. As noted above, most procedures in the NCS would be minimal risk with potential exceptions as noted above. The requirements for informed consent in minimal risk research are the assent of the child/adolescent and the permission of one parent. Under subpart D, the IRB may waive parental permission for research involving children where parental permission is problematic. Parental permission may be waived under 45 CFR 46.116(d). Section 46.408(c) states:

> [I]f an IRB determines that a research protocol is designed for conditions or a subject population for which parental permission is not a reasonable requirement to protect subjects (e.g., neglected or abused children), it may waive consent requirements provided an appropriate mechanism for protecting the children who will participate as research subjects is substituted and provided the waiver is not inconsistent with federal, state, or local law.

Children who are pregnant constitute a special case under subpart B. Subpart B refers readers to subpart D for a determination of whether an adolescent is defined as a child or as an adult under the federal regulations. This issue is addressed in 46.204(g), which reads: "For children as defined in 46.402(a) who are pregnant, assent and permission are obtained in accord with the provisions of subpart D."

Subpart B of the federal regulations addresses additional protections for pregnant women and the fetus. The father's permission under subpart B depends on who benefits from the research and the level of risk to the fetus. The NCS would seem to involve little or no risk to the fetus and would therefore be classified under 46.204(d):

> If the research holds out the prospect of direct benefit to the pregnant woman, the prospect of a direct benefit both to the pregnant woman and the fetus, or no prospect of benefit for the woman nor the fetus when risk to the fetus is not greater than minimal and the purpose of the research is the development of important biomedical knowledge that cannot be obtained by any other means, her consent is obtained in accord with the informed consent provisions of subpart A of this part.

As such, the father's permission would not be required for enrollment in the NCS. However, this may change if specific substudies involving the fetus are judged to be greater than minimal risk.

The involvement of the fathers of adolescent mothers in the life of their children and in the life of the teen mother will vary considerably. Men who father a child with teen women often suffer the same circumstances of socioeconomic deprivation as the teen mother (Anda et al., 2001). While most teen mothers are not married to the father, some will be cohabitating and many will maintain long-term relationships with the father. Often, fathers are not actively involved. In some cases, fathers will become the guardians of the children.

Appropriate Protections, If Minor Adolescents Are Included

Any decision on informed consent procedures for minor adolescents within the NCS should consider the ethical risks and benefits of each alternative and how these procedures can be justified within the framework of the federal regulations and the legal status of the adolescent under state law. Given inconsistencies in state laws, the NCS may find it helpful to develop a uniform approach to obtaining informed consent that would be consistent with the federal regulations and these different state laws. This, in turn, would avoid having different recruitment practices in different states which could limit the generalizability of the data from the NCS.

Ethical considerations here include the decision-making capacity of the pregnant adolescent to provide informed consent and the risks and benefits of requiring parental permission. As noted above, adolescents display considerable capacity to make decisions about minimal risk research. The informed assent of the pregnant adolescent is essential to respecting her emerging personhood. Her assent is also essential, because she will shoulder many of the burdens of research procedures.

Given the cognitive capacity of the typical adolescent, the consent/assent form document for a pregnant adolescent should closely resemble the informed consent document for women younger than 18 years. IRBs and investigators normally recognize the need to scale the reading level of consent forms to the expected reading levels of adult subjects (Hochhauser, 1999). Likewise, consent forms for adolescent subjects should be easily understood and complete to the criteria of the federal regulations in §46.116. However the reading skills of adolescents and adults vary widely and NCS investigators should be prepared to deal with subjects who are poor readers and those who are functionally illiterate. The consent process will need to consider the primary language of adolescent subjects. In the consent document, adolescents will be particularly concerned about confidentiality of data and the circumstances that may trigger disclosure, such as physical abuse.

In deciding about the need for parental permission, family dynamics and functionality are critical factors. Many adolescents will be continuing to live with their parents, but many will be living independently or with other relatives. Even when living independently from their parents, adolescent mothers may draw significant social support from the extended family. Many adolescents will come from dysfunctional families, but many will have parents who are conscientious but also socially disadvantaged themselves (Alan Guttmacher Institute, 1994; Hofferth, 1987; Moore et al., 1995). It will be difficult if not impossible to obtain full informed permission from parents in dysfunctional families. Correspondingly, requiring parental permission of all participants would likely create lower participation rates and perhaps differential participation, with higher risk adolescents being less likely to enroll (Santelli, 1997). Even if parental permission was not a requirement, most intact families will be cognizant of the adolescent mother's participation. Many young women would still turn to parents for advice before deciding about enrollment. Thus, support of the teen's family would be an asset in retaining the teen in a longitudinal study. Finally, in many cases grandmothers or other family members are the de facto guardians when it comes to the health and social needs of the adolescent's baby.

These considerations suggest that the IRBs reviewing the NCS should show some flexibility in requiring or waiving parental permission and in structuring informed consent procedures. The adolescent's consent (assent) should be primary, but the teenager should be encouraged to fully involve her own parents as appropriate and where possible. NCS investigators should be sensitive to the variety of families involved in the study. Assessment of family dynamics and teenager's social circumstances should be an essential part of study enrollment. If parental permission is not a requirement, the NCS should nonetheless develop procedures for involving grandparents and informing the extended family about the study with the prior permission of the adolescent subject. The NCS should also offer adolescents the counsel of a social worker or nurse, who is not involved in study recruitment, to provide advice on potential study enrollment. Whether the IRB decides to waive parental permission or declares that the teenager is not a child under state law and the federal definition of children, is probably less important than that the study develop consent procedures that are sensitive to the multiple kinds of family realities that will likely occur.

CONCLUSIONS/RECOMMENDATIONS

Returning to our two case studies and ethical questions, we believe that a strong case can be made for inclusion of pregnant adolescents who are minors in the NCS; the case for inclusion of minor adolescents at risk of pregnancy is more problematic. For pregnant teens, the risks are low and several inclusion benefits are suggested. The potential involvement of teens at risk of pregnancy, however, raises difficult operational and ethical issues including investigator responsibilities to prevent pregnancy and difficulties with either obtaining or waiving parental permission. An ethical case can be made for excluding teens at risk of pregnancy given their vulnerabilities and the specific risks to inclusion for this group.

This review suggests that in recruiting adolescents who are pregnant, research participation will require the adolescent's informed assent/consent and the adolescent's permission for the fetus. Most pregnant adolescents who would be recruited into the NCS would be capable of making decisions about research participation. Within a few years, all will become adults and will be fully responsible for health and research decisions for their offspring. State laws addressing pregnant teenagers vary but these generally recognize a teenager's rights to make independent decisions about prenatal care and care for their newborn. Given the definition of children in the federal regulations on research, consent for research is tied to state laws on clinical care and emancipation status.

We also believe it will be important to involve the adolescent's parents in helping the adolescent with the decision to join and with retention in the NCS. In many cases, the pregnant or parenting adolescent will be living with parents who are actively involved in the care of the child. This involvement of parents does not necessarily translate into a requirement for parental permission, and NCS investigators should be provided discretion in how to best involve parents. Likewise, permission of fathers of the teen mothers' child generally will not be a requirement, but NCS investigators should consider how to involve fathers. The involvement of parents and fathers should be negotiated with the teenagers— based on the adolescent's preferences and specific circumstances. Where parents are absent or dysfunctional or where the adolescent is functioning independently, parental permission should be waived. Where the parents are functional and providing important support to the pregnant teen, their involvement in the research process should be actively fostered by NCS investigators. An integral part of the informed consent and recruitment process should be an assessment of family dynamics in the extended family. The NCS should also offer adolescents the counsel of an independent social worker or nurse who can advise on study enrollment.

The NCS will likely involve review by multiple IRBs. The federal regulations allow investigators and IRBs broad latitude in designing consent procedures, as long as these procedures are consistent with the principles espoused in the *Belmont Report* (National Commission, 1978) and are not inconsistent with state and federal laws. Given the broad variation in state laws regarding pregnant and parenting adolescents, the NCS should develop a uniform approach to informed consent that can be justified under these varied laws and that is consistent with the federal regulations. Such procedures need to be sensitive to the cognitive capacity and changing legal status of the adolescent. These procedures should promote the inclusion of pregnant and parenting adolescents while providing robust protection from research risk. We hope the NCS will be a demonstration of our collective ability to achieve the very best ethical practices when engaged in the complex but important task of involving adolescents in research.

Questions for Discussion

1. What are the ethical issues raised by the NCS? How does the longitudinal, multisite, extensive and intensive nature of the study impact these ethical implications?

2. How might a change in the legal status of adolescents improve the problem of teen pregnancy in the United States? If you were a policy maker, would you try to change the current legal status quo? What kind of change would you advocate?

3. Which ethical and scientific criteria should determine the inclusion of specific groups within a research study? Are these criteria found in the

applicable federal and states laws regarding the participation of pregnant adolescents in research?

4. Do you hold the position that mothers younger than 18 years are important to the research questions of NCS or do you claim that they should be excluded from the study? In your answer, be sure to discuss the risk: benefit ratio and the criteria set forth in the NIH policy on inclusion of children.

5. What are the unique vulnerabilities of teenage mothers? How should the special needs of teenage mothers be addressed by NCS researchers while they attempt to recruit them to the study?

6. Should the NCS be responsible for efforts to prevent pregnancy in teens that might participate in the study? Should NCS investigators avoid influencing decisions about termination of pregnancy?

7. Do you support the authors' recommendation to include pregnant teenagers in the NCS with appropriate safeguards, but to exclude teenagers at risk of pregnancy? Why or why not?

   a. What are the implication of adolescents' emerging cognitive abilities and decision making capacity (the ability to provide informed consent) on their right to participate in research?

   b. How should these characteristics reflect on the legal status of adolescents?

   c. How can you reconcile empowering adolescents to provide consent while maintaining the role of parental permission in cases like this?

8. What are the current informed consent requirements and the legal status of adolescents according to the federal regulations on research (45 CFR 46) and according to states laws? What are the key differences between the state and federal levels?

——

References

Abma, J., Driscoll, A., & Moore, K. (1998). Young women's degree of control over first intercourse: An exploratory analysis. *Family Planning Perspectives, 30,* 12–18.

Alan Guttmacher Institute. (1994). *Sex and America's teenagers.* Washington, DC: Alan Guttmacher Institute.

Anda, R. F., Felitti, V. J., Chapman, D. P., Croft, J. B., Williamson, D. F., Santelli, J., et al. (2001). Abused boys, battered mothers and male involvement in teen pregnancy. *Pediatrics, 107,* e19.

Brewster, K. L. (1994). Neighborhood context and the transition to sexual activity among young black women. *Demography, 31,* 603–614.

Department of Health and Human Services, National Institutes of Health, Office for Protection from Research Risks. (2001). Code of Federal Regulations: Title 45-Public Welfare; Part 46: Protection of Human Subjects. Retrieved September 25, 2003 from http://ohrp.osophs.dhhs.gov/humansubjects/guidance/45cfr46.htm

Elster, A. B., & Kuznets, N. J. (1994). *American Medical Association guidelines for adolescent preventive services (GAPS): Recommendations and rationale.* Baltimore: Williams & Wilkins.

English, A., Kenney, K. E. (2003). *State minor consent laws: A summary.* 2nd edition. Chapel Hill, NC: Center for Adolescent Health & the Law

Hochhauser, M. (1999). Informed consent and patient's rights documents: A right, a rite, or a rewrite? *Ethics and Behavior, 9,* 1–20.

Hofferth, S. L. (1987). Influences on early sexual and fertility behavior. In S. L. Hofferth & C. D. Hayes (Eds.), *Risking the future: Adolescent sexuality, pregnancy, and childbearing: Vol. 2. Working papers and statistical appendices* (pp. 7–35). Washington, DC: National Academy Press.

Hogan, D. P., Astone, N. M., & Kitagawa, E. M. (1985). Social and environmental factors influencing contraceptive use among black adolescents. *Family Planning Perspectives, 17,* 165–169.

Kodish, F. D. (1999). Testing children for cancer genes: The rule of earliest onset. *Journal of Pediatrics, 135,* 390–395.

Leikin, S. L. (1983). An ethical issue in biomedical research: The involvement of minors in informed and third party consent. *Clinical Research, 31,* 34–40.

Levine, R. J. (1995). Adolescents as research subjects without permission of their parents or guardians: Ethical considerations. *Journal of Adolescent Health, 17,* 287–297.

Mastrionni, A. C., Faden, R., & Federman, D. (eds.) (1994). *Women and health research: Ethical and legal issues of including women in clinical studies* (Vol. 1). Washington, DC: Institute of Medicine, National Academy Press.

Melton, G. B. (1983). Toward "personhood" for adolescents. Autonomy and privacy as values in public policy. *American Psychologist, 38,* 99–103.

Moore, K. A., Miller, B. C., Glei, D., & Morrison, D. R. (1995). *Adolescent sex, contraception, and childbearing: A review of recent research.* Washington, DC: Child Trends, Inc.

National Children's Study. (2003, May 25). What is the National Children's Study? Retrieved May 25, 2003 from http://nationalchildrensstudy.gov/about/index.cfm.

National Commission for the Protection of Human Subjects of Biomedical and Behavioral Research. (1977). *Report and recommendations: Research involving children.* Washington, DC: US Government Printing Office. DHEW publication no. (OS) 77–0004.

National Commission for the Protection of Human Subjects of Biomedical and Behavioral Research. (1978). *The Belmont report: Ethical principles and guidelines for the protection of human subjects of research.* Washington, DC: US Government Printing Office. DHEW publication no. (OS) 78-0012.

National Institutes of Health. (2003, January 9). *NIH policy and guidelines on the inclusion of children as participants in research involving human subjects.* Retrieved January 9, 2003 January 9, 2003 from http://grants1.nih.gov/grants/guide/notice-files/not98-024.html

Petersen, A. C., & Leffert, N. (1995). Developmental issues influencing guidelines for adolescent health research: A review. *Journal of Adolescent Health, 17,* 298–305.

Reddy, D. M., Fleming, R., & Swain, C. (2002). Effect of mandatory parental notification on adolescent girls' use of sexual health care services. *Journal of the American Medical Association, 288,* 710–714.

Resnick, M. D., Bearman, P. S., Blum, R. W., Bauman, K., Harris, K., Jones, J., Tabor, J., Beohring, T., Seiring, R., Shaw, M., Ireland, M., Bearinger, L., Udray, R. (1997). Protecting adolescents from harm. Findings from the national longitudinal study of adolescent health. *Journal of the American Medical Association, 278,* 823–832.

Santelli, J. S. (1997). Human subjects protection and parental permission in adolescent health research. *Journal of Adolescent Health, 21,* 384–387.

Santelli, J. S., Lindberg, L. D., Abma, J., McNeely, C., & Resnick, M. (2000). Adolescent sexual, behavior, estimates and trends from four nationally representative surveys. *Family Planning Perspectives, 32,* 156–165, 194.

Santelli, J. S., Rochat, R., Hatfield-Timajchy, K., Colley Gilbert, B., Curtis, K., Cabral, R., & other members of the Unintended Pregnancy working group. (2003). The measurement and meaning of unintended pregnancy. *Perspectives on Sexual and Reproductive Health, 35,* 94–101.

Shearer, D. L., Mulvihill, B. A., Klerman, L. V., Wallander, J. L., Hovinga, M. E., & Redden, D. T. (2002). Association of early childbearing and low cognitive ability. *Perspectives on Sexual and Reproductive Health, 34,* 236–243.

Society for Adolescent Medicine. (2003). Guidelines for adolescent health research (a position paper of the society for adolescent medicine). Prepared by Santelli, J. S., Rogers, A. S., Rosenfeld, W. D., DuRant, R. H., Dubler, N., Morreale, M., et al. *Journal of Adolescent Health, 33*(5), 396–409.

Speers, M., Santelli, J. S., Rhoden, R., Reza, A., & Nieburg, P. (2000). *An evaluation of the participation of women, minorities and children in research conducted at the Centers for Disease Control and Prevention.* Office of Human Subjects Protection/Office of the Director, Centers for Disease Control and Prevention (unpublished manuscript).

Susman, E. J., Dorn, L. D., & Fletcher, J. C. (1992). Participation in biomedical research: The consent process as viewed by children, adolescents, young adults, and physicians. *Journal of Pediatrics, 121,* 547–552.

Thompson, R. A. (1980). Vulnerability in research: A developmental perspective on research risk. *Child Development, 61,* 1–16.

Ventura, S. J., Mosher, W. D., Curtin, S. C., Abma, J. C., & Henshaw, S. (2001). Trends in pregnancy rates for the United States, 1976–97: An update. *National Vital Statistics Reports, 49*(4), 1–9.

Weithorn, L. A. (1983). Children's capacities to decide about participation in research. *IRB: A Review of Human Subjects Research, 5*(2), 1–5.

Weithorn, L. A., & Scherer, D. G. (1994). Children's involvement in research participation decisions: Psychological considerations. In M. A. Grodin & L. H. Glanz (Eds.), *Children as research subjects: Science, ethics, and law* (pp. 133–179). New York: Oxford University Press.

II

Research Involving At-Risk Children

7

The Ethics of Newborn Screening Diabetes Research

Lainie Friedman Ross

CASE DESCRIPTION

In January 2002, a Florida newspaper proclaimed that "Florida had taken a progressive step in becoming the first state offering to screen newborns for the risk of developing juvenile diabetes" (Infant diabetes, 2002). Screening involves identifying children with a genetic predisposition to type 1 diabetes. It is offered as a voluntary test in conjunction with the mandatory newborn metabolic screening. Infants discovered to be at increased risk are being recruited for follow-up studies to determine if and when the child develops autoantibodies (preclinical disease) or overt diabetes. No therapies to prevent or retard the development of type 1 diabetes exist, and no experimental therapies are part of the research proposal. Is the research proposal ethical?

Newborn screening for diabetes raises ethical issues at two levels. At the primary level, one asks whether an informed parent should give permission for her child's participation. This type of ethical inquiry focuses on what information is needed for informed consent, who is the proper person to grant permission for enrollment, and whether subjects are being recruited fairly. At the secondary or meta-ethical level, one asks whether parents should be asked to enroll their newborns. This type of ethical inquiry focuses on whether healthy newborns are the appropriate population for predictive genetic screening for conditions (1) in which testing only leads to knowledge of increased susceptibility and (2) for which no therapies exist.

If the meta-ethical question is answered affirmatively, one must examine the primary-level concerns. However, if the meta-ethical question is answered in the negative, then the first level concerns become moot. If the research protocol does not pass ethical research standards, then parental permission should not be sought. This is true regardless of how many parents might consent. In this chapter I will focus on the meta-ethical question. Although I answer it negatively, I will address the issue of parental permission because there are data to show that more than 90% of parents give permission for diabetes screening of their newborns in the United States and abroad (Flanders, Graves, & Rewers, 1999; Kimpimaki et al., 2001). This concept reinforces the importance of sequence in the protection of children from research risk. Thoughtful reflection by investigators and careful scrutiny by institutional review boards must precede the recruitment of children and the informed consent process for research studies, and the fact that many parents would permit their children to be subjects in a study does not provide automatic or inherent ethical justification for the research.

Diabetes Prediction Studies in Newborns

In the United States, type 1 diabetes has an annual incidence of 15 per 100,000 in children and adolescents younger than 18 years, making it the most common metabolic disease of childhood (American Diabetes Association, 2002). Of major concern is that type 1 diabetes is increasing at a yearly rate of 2.5% throughout the world (Heine, 1999). As such, Florida's interest in diabetes prediction research in newborns is not unique. The BABY-DIAB studies in Germany and Australia are prospective studies from birth of children with at least one parent with diabetes mellitus. The studies are designed to perform serial blood tests on the children for evidence of autoantibody development (Colman et al., 2000; Couper, 2001; Hummel, Fuchtenbusch, Schenker, & Ziegler, 2000; Roll et al., 1996; Ziegler, Hummel, Schenker, & Bonifacio, 1999) and its relationship with environmental triggers (Couper, 2001; Roll et al., 1996).

Although newborns with an affected first-degree relative have a 10-fold higher incidence of developing type 1 diabetes (Buzzetti, Quattrocchi, & Nistico, 1998), most newborn studies do not focus on these children because they only account for 10% of type 1 diabetes cases (Dahlquist, 1999; Flanders et al., 1999). The DIPP (Diabetes Prediction and Prevention study) in Finland seeks to identify all newborns with HLA-DQB1 genotypes that confer a high (~8%) or moderate risk (1.7–2.6%) of developing type 1 diabetes (compared with a national average risk of 0.7%; Kimpimaki et al., 2001). Approximately 94.4% of parents consent to genetic screening and 14.8% of the children are found to be at some degree of increased risk (Ronningen, 1997). The Norwegian Babies against Diabetes (NOBADIA) seeks to identify the 4% of newborns in the general population with the highest genetic risk (12%) for developing type 1 diabetes (Kimpimaki et al., 2001). Begun in 1998, this study will follow these infants for 15 years. In Colorado, the Diabetes Autoimmunity Study in the Young (DAISY) seeks to identify newborns with the highest genetic risk alleles (2.3%) to participate in serial antibody screening (Flanders et al., 1999). Ninety-four percent of mothers consent (Flanders et al., 1999). The Florida newspaper report (Infant diabetes, 2002) refers to the Prospective Assessment in Newborns for Diabetic Autoimmunity (PANDA) study in which infants at increased genetic risk will be followed for antibody development to uncover possible environmental triggers such as breast-feeding, immunizations, and viral infections (Greener, 2000).

Of all the studies being done in the general newborn population, only DIPP in Finland includes a prevention component. Children who develop diabetes-associated autoantibodies are offered participation in a prevention trial with intranasally applied human insulin (Kupila et al., 2001). Of note, a safety study of intranasal administered insulin was only recently published (Kupila et al., 2003) and safety and efficacy data from DIPP are not yet available. Intranasal insulin was shown to be effective in NOD mice (Harrison, Dempsey-Collier, Kramer, & Takahashi, 1996). A second prediction-prevention study being done in Finland involves infants with an affected first-degree relative. The results of a pilot study of the Trial to Reduce IDDM (insulin dependent diabetes mellitus, or type 1 diabetes) in the Genetically at Risk (TRIGR) were reported in 1992–1993 (American Diabetes Association, 2002) were encouraging, and the second TRIGR study was launched in 1995 to examine whether avoiding cow's milk protein for the first 6–8 months of life prevents diabetes in infants with an affected first-degree relative (Paronen et al., 2000). The diet was effective in NOD mice (Karges et al., 1997), although there are some preliminary data to suggest it is ineffective in humans (Norris et al., 1996, Couper et al., 1999). After weaning from breast milk, infants enrolled in TRIGR were randomized to receive either Nutramigen (a casein-hydrolysate formula that lacks intact cow's milk) exclusively or Enfamil (a cow's milk based formula) mixed with 20% Nutramigen to control for taste and smell) (Paronen et al., 2000). No results are available yet.

It is noteworthy that all of the studies described above include disclosure of the child's genetic risk to the parents. Contrast such disclosure with the general consensus in the medical and medical ethics communities against clinical predictive genetic testing of children when no treatment exists (American Academy of Pediatrics, 2001; ASHG/ACMG, 1995; Institute of Medicine, 1994; Working Party of the Clinical Genetics Society, 1994). And yet, despite the medical and ethical consensus against clinical predictive testing, more than 90% of parents consent to research that involves predictive screening of their newborns for diabetes. In the next three sections, I address three questions: (1) What are the risks and benefits of such newborn research screening? (2) What is required for newborn research screening to be ethical? (3) Do current newborn diabetes research screening projects fulfill these ethical requirements? I then consider whether the high rate of parental permission successfully challenges the ethical problems raised by this screening research.

—

ETHICAL ANALYSIS AND DISCUSSION

The Risks and Benefits of Diabetes Susceptibility Research in Newborns

The expert consensus against isolated predictive identification of newborns and children for increased genetic susceptibilities when no preventive measures are available is based on the lack of therapeutic benefit (American Academy of Pediatrics, 2001; ASHG/ACMG, 1995; Institute of Medicine, 1994; Nordenfelt, 1996; Kodish, 1999; Siegler, Amiel, & Lantos, 1992; Working Party of the Clinical Genetics Society, 1994). When psychosocial risks and benefits of predictive identification are mentioned, it is presumed that the risks outweigh the benefits (ASHG/ACMG, 1995; Institute of Medicine, 1994; Kodish, 1999).

However, there are scant empirical data regarding the psychosocial risks and benefits of predictive screening with disclosure of results of children generally (Broadstock, Michie, & Marteau, 2000; Michie, 1996), let alone for newborn screening for a specific condition like type 1 diabetes. Although NOBADIA plans to do extensive psychological follow-up (Ronningen, 1997), there are very little data on the psychosocial risks associated with identifying newborns for a genetic predisposition to diabetes (Yu et al., 1999). The data that do exist regarding predictive diabetes identification are from studies in families that were notified that children (beyond infancy) or adults had islet cell antibodies (ICAs; a marker of beta cell destruction; Carmichael et al., 2000; Johnson, 2001; Johnson, Riley, Hansen, & Nurick, 1990; Johnson & Tercyak, 1995; Weber & Roth, 1997). These studies found that families were initially quite anxious, but most of the anxiety dissipated by 4 months (Carmichael et al., 2000; Johnson, 2001; Johnson et al., 1990; Johnson & Tercyak, 1995; Weber &Roth, 1997). However, anxiety persisted in some subgroups (e.g., those who relied on self-blame and wishful thinking as coping strategies; Carmichael et al., 2000; Johnson, 2001; Weber & Roth, 1997), such that the researchers concluded that some participants may experience greater distress than others (Johnson, 2001; Weber & Roth, 1997).

In addition, whether the anxiety will remain low needs to be determined. Psychological follow-up from other newborn screening programs suggest that harms can accrue over a much longer period, and that they can wax and wane. Consider, for example, alpha-1 antitrypsin deficiency (alpha-1) screening begun in Sweden in the early 1970s (Heyerdahl, 1988; Thelin, McNeil, Aspegren-Jansson, & Sveger, 1985b). Alpha-1 is an autosomal recessive predisposition to chronic lung disease in young adulthood with variable penetrance and expressivity. Parents of at-risk children were counseled that smoking and smoky environments could hasten or worsen their children's pulmonary symptoms. Psychological data were procured for twenty years on a subset of families with a child who screened positive (Heyerdahl, 1988; McNeil, Harty, Thelin, Aspegren-Jansson, & Sveger, 1986; McNeil, Thelin, Aspegren-Jansson, & Sveger,1985; McNeil, Thelin,

Aspegren-Jansson, Sveger, & Harty, 1985; Thelin, McNeil, Aspegren-Jansson, & Sveger, 1985a, 1985b, 1985c, 1985d). The data showed that parents initially had strong negative emotional reactions to the diagnosis (Thelin et al., 1985b), and yet, despite negative attitudes, the majority of parents had a positive attitude about the screening program that had identified their child's risk (Thelin et al., 1985a).

The alpha-1 screening program was stopped after five years because of the psychological stress it had caused in some families who had tested positive (McNeil, Thelin, Aspegren-Jansson, Sveger, & Harty, 1985). Follow-up data found increased smoking by fathers of affected children (Thelin et al., 1985b), and negative long-term effects in the mental and physical health of the mother (McNeil et al., 1986; Sveger, Thelin, & McNeil, 1999; Thelin et al., 1985d), in mother–child but not father–child interactions (McNeil et al., 1986), in parents' long-term emotional adjustment to their children's alpha-1 status (McNeil, Thelin, Aspegren-Jansson, & Sveger, 1985), and in the parents' view of their children's health (McNeil, Thelin, Aspegren-Jansson, & Sveger, 1985), although this improved over time (Thelin et al., 1985c). However, the children, as young adults, were aware of the dangers of smoking and smoky environments and had a positive attitude about alpha-1 screening (Sveger, Thelin, & McNeil, 1997). In 1997, the World Health Organization reviewed the data and published a memorandum in support of implementing alpha-1 newborn screening (World Health Organization, 1997). Although Sweden remains somewhat ambivalent (Sveger & Thelin, 2000), Oregon had a similar program in the 1970s (O'Brien, Buist, & Murphey, 1978) and supports re-implementation (Wall, Moe, Eisenberg, Powers, Buist, & Buist, 1990).

The situations with alpha-1 and type 1 diabetes screening are not completely analogous. First, as noted by the alpha-1 researchers, some of the psychological stress might have been avoided if the parents had been informed about the testing and given the opportunity to consent or refuse testing, which was not the case when alpha-1 testing was incorporated into universal screening programs in the 1970s (Sveger & Thelin, 2000). All of the predictive diabetes newborn screening programs described above include a separate informed consent process. And yet, even if a special informed consent is required, it may not be enough in part because "the pressure of the hospital setting, the parents' physician and emotional condition immediately after birth, and the cultural belief that 'medical testing is good for you' will lead most parents to consent" (Wertz, 2002). A second dissimilarity between the two conditions is that there are preventive measures that can be taken for alpha-1 that improve the benefit/harm ratio for alpha-1 screening. One would hypothesize greater harm in predictive information about type 1 diabetes when subjects and their families have no control over the development of diabetes (Senior, Marteau, & Peters, 1999; Lefcourt, 1982). What, then, are the risks and benefits of predictive identification of newborns at increased risk for type 1 diabetes? One potential clinical benefit is that parents can be taught the signs and symptoms of clinical disease so that their children are diagnosed early, and avoid being diagnosed in the emergency setting of diabetic ketoacidosis. The risk, however, is that parents may overreact and interpret a child's normal urination habits as a sign of polyuria. A second potential clinical benefit is that the parents will be familiar with a diabetes center and will make the transition to clinical care easier. However, a high-risk allele does not confer certainty of disease, and parents may become very anxious and make life plans based on an increased susceptibility, a susceptibility that has less than a 20% probability of fruition; and a low risk allele may give parents false reassurance of their child's health because some children with low-risk genetic alleles develop diabetes.

The most serious clinical risk, however, is that parents will conflate the experimental and nontherapeutic nature of diabetes screening with the established public health newborn screening programs geared to detect metabolic and endocrine disorders that require immediate treatment. Parents may decide that all newborn screening is experimental and refuse the clearly effective public health screening for Phenylketonuria (PKU) and hypothyroidism when they decide to refuse the experimental diabetes screening. Alternately, parents may conflate the experimental and established public health screening programs and consent to both without understanding that the former is nontherapeutic. This will leave them unprepared for a positive test result. Data show that the receipt of a positive test result has more negative effects than anticipated in population-based screening (vs. less negative effects than anticipated in testing of high-risk families; Michie & Marteau, 1998).

There are also potential psychosocial benefits and risks raised by experimental screening of newborns for diabetes. One potential psychosocial benefit is that the parent can prepare. And yet, given the high rate of false positives (the highest risk allele confers less than a 20% risk of developing diabetes), many parents will prepare unnecessarily, and the danger is that they may begin treating their child as ill, when the child has at most an increased risk of becoming ill in the future (McNeil, Thelin, Aspegren-Jansson, & Sveger, 1985). This is particularly true when the genetic factor is but one contributor to a higher relative risk of an illness that also depends on unknown individual or environmental co-factors (Croyle & Lerman, 1995). It may also adversely affect the parent–child relationship (Clayton, 1999; Headings, 1980; McNeil et al., 1986). This risk may be exaggerated in the newborn period, which is a particularly vulnerable time in parent–child relationships (Clayton, 1999; Fyro, 1988). Even families who have received a positive screening test that is quickly confirmed to be negative (e.g., false-positive hypothyroid screen) report greater strain on marriage and difficulties in their relationships with their children (Tymstra, 1986). Imagine then a positive screening test that only reflects increased susceptibility over a lifetime! These children may spend their childhood as neither healthy nor ill but "at risk" (Davison, Macintyre,

& Smith, 1994). Such labeling may cause familial stress (Clayton, 1999; Headings, 1980; Thelin et al., 1985c) and may be stigmatizing for the family, reflected in difficulty procuring health insurance (Clayton, 1999; Croyle & Lerman, 1995; Rcilly, Boshar, & Holtzman, 1997).

The concerns about genetic discrimination in health insurance are serious. Several studies have documented that genetic information leads to discrimination in health insurance (Billings et al., 1992; Geller et al., 1996). The institutional review board guidebook prepared by the Office of Human Research Protections (1993) specifically states that subjects in genetic research must be made aware of the potential for discrimination in health and life insurance.

In summary, given the low sensitivity and specificity of predictive genetic screening for type 1 diabetes in newborns, the current potential medical benefits of such information for the child and family are minimal. They must be judged in light of the possible medical and psychosocial risks, and the possibility that such experimental screening programs will be confused with established public health screening programs. The federal regulations do not allow nontherapeutic research on children when the risks outweigh the benefits (Department of Health and Human Services, 1983). Researchers who seek to do such research need to show how the benefits outweigh the risks, or modify their study design to achieve a positive benefit:risk ratio.

Minimizing Risks to Children

Even if researchers could show that the risks outweigh the benefits, the research may still not pass muster. Although the diabetes community clearly supports diabetes research in the general population of newborns (Infant diabetes, 2002; Schatz, Krischer, & Syler, 2000), the question remains whether current study designs minimize risk, a requirement enumerated by various reports on what is required for research to be ethical in general (Medical Research Council of Canada, 2002; National Commission, 1979; Nuremberg Code, 1946; World Medical Association, 2002), as well as in reports focusing on research with children (National Commission, 1977; Nicholson, 1986). In the United States, this requirement was adopted into the federal regulations regarding the protection of human research subjects (§46.111; Department of Health and Human Services, 1981). Several reports also note that because of the vulnerability of children, research should be conducted when possible on animals, then adults, and then older children (National Commission, 1977; Nicholson, 1986; World Medical Association, 2002). Unfortunately, the demographics of type 1 diabetes (American Diabetes Association, 2002; EURODIAB ACE Study Group, 2000; Heine, 1999) and the increasing number of new cases of children younger than 4 years (EURODIAB

ACE Study Group, 2000; Feltbower, McKinney, & Bodansky, 2000) mean that such research must be done on young children.

One question is whether it matters if the research is done on newborns (vs. older infants). Newborns are attractive for population genetic screening research because (1) virtually all newborns in developed countries are born in hospitals (captive population), (2) virtually all undergo screening for PKU and hypothyroidism, making screening already accepted, and (3) large amounts of blood can be obtained from the placenta at delivery without any physical risk to the baby. A delay of 3 months would not interfere with predictive research because autoantibodies and overt disease rarely develop before then (Kimpimaki et al., 2001). The advantage of such a delay is that it would distinguish this research study from current metabolic newborn screening. The major drawback of such a study design would be lower participation. Attempting to enroll children at primary care clinics is much less efficient than enrollment in the hospital. It requires the active recruitment by many primary care physicians who may not have a vested interest in the project and may not be willing to spend the time to get consent from the parent. It would also require a separate blood sample which both increases the physical riskiness of the study (albeit minimally) but could result in lower parental consent.

Whether delaying enrollment until infants are 3 months serves a valid purpose depends on whether the increased vulnerability of newborns and the newborn–parent relationship (Clayton, 1999; Headings, 1980) is significantly reduced by 3 months. However, even if this is not the case, one could argue, at minimum, in support of decision aids to improve the consent process (Entwistle, 2001) or a more active parental consent process.

Another way to reduce risk in genetic susceptibility research is to design studies that do not require disclosure of individual results because nondisclosure eliminates the psychosocial harms of classifying an individual as "at risk." In such a study, one would request parental permission (1) to procure a blood sample of the infant and (2) to track whether or not the infant develops diabetes by annual contact with local hospitals, pediatric endocrinologists, diabetes registries, or the families themselves. In Sweden, long-term studies have been done in this way (Samuelsson, Sundkvist, Borg, Fernlund, & Ludvigsson, 2001).

Critics might object to this study design requirement for two reasons. First, they may object on the grounds that parents will not consent to genetic testing of their newborns under these conditions, but that is an empirical question for which there are no data. Second, critics might also object because a policy of nondisclosure in the general population means that follow-up autoantibody screening studies will be more expensive because the researchers cannot target those at high risk. This concern is valid and will require innovative study designs. At minimum, consent should be sought not only for procuring the initial blood sample but also for permission to be recontacted to obtain follow-up data without disclosure of genetic results.

If one assumes that the research has scientific merit, and that it is unrealistic to assume that it can be done without identifying those individuals "at risk," the question remains who is the appropriate subject population. Given the demographics of the disease, it will require the participation of young children. But there is also the question of whether such research should be done on the general population, or only in newborns from high-risk families (e.g., a family with an affected first-degree relative). The scientific advantage of screening the low-yield general population is that it will increase the number of infants identified. The advantage of selectively screening the high-risk community is that one will identify a larger number of individuals "at risk" with a smaller sample. The major disadvantages of only recruiting from high-risk families are that the total number identified may be too small for some research and there is fear that this sample population may be biased. For example, most studies have concluded that ICAs are less predictive in the general population than in high-risk families (Bingley et al., 1993; Landin-Olsson et al., 1992; Veijola et al., 1996), with the exception of Schatz et al. (1994) in the United States.

The difference between screening the general population versus testing the high-risk community should not be seen as a value-neutral design choice. While type 1 diabetes is a serious public health problem for which population screening of infants would be appropriate if and when preventive measures are developed, the question being raised here is how early research should progress, given the vulnerability of the infant population. The answer becomes clearer if one uses the criteria that research must be designed to minimize risks, including psychosocial risks. There is some empirical evidence to support restricting the identification of risk to children in high-risk families. Children in these families are often viewed as "at risk" even before genetic markers were discovered, and are often labeled as such by their families even if they do not undergo genetic testing (Marteau, 1994; Wagner et al., 1995). The parents' behavior is not without merit: siblings have a 15-fold increased chance of developing type 1 diabetes compared with an individual from the general population. In addition, although the data are anecdotal, parents in families in which either a parent or child has diabetes frequently do monitor their other children for signs of glycosuria or hyperglycemia (Lucidarme, Donmingues-Muriel, Castro, Czernichow, & Levy-Marchal, 1998; Shepherd, Hattersley, & Sparkes, 2000; Wagner et al., 1995). The exact percentage is unknown because this is rarely shared with physicians (Lucidarme et al., 1998). Given the baseline anxiety that already exists within these families, genetic and immunological testing do not induce the anxiety (Lucidarme et al., 1998; Nordenfelt, 1996; Ziegler et al., 1999), but rather, either confirm or refute these concerns, albeit only probabilistically.

Finally, one must consider prediction research that is coupled with prevention. Clearly, the children need to be identified in order to employ the prevention strategy. Both the concern of introducing the "at-risk" status into the healthy population and the high false positivity rate have led many ethicists to conclude that initial studies should be restricted to children from high-risk families, despite their therapeutic potential (Nordenfelt, 1996; Roth, 2001; Siegler et al., 1992).

Do Current Research Designs Minimize Risk?

Population studies are important to understand incidence, prevalence, and gene-environment interactions of type 1 diabetes in the general population. However, the identification of at-risk newborns in the general population and the disclosure of these results to unsuspecting parents fail to minimize risks, an ethical requirement for all research involving human subjects. Population studies that are designed to disclose the results to parents in order to follow subjects prospectively need to be redesigned. This includes many of the studies being done today, including DIPP, NOBADIA, DAISY, and PANDA.

If it is necessary to disclose the risk status of infants, the risks to the subjects and their families can be reduced if the study population is restricted to infants from families with an affected first-degree relative. But even if one focuses on infants from high-risk families, the ethical requirement to minimize risk would support designing predictive studies that do not require disclosure of the results. Virtually all of the German and Australian BABYDIAB data could have been procured without disclosing results (except for 13 children from whom the German researchers requested more frequent testing because they had more than one positive antibody [Roll et al., 1996]. While this additional information may have been valuable, it greatly increased the potential psychosocial harms of the research and could have been omitted.

If the research includes a prevention strategy, identification of at-risk children will be necessary. Given the potential harms of introducing at-risk status into the healthy population, initial studies should only recruit children from high-risk families as TRIGR did.

Parental Permission

Given my arguments that newborn population screening for diabetes is unethical at this time, the issue of parent permission is moot. However, critics may argue that my ethical analysis must be wrong given that over 90% of parents permit their newborns' participation or, if not wrong, at least overly paternalistic.

The critics' argument is this: If the benefits do not clearly outweigh the risks, how do we explain that 94% of parents consent to screening for type 1 diabetes? In part, the high uptake can be explained by our culture's unequivocal support of testing generally (Nelkin & Tancredi, 1989; Wertz, 2002). The low frequency of positive results in the general population makes it attractive to individuals who seek reassurance (Andrykowski, Lightner, Studts, & Munn, 1997; Marteau & Croyle, 1998). The high uptake may also be explainable, in part, because of how the test is offered. Data show that uptake is highest when requested in person and when testing can be done immediately (Clarke, 1997b). In the case of newborn screening for type 1 diabetes, the blood may have already been procured (DAISY) or will be procured for traditional newborn screening.

One solution, then, may be to require more active parental involvement. A voluntary newborn screening program for Duchenne muscular dystrophy (DMD), a progressive neuromuscular disorder for which no treatment exists, has been offered in Wales for the last decade and it also has a 94% uptake rate (Clarke, 1997b). Clarke, one of the principal investigators, has suggested requiring parents to mail the blood spot for the DMD screening in order to yield a lower "more appropriate" uptake rate. As Clarke (1997b) explains: "To suggest that a lower uptake rate for a screening test would be preferable, that we should set a threshold of motivation so that infants are not screened unless their parents actively choose it, is certainly unusual but is perfectly appropriate in the context of an untreatable disease." To this end, the researchers implemented a pilot project to determine the feasibility of providing newborn screening for DMD in a way that made the optional nature of the text explicit. The result was an uptake of 78%, significantly lower than the current methodology (Parsons, Clarke, Hood, & Bradley, 2000). The analogy is not perfect. DMD is uniformly fatal whereas type 1 diabetes is treatable, although currently no treatment exists for either condition that can be provided presymptomically that will prevent or delay the onset of the disease (Diabetes Prevention Trial, 2002; Escolar & Scacheri, 2001). DMD is also virtually 100% penetrant (the likelihood of developing the disease if one has the gene) in contrast with the genetic markers for type 1 diabetes, which only result in an increased susceptibility. This means that there are many newborns identified as being at increased risk for type 1 diabetes who will not develop the disease. There are many dangers with creating awareness and labeling individuals "at risk" in a low-risk population (Clarke, 1997b; Davison et al., 1994): leading to vulnerable child syndrome, inappropriately treating the child as "ill" even before symptoms develop, or trying unproven and potentially dangerous preventive measures (Burris & Gostin, 2002; Clarke, 1997a; Davison et al., 1994; Johnson & Tercyak, 1995). Thus, because the genetic markers for type 1 diabetes only offer predispositional information and no preventive measures are available, one could make an argument, similar to Clarke's, that infants should not be screened unless the parents actively choose it: 94% uptake seems too high.

Even if the uptake is higher than it would be if (1) parents truly understood the risks and benefits of such research or (2) active parental involvement were required, the critics' cry of paternalism must be addressed. Paternalism is "the intentional overriding of one person's known preferences or actions by another person, where the person who overrides justifies the action by the goal of benefiting or avoiding harm to the person whose will is overridden" (Beauchamp & Childress, 1994, p. 274). But the situation at hand is not about interfering with an individual's decision about whether or not to participate in research, but whether to interfere with a parent's autonomy about whether or not to enroll *her child* in research. The issue, then, is not about whether or not to respect individual autonomy, but parental autonomy. Proxy decision making is more restricted than individual autonomy because individuals may take risks that they cannot authorize others to take (Buchanan & Brock, 1989; Ross, 1998). As such, it is morally justifiable to require either (1) that risk status not be disclosed in order to minimize the research risks for individuals who cannot consent for themselves or (2) that only children of high-risk families be eligible for participation.

CONCLUSION

Type 1 diabetes is a significant health problem in children, and accurate prediction in infancy will be necessary to prevent or delay its onset. However, prediction research in the newborn period has potentially serious psychosocial implications, particularly when it is being introduced into the unsuspecting general population, and research designs must account for them. To minimize harm to infants and their families, I propose two recommendations. First, if the research is solely predictive (e.g., it does not incorporate a prevention strategy), studies should be designed, when possible, to avoid disclosure of increased susceptibility results. Second, if disclosure is necessary, then the research should be restricted to children with an affected first-degree relative, and this would hold even for prediction-prevention protocols. These recommendations are based on the fundamental ethical obligation to minimize risk to infants who are potential subjects in diabetes prediction and prevention research, while at the same time allowing for critical scientific investigation of this serious childhood disease. This balanced approach may serve as a model for other questions that will arise at the crossroads of pediatrics, genetics, and public health research.

Questions for Discussion

1. What are the ethical issues raised by newborn screening for diabetes? Discuss your answer at both the primary (individual) level and the secondary (meta-ethical) level?

2. Does the fact that the vast majority of the parents in the US and abroad (i.e., more than 90%) permit their children to be subjects in research about newborn screening for diabetes provide justification for conducting such research?

3. How would you explain the consensus in our society against allowing isolated predictive identification of newborns and children for increased genetic susceptibilities when no preventive measures are available? Are you a part of this consensus?

4. In the alpha-1 screening program parents of at-risk children were counseled that smoking and smoky environments could hasten or worsen their children's pulmonary symptoms. Psychological data were procured for twenty years on a subset of families with a child who screened positive. What is your opinion with regard to the alpha-1 screening program described in the chapter? Do the results that were obtained support continued newborn screening?

5. What are the psychosocial risks associated with identifying newborns for a genetic predisposition to diabetes? What are the ethical implications of these risks?

6. What are the risks and benefits of predictive identification of newborns at increased risk for type 1 diabetes? Do you think the benefits outweigh the risks, or vice versa?

7. Why is there risk associated with the possibility that "experimental" screening programs for diabetes will be confused with established public health screening programs? What are the ethical implications of conflating these distinct endeavors? Can you suggest modifications of the form the programs take currently that could serve to minimize the risk of confusion?

8. Young children are a vulnerable population at risk for research related harm. Accordingly, research should be conducted when possible on animals, then adults, and then older children. Do you agree with the logic of this order in general? Does this apply to the case of type 1 diabetes predisposition screening research? Within the pediatric population, does it make a difference if the research is done on newborns as opposed to older infants? How do the ethical and practical answers to this question conflict?

9. Do you support studies that are conducted without identifying those individuals "at risk" and therefore do not require disclosure of individual results, such as the long-term study from Sweden described in the chapter? What are the ethical issues raised by this type of study?

10. Do you agree with the conclusion that initial studies should be restricted to children from high-risk families (vs. studies of the general population) despite their therapeutic potential? What are the advantages and disadvantages of studies conducted on high-risk population only?

11. The author of this chapter concludes that that newborn population screening for diabetes is unethical at this time. However, a counterargument claims that this ethical analysis is flawed and overly paternalistic since more than 90% of parents permit their newborns' participation. What is your opinion?

12. What are the implications of the fact that decisions about newborn screening for diabetes programs are made by surrogates rather than the screened individual him or herself?

Acknowledgments

L.R.'s research on genetics is supported by a Harris Foundation grant "Ethical and Policy Implications of Genetic Testing of Children," and her research on children in research is funded by an NIH Grant (NLM 1 G13 LM07472–01). L.R is also a member of the Internal Organizational Advisory Group (IOAG) for the Policy and Ethics Section of the Collaborative Network for Clinical Research on Immune Tolerance," also known as the Immune Tolerance Network (ITN), sponsored by the NIH. The opinions expressed in this paper represent her own views and do not necessarily reflect the views of the NIH, the ITN, or the Harris Foundation.

This chapter is based on a previously published work: Lainie Friedman Ross, M.D., Ph.D., Minimizing Risks: The Ethics of Predictive Diabetes Screening Research in Newborns *Archives of Pediatrics and Adolescent Medicine*, 2003; 157: 89–95. *Copyright © 2003, American Medical Association*. All rights reserved. With permission.

References

American Academy of Pediatrics, Committee on Bioethics. (2001). Ethical issues with genetic testing in pediatrics. *Pediatrics, 107*, 1451–1455.

American Diabetes Association. (2002, June 18). Prevention of type 1 diabetes mellitus [Conference Summary]. Retrieved October 1, 2003 from http://www.diabetesforum.net/cgi-bin/display _engine.pl?category_id=15&content_id=230

Andrykowski, M. A., Lightner, R., Studts, J. L., & Munn, R. K. (1997). Hereditary cancer risk notification and testing: How interested is the general population? *Journal of Clinical Oncology, 15(5)*, 2139–2148.

ASHG/ACMG (American Society of Human Genetics/American College of Medical Genetics). (1995). Points to consider: Ethical, legal, and psychosocial implications of genetic testing in children and adolescents. *American Journal of Human Genetics, 57,* 1233–1241.

Beauchamp, T. L., & Childress, J. F. (1994). *Principles of biomedical ethics* (4th ed.). New York: Oxford University Press.

Billings, P. R., Kohn, M. A., de Cuevas, M., Beckwith, J., Alper, J. S., & Natowicz, M. R. (1992). Discrimination as a consequence of genetic testing. *American Journal of Human Genetics, 50,* 476–482.

Bingley, P. J., Bonifacio, E., Shattock, M., Gillmore, H. A., Sawtell, P. A., Dunger, D. B., et al. (1993). Can islet cell antibodies predict IDDM in the general population? *Diabetes Care, 16,* 45–50.

Broadstock, M., Michie, S., & Marteau, T. M. (2000). The psychological consequences of predictive genetic testing: A systematic review. *European Journal of Human Genetics, 8,* 731–738.

Buchanan, A. E., & Brock, D. W. (1989). *Deciding for others: The ethics of surrogate decision making.* New York: Cambridge University Press.

Burris, S., & Gostin, L. O. (2002). Genetic screening from a public health perspective: Three "ethical" principles. In J. Burley & J. Harris (Eds.), *A companion to genethics* (pp. 455–464). Oxford: Blackwell Publishers.

Buzzetti, R., Quattrocchi, C. C., & Nistico, L. (1998). Dissecting the genetics of type 1 diabetes: Relevance for familial clustering and differences in incidence. *Diabetes/Metabolism Reviews, 14,* 111–128.

Carmichael, S. L., Johnson, S. B., Weiss, A., Fuller, K. G., She, J. X., & Schatz, D. A. (2000). Psychological impact of screening programs in mothers of children at-risk for type 1 diabetes. *Diabetes 49*(Suppl. 1), A317.

Clarke, A. J. (1997a). The genetic dissection of multifactorial disease: The implications of susceptibility screening. In P. S. Harper & A. J. Clarke (Eds.), *Genetics, society and clinical practice* (pp. 93–106). Oxford: Bios Scientific Publishers.

Clarke, A. J. (1997b). Newborn screening. In P. S. Harper & A. J. Clarke (Eds.), *Genetics, society and clinical practice* (pp. 107–117). Oxford: Bios Scientific Publishers.

Clayton, E. W. (1999). What should be the role of public health in newborn screening and prenatal diagnosis? *American Journal of Preventive Medicine, 16,* 111–115.

Colman, P. G, Steele, C., Couper, J. J., Beresford, S. J., Powell, T., Kewming, K., et al. (2000). Islet autoimmunity in infants with a type 1 diabetic relative is common but is frequently restricted to one autoantibody. *Diabetologia, 43,* 203–209.

Couper, J. J. (2001). Annotation: Environmental triggers of type 1 diabetes. *Journal of Pediatrics and Child Health, 37,* 218–220.

Couper, J. J, Steele, C., Beresford, S. D., Powell, T., McCaul, K., Pollard, A., et al. (1999). Lack of association between duration of breast feeding or introduction of cow's milk and development of islet autoimmunity. *Diabetes, 48,* 2145–2149.

Croyle, R. T., & Lerman, C. (1995). Psychological impact of genetic testing. In R. T. Croyle (Ed.), *Psychosocial effects of screening for disease prevention and detection* (pp. 11–38). New York: Oxford University Press.

Dahlquist, G. G. (1999). Primary and secondary prevention strategies of pre-type 1 diabetes: Potentials and pitfalls. *Diabetes Care, 22*(Suppl. 2S), 4B–6B.

Davison, C., Macintyre, S., & Smith, G. D. (1994) The potential social impact of predictive genetic testing for susceptibility to common chronic disease: A review and proposed research agenda. *Sociology of Health and Illness, 16,* 340–371.

Department of Health and Human Services. (1983, revised 1991). 45 CFR 46 Subpart D. Additional

Protections for Children Involved as Subjects in Research. 48 *Federal Register* 9814-20 (1983). Revised 56 *Federal Register* 29,032 (1991).

Department of Health and Human Services. (1981) 45 CFR 46 Subpart A. Final Regulations Amending Basic HHS Policy for the Protection of Human Research Subjects—Department of Health and Human Services. *Federal Register.* 46(16 Pt 2):8366–91, 1981 Jan 26. Revised: Federal policy for the protection of human subjects. Final rule. *Federal Register.*

Diabetes Prevention Trial–Type 1 Diabetes Study Group. (2002). Effects of insulin in relatives of patients with type 1 diabetes mellitus. *New England Journal of Medicine, 346,* 1685–1691.

Entwistle, V. (2001). The potential contribution of decision aids to screening programmes. *Health Expectations, 4,* 109–115.

Escolar, D. M., & Scacheri, C. G. (2001). Pharmacologic and genetic therapy for childhood muscular dystrophies. *Current Neurology & Neuroscience Reports, 1,* 168–174.

EURODIAB ACE Study Group. (2000). Variation and trends in incidence of childhood diabetes in Europe. *Lancet, 355,* 873–876.

Feltbower, R. G., McKinney, P. A., & Bodansky, H. J. (2000). Rising incidence of childhood diabetes is seen at all ages and in urban and rural settings in Yorkshire, United Kingdom. *Diabetologia, 43,* 682–684.

Flanders, G., Graves, P., & Rewers, M. (1999). Review: Prevention of type 1 diabetes from laboratory to public health. *Autoimmunity, 29,* 235–246.

Fyro, K. (1988). Neonatal screening: Life-stress scores in families given a false-positive result. *Acta Paediatrica Scandinavia,77,* 232–238.

Geller, L. N, Alpler, J. S., Billings, P. R., Barash, C. I., Beckwith, J., & Natowicz, M. R. (1996). Individual, family, and societal dimensions of genetic discrimination: A case study analysis. *Science and Engineering Ethics, 2,* 71–88.

Greener, M. 2000. (PANDA) identifies babies at risk of developing type 1 diabetes. *Molecular Medicine Today, 6,* 3.

Harrison, L. C., Dempsey-Collier, M., Kramer, D. R., Takahashi, K. (1996). Aerosol insulin induces regulatory CD8 gamma delta T cells that prevent murine insulin-dependent diabetes. *Journal of Experimental Medicine 184,* 2167-74.

Headings, V. (1980). Counseling in a hospital-based newborn screening service. *Patient Counseling and Health Education, 2,* 80–83.

Heine, R. J. (1999). Diabetes in the next century: Challenges and opportunities. *Netherlands Journal of Medicine, 55,* 265–270.

Heyerdahl, S. (1988). Psychological problems in relation to neonatal screening programmes. *Acta Paediatrica Scandinavica, 77,* 239–241.

Hummel, M., Fuchtenbusch, M., Schenker, M., & Ziegler, A. G. (2000). No major association of breast-feeding, vaccinations, and childhood viral diseases with early islet autoimmunity in the German BABYDIAB study. *Diabetes Care, 23,* 969–974.

Infant diabetes test is good start [Editorial]. (2002, January 8). *St. Petersburg Times,* p. 8A.

Institute of Medicine. (1994). *Assessing genetic risks: Implications for health and social policy.* Washington, DC: National Academy Press.

Johnson, S. B. (2001). Screening programs to identify children at risk for diabetes mellitus: Psychological impact on children and parents. *Journal of Pediatric Endocrinology & Metabolism, 14,* 653–659.

Johnson, S. B., Riley, W. J., Hansen, C. A., & Nurick, M. A. (1990) Psychological impact of islet cell-antibody screening: Preliminary results. *Diabetes Care, 13,* 93–97.

Johnson, S. B., & K. P. Tercyak, M. A. (1995). Psychological impact of islet cell-antibody screening for IDDM on children, adults and their family members. *Diabetes Care, 18,* 1370–1372.

Karges, W., Hammond-McKibben, D., Cheung, R. K., Visconti, M., Shibuya, N., Kemp, D., & Dosch, H. M. (1997). Immunological aspects of nutritional diabetes prevention in NOD mice: A pilot study for the cow's milk based IDDM prevent trial. *Diabetes, 46,* 557–564.

Kimpimaki, T., Kupila, A., Hamalainen, A. M., Kukko, M., Kulmala, P., Savola, K., et al. (2001). The first signs of b-cell autoimmunity appear in infancy in genetically susceptible children from the general population: The Finnish type I diabetes prediction and prevention study. *Journal of Clinical Endocrinology & Metabolism, 86,* 4782–4786.

Kodish, E. (1999). Testing children for cancer genes: The rule of earliest onset. *Journal of Pediatrics, 135,* 390–395.

Kupila, A., Muona, P., Simell, T., Arvilommi, P., Savolainen, H., Hamalainen, A-M., et al. (2001). Feasibility of genetic and immunological prediction of Type 1 diabetes in a population-based birth cohort. *Diabetologia, 44,* 290–297.

Kupila, A., Sipila, J., Keskinen, P., Simell, T., Knip, M., Pulkki, K., Simmell, O. (2003). Intranasally administered insulin intended for prevention of type 1 diabetes—a safety study in healthy adults. *Diabetes/Metabolism Research and Reviews, 19,* 415–420.

Landin-Olsson, M., Palmer, J. P., Lernmark, A., Blom, L., Sundkvist, G., Nystrom, L., & Dahlquist. (1992). Predictive value of islet cell and insulin autoantibodies for type 1 (insulin-dependent) diabetes mellitus in a population-based study of newly-diagnosed diabetic and matched control children. *Diabetologia, 35,* 1068–1073.

Lefcourt, H. M. (1982). *Locus of control: Current trends in theory and research* (2nd ed.). New York: Halstead.

Lucidarme, N., Donmingues-Muriel, E., Castro, D., Czernichow, P., & Levy-Marchal, C. (1998). Appraisal and implications of predictive testing for insulin-dependent diabetes mellitus. *Diabetes & Metabolism, 23,* 550–553.

Marteau, T. M. (1994). Psychology and screening, narrowing the gap between efficacy and effectiveness. *British Journal of Clinical Psychology, 33,* 1–10.

Marteau, T. M., & Croyle, R. T. (1998). The new genetics: Psychological responses to genetic testing. *British Medical Journal, 316,* 693–696.

McNeil, T. F., Harty, B., Thelin, T., Aspegren-Jansson, E., & Sveger, T. (1986). Identifying children at high somatic risk: Long-term effects on mother-child interaction. *Acta Psychiatrica Scandinavica, 74,* 555–562.

McNeil, T. F, Thelin, T., Aspegren-Jansson, E., & Sveger, T. (1985). Identifying children at high somatic risk: Possible effects on the parents' views of the child's health and parents' relationship to the pediatric health services. *Acta Psychiatrica Scandinavica, 72,* 491–497.

McNeil, T. F., Thelin, T., Aspegren-Jansson, E., Sveger, T., & Harty, B. (1985). Psychological factors in cost-benefit analysis of somatic prevention. A study of the psychological effects of neonatal screening for alpha 1-antitrypsin deficiency. *Acta Paediatrica Scandinavica, 74,* 427–432.

Medical Research Council of Canada, Natural Science and Engineering Research Council of Canada, Social Science and Humanities Research Council of Canada. (2002, June 18). *Tri-Council Policy Statement. Ethical Conduct for Research Involving Humans.* Retrieved October 10, 2003 from http://www.nserc.ca/programs/ethics/English/ethics-e.pdf

Michie, S. (1996). Predictive genetic testing in children: Paternalism or empiricism. In T. Marteau and M. Richards (Eds.), *The troubled helix: Social and psychological implications of the new genetics* (pp. 177–183). Cambridge: Cambridge University Press.

Michie, S., & Marteau, T. M. (1998). Predictive genetic testing in children: The need for psychological research. In A. J. Clarke (Ed.), *The genetic testing of children* (pp. 169–181). Oxford: Bios Scientific Publishers.

National Commission for the Protection of Human Subjects of Biomedical and Behavioral Research. (1977). *Report and recommendations: Research involving children.* Washington, DC: U.S. Printing Office.

National Commission for the Protection of Human Subjects of Biomedical and Behavioral Research. (1979). *Belmont report: Ethical principles and guidelines for the protection of human subjects of research.* Washington, DC: U.S. Government Printing Office.

Nelkin, D., & Tancredi, L. (1989). *Dangerous diagnostics: The social power of biological information.* New York: Basic Books.

Nicholson, R. H. (ed.). (1986). *Medical research with children: Ethics, law and practice. The report of an Institute of Medical Ethics working group on the ethics of clinical research investigations on children.* Oxford: Oxford University Press.

Nordenfelt, L. (1996). Prevention and ethics in medicine: The case of diabetes prevention. *Journal of Pediatric Endocrinology & Metabolism, 9,* 381–386.

Norris, J. M., Beaty, B., Klingensmith, G., Yu, L., Hoffman, M., Chase H. P., et al. (1996). Lack of association between early exposure to cow's milk protein and beta-cell autoimmunity: Diabetes autoimmunity study in the young (DAISY). *Journal of the American Medical Association, 276,* 609–614.

Nuremberg Code, principle 1, (1946). Reprinted in W. T. Reich (Ed.), *Encyclopedia of bioethics* (1978, Vol. 4, p. 1764). New York: Free Press.

O'Brien, M. L, Buist, N. R. M., & Murphey, W. H. (1978). Neonatal screening for alpha$_1$-antitrypsin deficiency. *Journal of Pediatrics, 92,* 1006–1010.

Office for Human Research Protections. (1993). *Institutional review board guidebook, chapter 5, part H: Human genetic research.* Retrieved July 26, 2004 from http://www.hhs.gov/ohrp/irb/irb_chapter5ii.htm#h12

Paronen, J., Knip, M., Savilahti, E., Virtanen, S. M., Illonen, J., Akerblom, H. K., Vaarala, O., (2000). Effect of cow's milk exposure and maternal type 1 diabetes on cellular and humoral immunization to dietary insulin in infants at genetic risk for type 1 diabetes. *Diabetes, 49,* 1657–1665.

Parsons, E. P., Clarke, A. J., Hood, K., & Bradley, D. M. (2000). Feasibility of a change in service delivery: The case of optional newborn screening for duchenne muscular dystrophy. *Community Genetics, 3,* 17–23.

Reilly, P. R., Boshar, M. F., & Holtzman, S. H. (1997). Ethical issues in genetic research: Disclosure and informed consent. *Nature Genetics,15,* 16–20.

Roll, U., Christie, M. R., Fuchtenbusch, M., Payton, M. A., Hawkes, C. J., & Ziegler, A. G. (1996). Perinatal autoimmunity in offspring of diabetic parents: The German multicenter BABY-DIAB study: Detection of humoral immune responses to islet antigens in early childhood. *Diabetes, 45,* 967–973.

Ronningen, K. S. (1997). Genetics in the prediction of insulin-dependent diabetes mellitus: From theory to practice. *Annals of Medicine, 29,* 387–392.

Ross, L. F. (1998). *Children, families, and health care decision making.* Oxford: Oxford University Press.

Ross, L. F. (2003). The ethics of type 1 diabetes prediction and prevention research. *Theoretical Medicine and Biology, 24,* 177–197.

Roth, R. (2001). Psychological and ethical aspects of prevention trials. *Journal of Pediatric Endocrinology and Metabolism, 14,* 669–674.

Samuelsson, U., Sundkvist, G., Borg, H. Fernlund, P., & Ludvigsson, J. (2001). Islet autoantibodies in the prediction of diabetes in school children. *Diabetes Research and Clinical Practice, 51,* 51–57.

Schatz, D., Krischer, J., Horne, G., Riley, W., Spillar, R., Silverstein, J., et al. (1994). Islet cell antibodies predict insulin-dependent diabetes in United States school age children as powerfully as in unaffected relatives. *Journal of Clinical Investigation, 93,* 2403–2407.

Schatz, D. A., Krischer, J. P., & Syler, J. S. (2000). Therapeutic controversy: Now is the time to prevent type 1 diabetes. *Journal of Clinical Endocrinology and Metabolism, 85,* 495–498.

Senior, V., Marteau, T. M., & Peters, T. J. (1999). Will genetic testing for predisposition for disease result in fatalism? A qualitative study of parents responses to neonatal screening for familial hypercholesterolaemia *Social Science and Medicine, 48,* 1857–1860.

Shepherd, M., Hattersley, A. T., & Sparkes, A. C. (2000). Predictive genetic testing in diabetes: A case study of multiple perspectives. *Qualitative Health Research, 10,* 242–259.

Siegler, M., Amiel, S., & Lantos, J. (1992). Scientific and ethical consequences of disease prediction. *Diabetologia, 35*(Suppl. 2), S60–S68.

Sveger, T., & Thelin, T. (2000). A future for neonatal alpha1-antitrypsin screening? *Acta Paediatrica, 89,* 628–631.

Sveger, T., Thelin, T., & McNeil. T. F. (1997). Young adults with alpha$_1$-antitrypsin deficiency identified. *Acta Paediatrica, 86,* 37–40.

Sveger, T., Thelin, T., & McNeil. T. F. (1999). Neonatal alpha1-antitrypsin screening: Parents' views and reactions 20 years after the identification of the deficiency state. *Acta Paediatrica, 88,* 315–318.

Thelin, T., McNeil, T. F., Aspegren-Jansson, E., & Sveger, T. (1985a). Psychological consequences of neonatal screening for alpha-1-antitrypsin deficiency. Parental attitudes toward "ATD-check-ups" and parental recommendations regarding future screening. *Acta Paediatrica Scandanavica, 74,* 841–847.

Thelin, T., McNeil, T. F., Aspegren-Jansson, E., & Sveger, T. (1985b). Psychological consequences of neonatal screening for alpha-1-antitrypsin deficiency. Parental reactions to the first news of their infants' deficiency. *Acta Paediatrica Scandanavica, 74,* 787–793.

Thelin, T., McNeil, T. F., Aspegren-Jansson, E., & Sveger, T. (1985d). Identifying children at high somatic risk: Parents' long-term emotional adjustment to their children's alpha-antitrypsin deficiency. *Acta Psychiatrica Scandanavica, 72,* 323–330.

Thelin, T., McNeil, T. F., Aspegren-Jansson, E., & Sveger, T. (1985c). Identifying children at high somatic risk: Possible long-term effects on the parents' view of their own health and current life situation. *Acta Psychiatrica Scandanavica, 71,* 644–653.

Tymstra, T. (1986). False positive results in screening test: Experience of parents of children screened for congenital hypothyroidism. *Family Practice, 3,* 92–96.

Veijola, R., Reijonen, H., Vahasalo, P., Sabbah, E., Kulmala, P., Ilonen, J., et al. (1996). HLA-DQB1-defined genetic susceptibility, beta cell autoimmunity, and metabolic characteristics in familial and nonfamilial insulin-dependent diabetes mellitus. *Journal of Clinical Investigation, 98,* 2489–2495.

Wagner, A., Tibben, A., Bruining, G. J., Aanstoot, H. J., Tiems, I., Blondeau, M. J. C. E., & Niermeijer, M. F. (1995). Preliminary experience with predictive testing for insulin-dependent diabetes mellitus. *Lancet, 346,* 380–381.

Wall, M., Moe, E., Eisenberg, J., Powers, M., Buist, N., & Buist, A. S. (1990). Long-term follow-up of a cohort of children with alpha-1-antitrypsin deficiency. *Journal of Pediatrics, 116,* 248–251.

Weber, B., & Roth, R. (1997). Psychological aspects in diabetes prevention trials. *Annals of Medicine, 29,* 461–467.

Wertz, D. (2002). Testing children and adolescents. In J. Burley & J. Harris (Eds.), *A companion to genethics* (pp. 92–113). Oxford: Blackwell Publishers.

Working Party of the Clinical Genetics Society [UK]. (1994). The genetic testing of children. *Journal of Medical Genetics, 31,* 785–797.

World Health Organization. (1997). Alpha₁-antitrypsin deficiency: Memorandum from a WHO meeting. *Bulletin of the World Health Organization, 75,* 397–415.

World Medical Association. (2002, March 17). Declaration of Helsinki. Ethical principles for medical research involving human subjects. Washington, DC: Author. Retrieved July 26, 2004 from http://www.wma.net/e/policy/b3.htm

Yu, M. S., Norris, J. M., Mitchell, C. M., Butler-Simon, N., Groshek, M., Follansbee, D., et al. (1999). Impact on maternal parenting stress of receipt of genetic information regarding risk of diabetes in newborn infants. *American Journal of Medical Genetics, 86,* 219–226.

Ziegler, A. G., Hummel, M., Schenker, M., & Bonifacio, E. (1999). Autoantibody appearance and risk for development of childhood diabetes in offspring of parents with type 1 diabetes: The 2-year analysis of the German BABYDIAB study. *Diabetes, 48,* 460–468.

8

Payments for Participation
of Children in Research

Douglas S. Diekema

CASE DESCRIPTION

In order to determine how mucin quantity differs before the onset of infection and after onset of infection, the investigators propose to perform bronchoalveolar lavage in infants diagnosed with cystic fibrosis during the first month of life. Participation in this research will require a procedure called bronchoscopy that would not be otherwise clinically indicated. Bronchoalveolar lavage fluid would be obtained from these infants at three time points: following diagnosis but before 6 weeks of age, at 6 months of age, and at 12 months of age. The mucin quantity in the fluid would be studied to determine its relationship to the onset of infection.

The investigators propose to reimburse parents for travel and parking, pay subjects $100 for each bronchoscopy completed plus another $50 for completing the entire series of three procedures (total $350 for completion of study), and pay parents of subjects $50 for each bronchoscopy visit completed and an additional $50 for completion of the entire series of three visits (total $200 for completion of study).

Providing payment to those who participate is common practice for research studies involving both children and adults. While there may be good reasons for providing payment for research participation, there are also reasons to be concerned about the practice, especially when the subjects are children. This chapter will examine the ethical implications of providing payment to children and their parents for participation in research. After a brief survey of current practices regarding payments to research participants, this chapter examines the distinct kinds of payments offered to research participants and their parents, evaluates the ethical considerations relevant to each kind of payment, and makes some final recommendations concerning the provision of payments for research involving children.

ETHICAL ANALYSIS AND DISCUSSION

The Practice of Paying Research Subjects

Offering payment to entice humans to participate as experimental subjects is not a new practice. In experiments conducted in the early 1800s, army physician William Beaumont provided Alexis St. Martin with lodging, food, and $150 a year for the right to use him as an experimental subject (Rothman, 1995; Selzer, 1998). During the latter half of the 19th century, Walter Reed paid volunteers $100 in gold to participate in experiments investigating the transmission of yellow fever. Those who contracted yellow fever received an additional $100 (which would be paid to their heirs in the event of the volunteer's death; Rothman, 1995; Tishler & Batholomae, 2002).

In the present day, the practice of offering payment as an enticement to participate in clinical trials is common, especially for interventional and drug trials (Dickert, Emanuel, & Grady, 2002; Latterman & Merz, 2001). Moreover, the practice of payment in exchange for research participation is not limited to studies involving adults. Weise, Smith, Maschke, and Copeland (2002) found that 66% of surveyed institutional review boards (IRBs) reported approval of at least one pediatric protocol that offered payment for participation. Only 11% of IRBs reported not having approved pediatric trials that offered payment.

Financial inducements are considered essential for many research studies to achieve their recruitment goals. Among adults, financial inducements have been shown to significantly motivate healthy volunteers to participate as research subjects (Bigorra & Banos, 1990; Hassar et al., 1977; Novak, Seckman, & Stewart, 1977; Tishler & Batholomae, 2002; van Gelderen, Savelkoul, van Dokkum, & Meulenbelt, 1993). Money provided at completion of a study appears to be more effective at achieving retention of study subjects than gifts of similar value provided at regular intervals throughout a study (Rudy, Estok, Kerr, & Menzel, 1994). One survey of factors influencing parental permission for enrollment of children in clinical research found that although financial benefit was not the most important factor influencing a parent's decision to enroll a child in clinical research, it did positively influence parental consent (Rothmier, Lasley, & Shapiro, 2003).

The practice of offering payment in research studies that enroll children is a controversial one that requires parents, investigators, and IRBs to weigh the importance of several competing values. On one hand, inducement payments may be essential to the recruitment and retention of research subjects, and prohibiting payments might jeopardize some important research. In addition, the obligation to treat research subjects fairly might include compensating them for time, effort, and discomfort as well as compensating them for their contribution to the social good. These important objectives must be balanced against the need to protect children from the potential harms of research participation and to ensure that parents remain free of influences that might tempt them to enroll a child in a research protocol that is not consistent with the best interests of their child.

Types of Payment for Research Participation

Not all payments to research subjects or their parents carry the same ethical implications, and it therefore becomes important to distinguish various kinds of payments. Payments may fall into two general categories: payments that remove impediments or barriers to research participation (reimbursement) and payments that provide inducements to participate in research. For the remainder of this chapter, I will refer to the former as reimbursement and the latter as inducement. While both types of payment are intended to increase the likelihood that persons will enroll in research, they operate differently and carry different ethical implications.

Reimbursement refers to payments intended to compensate for out-of-pocket expenses directly related to participation in the research project. These might include costs of parking, travel, meals, overnight lodging, phone calls, and child care that a family might incur because of research participation. Each of these represents an expense that would not have occurred if the parents or child had chosen not to participate. Reimbursements reflect the view that participation in research ought not require cost on the part of the subject or family, but should be "revenue-neutral" (Dickert & Grady, 1999). Reimbursement might also include payments intended to replace lost wages, but such payments function as reimbursement (vs. inducement) only if the recipient has lost income because of the need to miss time at work and the payment does not exceed the amount actually lost because of involvement in the research project. In the clinical trial proposed in the case description above, the investigators intend to reimburse only the costs of travel and parking. If families will be recruited from a distance, they should also consider reimbursing the cost of overnight lodging and meals. Most investigators choose not to reimburse lost wages because the complex accounting (determining which parents had to skip work to participate and how much wage was lost) makes it impractical. This decision is justified as long as parents are made aware that lost wages will not be reimbursed.

Inducements are payments or goods provided to research subjects or their parents to encourage them to enroll in a research project. Wendler, Rackoff, Emanuel, and Grady (2002) have described three kinds of inducement payments that may be provided to children or their parents: compensation payments, appreciation payments, and incentive payments. Compensation payments are intended to pay parents and children for the time and inconvenience of participation in research. As discussed above, this form of payment is not intended to replace lost wages, but rather to provide a payment for time and effort that is independent of whether the parent or participant has suffered a loss of income in order to participate. Others have characterized this as paying a wage to those who "labor" as research subjects (Ackerman, 1989; Dickert & Grady, 1999). Appreciation payments are bonuses given after a child has completed research procedures that are intended to thank the child for participating. Finally, incentive payments are intended to encourage enrollment in the research project (Wendler et al., 2002). Compensation, appreciation, and incentive payments can be difficult to differentiate, and a payment scheme may serve multiple purposes. Appreciation and incentive payments are more likely to exert undue influence than compensation inducements. What all three types of inducement have in common, however, is that they go beyond simple reimbursement (removing barriers to research participation) and provide a positive incentive to enroll.

In the infant bronchoscopy study, the investigators propose to pay research subjects $100 and parents $50 for each of three bronchoscopies. These payments constitute inducement payments because they exceed the reimbursement level (i.e., the family's actual expenses resulting from participation in the research). The suggested payments might reasonably be considered compensation for the time expended by parents and for the discomfort experienced by the infants who participate. The payments may also act as incentives by making enrollment more appealing. Finally, the investigators propose to pay parents and subjects each an additional $50 at the end of the study for completion of the entire series of three visits. While this might be considered an appreciation payment, it also functions as an incentive payment intended to encourage subjects and their parents to complete the entire study.

Ethical Guidelines and Policies Related to Payment

As the research team and IRB grapple with whether these payments should be allowed, they may seek guidance from a number of sources including codes of research ethics, federal regulations and guidelines, and professional society guidelines. With regard to the issue of payments to subjects in pediatric research, these sources offer general guidance that is often vague, subject to a wide range of interpretation, and not always consistent.

Looking first to the historically important codes of research ethics, neither the Nuremberg Code nor the *Declaration of Helsinki* directly addresses the issue of payment to research subjects. The *Belmont Report* indirectly addresses the issue in its discussion of voluntariness in informed consent:

This element of informed consent requires conditions free of coercion and undue influence. Coercion occurs when an overt threat of harm is intentionally presented by one person to another in order to obtain compliance. Undue influence, by contrast, occurs through an offer of an excessive, unwarranted, inappropriate or improper reward or other overture in order to obtain compliance. Also, inducements that would ordinarily be acceptable may become undue influences if the subject is especially vulnerable. (National Commission, 1979)

In its report on IRBs, the National Commission for the Protection of Human Subjects of Biomedical and Behavioral Research elaborated on the concept of undue influence and recommended that in order to prevent undue influence during the consent process, IRBs might limit "remuneration to payment for the time and inconvenience of participation and compensation for any injury resulting from participation" (National Commission, 1978).

More recently, the National Bioethics Advisory Commission briefly addressed the issue in their report on ethical and policy issues in research involving human participants by recognizing that potential benefits of research participation (including monetary incentives) might create undue influence on economically disadvantaged persons, even those possessing the cognitive capacity to provide consent. This might threaten the voluntariness of consent:

For example, offers of large sums of money as payment for participation or access to free health care services (for conditions not related to the research) could lead some prospective participants to enroll in a research study when it might be against their better judgment and when otherwise they would not do so. (National Bioethics Advisory Commission, 2001)

The report recommends that IRBs make certain that research offers a "reasonable choice" to prospective enrollees, which might require reducing the amount of payment offered to participants.

The Code of Federal Regulations governs research involving human subjects (45 CFR 46) in the United States. These federal regulations make no direct reference to payment of research subjects other than stating that an investigator should seek consent under circumstances "that minimize the possibility of coercion or undue influence" and to require that "for research involving more than minimal risk, an explanation as to whether any compensation and an explanation as to whether any medical treatments are available if injury occurs and, if so, what they consist of, or where further information may be obtained" (45 CFR 46.116(a(6))). Unfortunately, this legal manifestation of research ethics is remarkably silent on the critical issue of subject payment, leaving wide discretion for interpretation by investigators and IRBs.

Federal agencies responsible for the enforcement of the regulations governing human subjects research may also offer official guidance, though this guidance does not carry the force of law. The Office for Human Research Protections, the federal agency responsible for enforcing the federal regulations related to human subjects research, offers brief guidance in their *Tips on Informed Consent* (Office for Human Research Protections, 1993): "If payment is given to defray the incurred expense for participation, it must not be coercive in amount or method of distribution." The Food and Drug Administration (FDA) offers further guidance explicitly related to the payment of research subjects (Food and Drug Administration, 1998). This guidance includes several components. First, payment to research subjects for participation in studies is not to be considered a benefit of research participation by the IRB. Second, the amount and schedule of all payments should be presented to the IRB at the time of initial review. Third, the IRB should review both the amount of payment and proposed method and timing of disbursement to assure that neither are coercive or present undue influence. The FDA further expands on the latter point:

> Any credit for payment should accrue as the study progresses and not be contingent upon the subject completing the entire study. Unless it creates undue inconvenience or a coercive practice, payment to subjects who withdraw from the study may be made at the time they would have completed the study (or completed a phase of the study) had they not withdrawn. For example, in a study lasting only a few days, an IRB may find it permissible to allow a single payment date at the end of the study, even to subjects who had withdrawn before that date. While the entire payment should not be contingent upon completion of the entire study, payment of a small proportion as an incentive for completion of the study is acceptable to FDA, providing that such incentive is not coercive. The IRB should determine that the amount paid as a bonus for completion is reasonable and not so large as to unduly induce subjects to stay in the study when they would otherwise have withdrawn. All information, including the amount and schedule of payment(s), should be set forth in the informed consent document. (Food and Drug Administration, 1998)

While neither federal regulation nor guidance addresses the issue of payments to minors explicitly, the European community has banned the use of incentives or financial inducements (with the exception of compensation) in medicinal clinical trials involving minors (European Parliament and the Council of the European Union, 2001).

Finally, the Committee on Drugs of the American Academy of Pediatrics has also addressed the issue of payment for participation in clinical research involving children. Compensation of child or family for direct or indirect costs incurred because of the child's involvement in the study is considered appropriate as long as the amount does not become an inducement for the participation of the child subject. Beyond compensation, the academy states:

> It is in accord with the traditions and ethics of society to pay people who participate and cooperate in activities that benefit others. However, serious ethical questions arise when payment is offered to adults acting on behalf of minors in return for allowing minors to participate as research subjects. The remuneration should not be beyond a token gesture of appreciation for participation. If remuneration is to be provided to the child, it is best if it is not discussed before the study's completion. This will help assure that the remuneration is not part of the reasons that a child volunteered or is volunteered for a study. . . . The IRB should review any proposed remuneration to assure that the possibility for coercion has been avoided. (American Academy of Pediatrics Committee on Drugs, 1995)

The American Academy of Pediatrics recommendation that remuneration not be discussed prior to a study's completion is notable because it seems to conflict with FDA guidance that all information including amount and schedule of payments be set forth in the informed consent document.

What seems to tie all these sources together is the claim that coercion and undue influence should be avoided. Coercion by definition is a credible threat of harm or force to control another person (Beauchamp & Childress, 2001). Offers of payment are different than threats of punishment or harm and therefore should not be characterized as coercive. They may, however, represent an undue influence. Unfortunately, the notion of undue influence is a vague and controversial one. The case presented at the beginning of this chapter raises the question of whether the offer to pay children $350 and parents of those children $200 to participate in research procedures represents an undue influence.

Both FDA guidance and the American Academy of Pediatrics imply that undue influence exists when the presence of financial incentive causes the decision maker to choose differently than they would have without the presence of the financial inducement. Others have taken issue with that notion on the grounds that it does not show sufficient respect for the autonomy of the decision maker. In the case of surrogate decision makers, however, appeals to autonomy carry limited weight. Respect for autonomy recognizes that we should respect a person's right to make decisions regarding his or her own welfare. However, a surrogate decision maker makes decisions regarding the welfare of someone other than him or herself. While parents (as surrogate decision makers) should be given freedom to make decisions for their children, those decisions can be challenged if other interests interfere with their ability to protect the welfare of their children. What is important to recognize at this point is that what represents an inappropriate or undue inducement for a competent adult making a decision about his or her own participation in research may differ from what is inappropriate for someone making a decision on behalf of another, as is the case with pediatric research.

Ethical Concerns Regarding Payments in Pediatric Research

Research involving children raises distinctly different ethical concerns than research that involves competent adults. The proposed bronchoscopy study intends to enroll infants, who are completely unable to participate in decision making. If this study were being performed in adults, an analysis of payments for research participation would focus on the balance between respecting the autonomy of individual persons by allowing them to make decisions for themselves and the need to protect research subjects from unnecessary or excessive harms. Some would further argue that research participants deserve to be paid for the time, effort, and risk involved in research participation. Dickert and Grady (1999) argue that the principle of autonomy supports payment of competent adults for research participation and suggest a "wage-payment" model based upon the notion that since research participation requires time, effort, and occasionally discomfort, persons ought to be compensated as they would be for a low-wage job. Just as someone might choose to take a high-risk job working in a mine or logging forests, a person should be free to assume the risks of research participation if they feel the risks and effort are justified by the payment being offered (Siminoff, 2001). In other words, respecting autonomy requires allowing a competent person to make his or her own judgment about risks and benefits. To remove the possibility of payment would be to rob the person of choice, a paternalistic action contrary to the principle of respect for autonomy. This argument carries little weight in research with children, however, where appeal to the principle of autonomy makes little sense.

An essential difference between the bronchoscopy study as proposed and a bronchoscopy study with adult subjects is that children are not fully autonomous, cannot provide valid consent, and, with the possible exception of some adolescents, are not capable of protecting their own interests. Payments for research participation require caution when the participants (children) are not in a position to provide valid consent.

Children must rely on others to guard their interests. Whereas an adult can decide whether to assume certain risks in order to receive certain benefits (i.e., payment), a parent makes decisions about what risks will be assumed by the child. The fundamental ethical concern that should guide research involving children is that their well-being be the primary interest, placed ahead of the interests of society and others in research participation decisions. Parents or guardians are assumed to act in the best interest of their children when making decisions regarding research participation. Anything that subverts that goal should be considered suspect. Payments for research participation in pediatric studies raise concerns when they have the potential to distort decision making, tempting parents to consider issues other than the welfare of the child as they consider enrollment (Wendler et al., 2002).

In the case of research, the federal regulations (45 CFR 46, subpart D), the local IRB, and the child's parent or legal guardian provide three mechanisms for protecting the interests of children. While the federal regulations provide no specific guidance regarding payments to children or their parents for research participation, they do restrict the level of risk to which a child can be subjected. The level of risk to which a child is exposed in the proposed research study is an important factor in determining the appropriateness of payment. Since the primary ethical aim is to ensure the well-being of the child and avoid causing harm, studies that are minimal risk pose fewer concerns than those which might subject a child to greater than minimal risk. Studies involving greater than minimal risk will require more attention to the impact of payment on the parent's ability to protect the well-being of a child. Even in research that offers the prospect for direct benefit to the child, inducement payments can distort a parent's assessment of possible benefits and harms, and such payments should be evaluated for their potential to do so.

The IRB is charged with determining whether the level of risk is approvable under the federal regulations, assuring that risk has been minimized, and evaluating the potential for payment to distort the decision making of a child's parents. In evaluating whether payments are permissible, the level of risk to which a child will be exposed in a given research project and the degree to which the proposed payments affect a parent's ability to focus exclusively on the interest of the child are both important considerations. Certain payments may serve to focus the parent's attention inappropriately on financial gain rather than the risk of the research procedures. The degree to which financial gain may influence parents' judgment can be affected by many variables. Even individuals at the same economic level may value risk exposure and financial benefits of participation differently. This concern may be particularly acute for a family with limited or no income, for whom the prospect of some financial benefit could become an overwhelming factor in deciding about research procedures. IRBs must be careful to prohibit payments that may distort the decision making of parents in this way. While an IRB that prohibits payments can be accused of acting in a manner that is overly paternalistic, it must be remembered that these are not situations in which potential research subjects are making decisions regarding their own welfare. While parents are given a wide range of decision-making discretion on behalf of their children, it may be appropriate for IRBs to err on the side of protecting children by assuring that parents are not tempted to make decisions regarding the welfare of a child on the basis of financial remuneration rather than the potential risk and benefit posed by the study in question.

The proposed bronchoscopy study offers several different kinds of payments, each of which has different potential to distort parental decision making. Having discussed the relevant ethical features, we will now turn to a discussion of the appropriateness of various kinds of payments in pediatric research.

Reimbursement Payments

The investigators of the infant bronchoscopy study propose to reimburse parents for travel and parking. This appears to be ethically acceptable, and some would argue that it should be required. Reimbursement payments serve to repay parents or participants for the out-of-pocket expenses they have incurred in order to participate in the research project. A reasonable argument can be made that reimbursement should always be offered on the grounds that persons should not be made worse off because of their willingness to contribute their time and effort as research subjects. In the event that reimbursement is not offered, the consent form and process should make it clear that costs associated with research participation will not be reimbursed.

At the same time, reimbursement payments serve only to reduce barriers to research participation and do not provide any incentive likely to distort parental decision making. Reimbursement of actual costs does not tempt a parent to consider issues beyond the welfare of the child as they make decisions regarding research participation and is therefore an appropriate payment.

Reimbursement payments should be directed toward the person who bore the costs being reimbursed. In most pediatric studies, this will be the parent or guardian. Furthermore, reimbursement should not be contingent upon anything other than having incurred costs associated with the research project. For example, if parents travel to the study site and decide not to enroll their child or decide to drop out of the study after the first bronchoscopy, reimbursement of incurred expenses should still be provided.

Inducement Payments

The investigators of the infant bronchoscopy study also propose to pay subjects $100 for each bronchoscopy completed plus another $50 bonus for completing the entire series of three procedures (total $350 for completion of study) and pay parents of subjects $50 for each bronchoscopy visit completed and an additional

$50 for completion of the entire series of three visits (total $200 for completion of study). These payments exceed the study-related out-of-pocket costs to the family. In assessing the appropriateness of this payment plan, several factors require attention.

First, the level of risk to which infants will be subjected represents an important factor. For research projects involving no greater than minimal risk, the likelihood of harm to the child should not be any greater than that encountered during routine events and activities regularly experienced by the child. In such research, even payments that might distort parental decision making would be unlikely to result in significant harm to the child. On the other hand, large payments would nonetheless tempt some parents to pay less attention to the well-being of their child. Even when harm is unlikely to result, it seems wrong to intentionally encourage a surrogate decision maker to base a decision regarding a child's research participation on financial gain rather than the child's well-being. Therefore, while payments to induce participation in minimal risk studies may be appropriate, the amounts should be modest enough that parents are not tempted to "use" their child as a means to the end of financial benefit.

Even modest payments, however, may raise concerns that require careful consideration. Some commentators have suggested that payments not exceeding the minimum wage for time expended on research-related tasks are unlikely to exert undue influence on potential participants (Dickert & Grady, 1999; Macklin, 1981) and in the context of minimal risk research might be appropriate. On the other hand, it is important to recognize that the offer of inducement payments will almost inevitably create recruitment issues that raise questions of justice. These will be difficult to address without also creating undue influence on some parents. While inducement payments limited to a minimum wage level minimize undue influence, they are more likely to attract volunteers from lower socioeconomic groups, thus creating an unfair distribution of the risks and burdens of research participation (Macklin, 1981; Reame, 2001). In addition, such recruitment bias might limit the generalizability of study results. Since large payments are more likely to attract persons from a broad range of socioeconomic situations, they are more likely to assure that the burden of research is distributed evenly across society, thus satisfying the requirements of justice in recruitment. However, large payments may represent an undue influence on those of minimal economic means, thus compromising the ability of lower income parents to focus primarily on the best interests of a child. This tension might argue for the elimination of all inducement payments in pediatric research. The only way to successfully eliminate both the distorting influence in decision making and any incentive that might be more favorably perceived by one socioeconomic group over others would be to completely prohibit inducement payments in pediatric research, as the European community has done.

Second, the amount of payment must be evaluated for its likelihood to distort parental decision making. For studies involving greater than minimal risk, amounts that could potentially distort decision making of any parent who might be considering enrollment of an infant in the study should be reduced or eliminated. The infant bronchoscopy study involves greater than minimal risk. In this case, it becomes very important that parents be able to focus on the well-being of their infant as they consider enrollment, and not be tempted to minimize their risk assessment because of the potential for financial gain. While some would argue that this implies avoiding payments that exceed a minimum wage, others would argue that even minimum wage payments can be influential for a family with desperate need and no employment opportunities. In order to avoid the risk of creating a moral hazard for these parents, some would argue that no payment beyond reimbursement should be offered to parents where the risk of the research exceeds minimal risk (Moreno, 2001; Resnik, 2001).

In this particular case, parents stand to earn $200 by enrolling their child in a study that clearly presents the potential for greater than minimal risk. This represents a substantial amount of money for some parents, who might otherwise need to work for a week to earn that amount. In addition, their child stands to earn $350 over the course of the study, an even greater amount. Since the child is younger than 1 year, the parent will inevitably control that money as well, since there is no way to guarantee that the child ultimately receives the money or even benefits from it. Thus, the parent is effectively being offered $550 to enroll their child in a study that presents risk to the child. This is not an acceptable situation, creating a moral hazard in requiring parents to weigh significant financial benefit to themselves against risk assumed by their child. Whenever the risk of harm accrues to one individual and the benefit goes to someone else, there is a clear need to protect the vulnerable party.

Third, the schedule of payments must be carefully examined to determine whether it treats all participants fairly, and whether it may create a distorting influence on parental decision making at any point in the course of the research protocol. The bronchoscopy payment schedule calls for payments to be delivered after each procedure and for a payment following completion of all three procedures. The timing of the first three payments seems appropriate in that the payment is directly related to each procedure, thus compensating the subjects and parents each time they must expend effort or suffer discomfort. However, the intention of the final payment is clearly to reward subjects and their parents for remaining in the study. The problem with this payment is that it provides an incentive for a parent to keep their child in the study through all three procedures in order to receive that final bonus payment. Following the initial procedure a parent may decide that they do not wish to subject their child to two more procedures and consider withdrawing. However, knowing that they will receive the bonus payment only if they carry through with all three procedures, some parents might decide otherwise. Even if the total payment amount did not create a distorting influence on parental decision making, making receipt of a payment contingent upon remaining in the study until its completion may distort decision making in undesirable ways and should be discouraged. While payments may be distributed throughout a study as compensation for time and effort expended, payments should not be dependent on completing all study procedures. This is the only way that the prerogative of study withdrawal can be fully protected.

Finally, payments must be directed toward the appropriate recipients. As discussed above, reimbursement payments are usually directed toward the person who bears the costs associated with research participation. However, while it might be reasonable to provide parents with some payment to compensate for time and effort in bringing their child to the study site, it is the child who bears the burden, discomfort, and risk of harm associated with research procedures. On the other hand, if parents are being asked to fill out questionnaires or participate in interviews, for example, compensation for those efforts that approximates minimum wage might be reasonable. In general, compensation for discomfort, risk, effort, or inconvenience should be directed toward the person bearing those burdens. Because nonmonetary forms of compensation such as gift certificates, a video, or a toy appear less likely to distort decision making and can more easily be directed toward a child, these forms of compensation should be considered in place of cash payments (Fernhoff, 2002; Wendler et al., 2002). At the same time, gifts must be carefully considered for the burden they might place on parents. A video, for example, requires that the parent have a video player at home and can create an awkward situation for those who do not. Likewise, a gift certificate to a toy store can create a difficult situation for parents who are limited in their ability to travel to get to the store.

Small incentives present less concern when directed at children than at the adult decision maker. It seems reasonable to offer a small toy or payment to a child in order to convince them to cooperate with minimal risk procedures, like completing a questionnaire or having blood drawn on a single occasion, as long as the value is not significant enough to cause a child to participate in an activity that might do them harm (Wendler et al., 2002). Investigator integrity, risk assessment by the IRB, and parental permission are the primary protections in place to guard the well-being of children in research. The purpose of assent is not to provide an additional protective mechanism, but rather to provide a way for children to voice their preferences. Therefore, the offer of a gift of modest value to a child may be used to make involvement in the research more appealing to the child without compromising the protection of the child.

Disclosure of Payment

If the IRB has determined that reimbursement or inducement payments are justified and an ethically appropriate schedule for disbursement of payment has been developed, we must determine what information concerning research payment should be disclosed to families and children prior to enrollment. The American Academy of Pediatrics suggests that nondisclosure of payments other than reimbursement might be a solution to the problem of payments distorting judgment in the consent process: "If remuneration is to be provided to the child, it is best if it is not discussed before the study's completion. This will help assure that the remuneration is not part of the reasons that a child volunteered or is volunteered for a study" (American Academy of Pediatrics Committee on Drugs, 1995). On the other hand, this practice eliminates the incentive value of payments, thus removing the reason many investigators have for offering them. It may also place investigators in an awkward position when parents ask whether payment is being offered, and families might learn about payments in other ways (through others enrolled in the study, websites, etc.; Wendler et al., 2002). Finally, it can be argued that if the investigator and IRB have taken their responsibility seriously with regard to payments, paid careful attention to the risk level of the study, reduced or eliminated inducement payments to a level that will not distort parental decision making, and eliminated payments that reward parents or subjects for completion of the study, then nondisclosure offers little additional protection, and the full payment schedule should be disclosed in the consent form and during the consent process.

Compensation for Research Harms

One further issue requires discussion. Despite the protections in place to protect children who participate in research, occasionally a child will suffer injury as a result of their research participation. The infant bronchoscopy study carries the potential risk that a serious complication could occur as a result of the procedure or the anesthesia that accompanies it. The principle of justice requires that a mechanism exist so that the child and his or her parents do not become burdened with the costs associated with medical care or rehabilitation that results from a research related injury (National Bioethics Advisory Commission, 2001). Ideally, no research subject should be left worse off than if he or she had not participated in research. Even if informed about the potential risks of research participation in the consent/permission process, the act of research participation is predominantly one of contribution to the benefit of others. Those who participate in research should not be left to suffer consequences that directly result from that participation. This seems particularly true when the subject is a child who has not freely chosen to participate in the research yet might be the victim of unforeseen adverse consequences. While it might be argued that research offering the prospect of direct benefit to the child should be exempt from this requirement since the overall likelihood of benefit justifies the potential risks, it still seems reasonable that parents should not have to assume responsibility for costs related to injury resulting from procedures or aspects of the protocol that are not potentially therapeutic or for injuries from nonvalidated therapies that are more serious than those encountered when pursuing conventional treatment for the same condition (Ackerman, 1989). The investigator, sponsor, and IRB should assume responsibility for assuring that a mechanism for compensation for research related injury exists prior to the enrollment of subjects in any research project.

SOME CONCLUDING THOUGHTS

Payments offered to children or their parents for research participation must be considered very carefully. Children cannot adequately protect their own interests and must rely on others, primarily their parents to look after those interests. When children are enrolled in research projects, any financial incentive that has the potential to distort parental decision making by tempting parents to consider issues other than the welfare of their child as they consider enrollment should be eliminated.

Reimbursement for out of pocket costs associated with research participation (i.e., meals, parking, travel to and from the research site, lodging for studies requiring an overnight stay, etc.) will eliminate at least some of the barriers to research participation without altering a parent's ability to consider a child's welfare above other interests. These payments should be directed to the person bearing responsibility for those costs. If for some reason, research-related expenses cannot be reimbursed, the consent form should make this clear.

Inducement payments may place undue pressure on parental decision makers, and must be carefully examined for their potential to distort parental decision making among potential research enrollees. They should be limited to an amount that will not distort the decision making of the parent. These payments should be directed to the person bearing the burdens of the research, and should be related to time and effort expended. Payments that require completion of all research procedures are almost always inappropriate. Consideration should be given to providing inducements to children in nonmonetary forms to enhance the likelihood that they will ultimately be enjoyed by the child.

Finally, justice demands that children and their parents not be made worse off as a result of research related injuries, and that some process exist for compensation of medical or rehabilitation costs that result directly from research participation prior to enrollment in the study. Investigators, IRB members, and parents must remain vigilant in their efforts to protect children from exploitation in research studies, but retain balance so that progress in our understanding of childhood health and disease moves forward.

Questions for Discussion

1. Is it ethically appropriate for payments to be provided to participants and parents who enroll in pediatric research studies? If so, what form should compensation take? To whom should payment be directed?

2. Considering the ethical principles of beneficence, nonmaleficence, and justice and the pediatric population being discussed which of the two types of payment is more problematic, reimbursement payment or inducement payment?

3. The author of this chapter argues that coercion and undue influence must be avoided when offering payments to competent, adult research participants. Do you find these criteria clear and appropriate? Can they be applied to research involving children?

4. Discuss the appropriateness of various types of payments in pediatric research (reimbursement payment, inducement payments).

5. What are the ethical concerns relating to the acceptance of inducement payments in pediatric research? Should the amount, the timing, or the type of the payment (i.e., cash money vs. gift) make a difference?

6. In your view, should inducement payments in pediatric research be completely prohibited? Defend your answer.

7. If payments for pediatric research participation are ethically permissible, what payment schedule is most consistent with the important moral considerations?

8. Should payments be prospectively disclosed to participants? Ethically speaking, do the advantages of nondisclosure of inducement payment outweigh the disadvantages?

9. What is the ethical justification for creating a mechanism for compensation for research related injury prior to the enrollment of subjects in any research project?

References

Ackerman, T. F. (1989). An ethical framework for the practice of paying research subjects. *IRB: A Review of Human Subjects Research, 11*, 1–4.

American Academy of Pediatrics Committee on Drugs. (1995). Guidelines for the ethical conduct of studies to evaluate drugs in pediatric populations. *Pediatrics, 95*(2), 286–294.

Beauchamp, T. L., & Childress, J. F. (2001). *Principles of biomedical ethics* (5th ed.). New York: Oxford University Press.

Bigorra, J., & Banos, J. E. (1990). Weight of financial reward in the decision by medical students and experienced healthy volunteers to participate in clinical trials. *European Journal of Clinical Pharmacology, 38*, 436–443.

Dickert, N., Emanuel, E., & Grady, C. (2002). Paying research subjects: an analysis of current policies. *Annals of Internal Medicine, 136*(5), 368–373.

Dickert, N., & Grady, C. (1999). What's the price of a research subject? Approaches to payment for research participation. *New England Journal of Medicine, 341*, 198–203.

European Parliament and the Council of the European Union. (2001). Directive 2001/20/EC of the European Parliament and the Council of 4 April (2001) on the approximation of the laws, regulations and administrative provisions of the member states relating to the implementation of good clinical practice in the conduct of clinical trials on medicinal products for human use. *Official Journal of the European Communities, L 121*, 34–44.

Fernhoff, P. M. (2002). Paying for children to participate in research: a slippery slope or an enlightened stairway? *Journal of Pediatrics, 141*(2), 153–154.

Food and Drug Administration. (1998). *Information Sheets: Guidance for institutional review boards and clinical investigators.* Retrieved July 22, 2004 from http://www.fda.gov/oc/ohrt/irbs/toc4.html

Hassar, M., Pocelinko, R., Weintraub, M., Nelson, D., Thomas, G., & Lasagna, L. (1977). Free living volunteer's motivations and attitudes toward pharmacologic studies in man. *Clin Pharmacol Ther, 21*, 515–519.

Latterman, J., & Merz, J. F. (2001). How much are subjects paid to participate in research? *American Journal of Bioethics, 1*(2), 45–46.

Macklin, R. (1981). On paying money to research subject. *IRB: A Review of Human Subjects Research, 3*, 1–6.

Moreno, J. D. (2001). It's not about the money. *American Journal of Bioethics 1*, (2), 46–47.

National Bioethics Advisory Commission. (2001). *Ethical and policy issues in research involving human participants.* Washington, DC: Government Printing Office.

National Commission for the Protection of Human Subjects of Biomedical and Behavioral Research. (1978). *Report and recommendations on institutional review boards.* Washington, DC: Government Printing Office.

National Commission for the Protection of Human Subjects of Biomedical and Behavioral Research. (1979). *The Belmont report: Ethical principles and guidelines for the protection of human subjects of research.* Washington, DC: Government Printing Office.

Novak, E., Seckman, C. E., & Stewart, R. D. (1977). Motivations for volunteering as research subjects. *Journal of Clinical Pharmacology, 17*, 365–371.

Office for Human Research Protections. (1993). *Tips on informed consent.* Retrieved July 22, 2004 from http://www.hhs.gov/ohrp/humansubjects/guidance/ictips.htm

Reame, N. K. (2001). Treating research subjects as unskilled wage earners: A risky business. *American Journal of Bioethics, 1*(2), 53–54.

Resnik, D. B. (2001). Research participation and financial inducements. *American Journal of Bioethics, 1*(2), 54–56.

Rothman, D. J. (1995). Human research: Historical aspects. In W. T. Reich (Ed.), *Encyclopedia of bioethics* (pp. 2248–2258). New York: Simon & Schuster MacMillan.

Rothmier, J. D., Lasley, M. V., & Shapiro, G. C. (2003). Factors influencing parental consent in pediatric clinical research. *Pediatrics, 11*(5), 1037–1041.

Rudy, E. B., Estok, P. J., Kerr, M. E., & Menzel, L. (1994). Research incentives: Money versus gifts. *Nursing Research, 43,* 253–255.

Selzer, R. (1998). Alexis St. Martin. In *The Doctor Stories* (pp. 209–223). New York: Picador.

Siminoff, L. A. (2001). Money and the research subject: a comment on Grady. *American Journal of Bioethics, 1*(2), 65–66.

Tishler, C. L., & Batholomae, S. (2002). The recruitment of normal healthy volunteers: a review of the literature on the use of financial incentives. *Journal of Clinical Pharmacology 42,* (4), 365–375.

van Gelderen, C. E., Savelkoul, T. J., van Dokkum, W., & Meulenbelt, J. (1993). Motives and perception of healthy volunteers who participate in experiments. *European Journal of Clinical Pharmacology, 45,* 15–21.

Weise, K. L., Smith, M. L., Maschke, K. J., & Copeland, H. L. (2002). National practices regarding payment to research subjects for participating in pediatric research. *Pediatrics, 110*(3), 577–582.

Wendler, D., Rackoff, J. E., Emanuel, E., & Grady, C. (2002). The ethics of paying for children's participation in research. *Journal of Pediatrics, 141*(2), 166–171.

9

Justice, Lead, and Environmental Research Involving Children

Robert M. Nelson

CASE DESCRIPTION

The Lead-based Paint Abatement and Repair and Maintenance Study in Baltimore (hereafter referred to as the Baltimore lead abatement study) was conducted between 1992 and 1996. The primary objective of the study was to determine the short-term (2–6 months) and long-term (12–24 months) efficacy of three different levels of "interim control interventions" in structurally sound housing where children were at risk of exposure to lead in settled house dust and paint. The three levels of intervention (referred to as low, intermediate, or high) were compared to two different control groups of either modern urban housing built after 1979 or housing that received comprehensive lead abatement between 1989 and 1991. The outcome measures included the analysis of lead in residential dust using two different collection methods (i.e., traditional wipe and experimental cyclone) and serial blood lead concentrations of young children living in the affected housing (EPA, 1997a, 1997b, 1997c, 1998; Farfel et al., 1996).

Any house (including the control groups) to be included in the 2-year study must have been the primary residence for at least one child who was between the age of 6 through 48 months at the time of enrollment. In addition, intervention (or noncontrol) houses must have had preintervention dust lead loadings that exceeded the Maryland postabatement clearance levels in order to be eligible for one of the three intervention groups. Eligible houses that were occupied at the time of enrollment were randomized to either the low or intermediate-level intervention. Eligible houses that were vacant were randomized to either the intermediate or high-level intervention. The randomization scheme was designed to assure an equal distribution of houses among the three groups, with the intermediate intervention evenly distributed between housing that was either occupied or vacant at enrollment. The cost of the low-, medium-, and high-level interventions were capped by the Maryland Department of

Housing and Community Development at $1650, $3500, and $6,000–7000, respectively, with financing available through a special loan program to low-income owner occupants and private property owners who rent their properties to low-income tenants. The interventions were designed in collaboration with a planning group that included local organizations experienced in lead abatement. The Maryland Department of the Environment required that the high-level intervention meet Maryland's interim postabatement lead clearance levels. It did not stipulate this requirement for the low- or medium-level interventions (EPA, 1997a, 1997b, 1997c).

The study found that all three levels of intervention were able to reduce house dust lead loadings to below preintervention levels, but to differing degrees (as would be expected from the study design). Partial reaccumulation of dust and dust lead loadings in all three intervention groups was the greatest during the first 2 months after intervention, with little subsequent reaccumulation through the second year of follow-up. Controlling for age and season, there was a significant relationship between young children's blood lead concentration and a composite measure of house dust lead, with children in the modern urban group having significantly lower blood lead concentrations, as would be expected. Children with baseline blood lead concentrations $\geq$ 15 µg/dL in each of the lead-affected (i.e., intervention) housing groups had a significant reduction in blood lead concentration during follow-up. Although there was no significant difference within each intervention group, children with baseline blood lead concentrations $<$ 15 µg/dL in the three intervention groups combined had a significant reduction in blood lead concentration over time. Examining the outcome of infants born into the lead-affected housing, the study found that the blood lead concentration of most children who reached the age of 6 months during follow-up increased over time yet remained $<$ 10 µg/dL (EPA, 1997b, 1997c).

After the study, at least three sets of parents brought suit against the organization that conducted the study, Kennedy Krieger Institute (KKI), claiming that KKI failed to inform the parent(s) either that lead remained a potential hazard in the home or that high lead dust levels were found in the home even as their child's blood lead levels rose. According to press reports, the blood lead levels of three of the involved children went from 6 to 21, from 9 to 32, and from 11 to 24 µg/dL (Roig-Franzia, 2001). The initial lawsuits were dismissed by a municipal court. On appeal, the Court of Appeals of Maryland reversed the lower court decision. In doing so, the Court of Appeals questioned whether parents have the authority to enroll healthy children in nontherapeutic research that presents any risk of injury or damage to the child's health (Maryland Court of Appeals, 2001a). This standard was later clarified to mean "any articulable risk beyond the minimal kind of risk that is inherent in any endeavor" (Maryland Court of Appeals, 2001b). Remanded back to the lower court for subsequent trial, the lawsuit was eventually dismissed with prejudice in favor of the defendant KKI (R. M. Nelson, personal communication, July 11, 2003).

Summary

This chapter examines the Baltimore lead abatement study as an example of environmental research on reducing the health risks from exposure to toxic compounds. The effort to reduce exposure to an environmental neurotoxin through partial lead abatement benefited many of the children in the study. Absent of information about available housing alternatives, some children may have been placed at risk by moving into lead-affected housing that had only been partially abated. Defining a child's condition (i.e., at risk from lead exposure) as a result of limited socioeconomic resources is problematic because it may justify both an increased risk exposure and limits on the locally available interventions. This may conflict with the fundamental ethical requirement for justice in research. The Baltimore lead abatement study can be compared to pesticide research using human subjects to determine the dosing level at which there are no observed adverse effects. Broadening the question to how one would conduct interventional research on reducing the impact of environmental neurotoxins, the model of community-based participatory research is offered as a promising option. This chapter concludes that interventional research designed to reduce exposure to environmental toxins can involve children and be conducted ethically under limited conditions.

___

ETHICAL ANALYSIS AND DISCUSSION

Applying the Existing Federal Guidelines

The Maryland Court of Appeals argued that parents do not have the legal authority to enroll their healthy children in nontherapeutic research that presents greater than minimal risk (Maryland Court of Appeals, 2001a). This argument is consistent with the categories that are already established within the federal regulations governing research involving children (Nelson, 2002). Following from the principle of nonmaleficence (or "do no harm"), when a research intervention or procedure does not offer the possibility of direct benefit to the children enrolled in the research, the risks associated with that intervention must be restricted to either minimal risk or a minor increase over minimal risk (if the research meets other stipulations). One of these other stipulations is that the research would be expected to yield vital information of importance in understanding or ameliorating the child's condition. In effect, a child must have a condition (and thus not be considered healthy) in order for the allowable risk associated with the research to be a minor increase over minimal risk. If a research intervention offers the prospect of direct benefit, the risks associated with the research may be greater than a minor increase over minimal risk provided that the risk is justified by the anticipated direct benefit to the child and that the risk/benefit relationship of the research is comparable to any and all available alternatives (U.S. Department of Health and Human Services, 1983). The principle of beneficence establishes both parental and societal responsibility to protect a child by assuring that the child is not placed at a disadvantage by being enrolled in research. Thus, to evaluate the Baltimore lead abatement study in the context of the existing federal guidelines for research involving children, at least three questions need to be addressed: (1) whether the research presented the prospect of direct benefit to the enrolled children, (2) whether the children enrolled in the research were healthy or had a condition, and (3) whether the research presented more than minimal risk.

The Prospect of Direct Benefit

The research appears to have been designed so that any child enrolled in the research would either not be exposed to high levels of environmental lead (i.e., the two control groups) or receive the benefit of at least partial lead abatement (i.e. the three intervention groups). The research design did not include a control group made up of children living in houses containing lead-based paint hazards. Although this may have improved the scientific quality of the study, investigators considered it unethical to simply monitor blood lead levels in the face of potentially high environmental lead levels (EPA, 1997b, 1997c). In effect, the control groups reflected the current understanding of the "established effective interventions" of either full lead abatement or the use of nonlead paint to prevent environmental lead poisoning. The three intervention groups sought to establish "locally available alternatives" in the face of economic disincentives to perform complete lead abatement on older lead-affected housing. All of the houses selected for one of the three levels of intervention had environmental lead levels that exceeded those that would otherwise be allowed after lead abatement (EPA, 1997c). At the time of the study, owners were not required to abate residential properties prior to children becoming poisoned regardless of the level of environmental lead, as health department inspections for hazards requiring abatement usually did not occur until after the report of a lead-poisoned child. Nevertheless, the lead-affected housing receiving the highest level intervention met the Maryland postabatement clearance standards, so that children moved into these houses were the beneficiaries of the same level of environmental cleaning that would otherwise have been received. However, occupied (and half of the unoccupied) houses at a time of enrollment were assigned to either the low or intermediate-level intervention, neither of which were designed to achieve postabatement clearance levels (EPA, 1997c). Thus, it would appear that the majority of children who were either living in or moved into lead-affected housing at enrollment received the potential benefit of a partial lead abatement intervention that they might not have otherwise received. However, the majority of children were known to be living in a lead-affected environment that had only been partially abated to less than the prevailing Maryland lead clearance standards. The key question is whether these children who were either living in or moved into housing that was only partially abated (i.e., the low or intermediate intervention groups) were placed at an unacceptable risk. In effect, were these children at risk and thus potentially benefited from the intervention or were they healthy children placed at risk by moving into lead-affected housing?

All but one of 30 children in the low-level intervention group had an initial blood lead concentration below 20 μg/dL, and one child developed a blood lead concentration of just greater than 20 μg/dL during the study. Three of the initial 25 homes in the low-level intervention group were subsequently cleaned to meet the Maryland postabatement clearance standards, but we do not know if any were the home of either child with an initial or subsequent blood lead concentration of greater than 20 μg/dL (EPA, 1997c). Setting data from the two children aside, the low-level intervention group appears to have met the "local" legal standard that requires lead abatement only after a child has been lead poisoned, usually defined as a blood lead concentration of greater than 20 μg/dL. However, 5 of 31 children who lived in houses that received the intermediate-level intervention had initial blood lead concentration levels of greater than 20 μg/dL (EPA, 1997c). It is not known whether one or more of these five children lived in owner occupied housing, occupied the affected housing at the time of enrollment or may have moved into housing that had received the intermediate-level intervention in spite of an elevated blood lead concentration level. In addition, three children living in intermediate-level housing developed blood lead concentrations of greater than 20 μg/dL, with the blood lead concentration of two of these children subsequently falling to below 20 μg/dL (EPA, 1997a). Thus, the children who either occupied or were moved into the intermediate-level housing, and had elevated blood lead concentrations of greater than 20 μg/dL, appear *not* to have received an intervention equivalent to the alternative that they may have received outside of the study (i.e., full lead abatement). In addition, the argument that the children who were moved into the lead-affected housing after the intermediate-level intervention benefited from the procedure assumes that the parents (if adequately informed) did not have the choice to move into housing that had previously undergone a full lead abatement or had been built after 1979 (i.e., the two control groups). Absent specific knowledge of the alternative housing available to each individual child who was moved into the housing that had undergone the intermediate-level abatement, it is not possible to draw any conclusions as to whether a given child stood to benefit from or was placed at greater risk by participation in the research study.

Having a Condition and Justified Risk Exposure

The suggestion that a child may benefit from an intervention implies that the child has a condition that the intervention may either ameliorate or correct. A child that is at risk for the development of an elevated blood lead concentration may benefit from the reduction of environmental lead. Thus, being at risk for the development of an elevated blood lead concentration can be considered a condition when evaluating the appropriateness of risk exposure within the Baltimore lead abatement study. Although the presence of a condition might justify exposure to a minor increase over minimal risk, all of the monitoring procedures included in the Baltimore lead abatement study could be considered minimal risk. Intermittent monitoring of blood lead concentrations is part of routine medical care and clearly fits even the most narrow interpretation of the definition of minimal risk.

But what about the risk of the interim or partial lead abatement procedures? Lead is a known neurotoxin. At the time of the Baltimore lead abatement study, the adverse impact of an elevated *blood* lead concentration on neurodevelopmental outcome was well established (Centers for Disease Control and Prevention, 1991). For a child to be in contact with any known level of *environmental* lead was to place that child at measurable risk of subsequent cognitive impairment. In fact, one commentator argued that the study failed to minimize risk by relying on measurements of blood lead concentrations rather than environmental lead exposure measured by skin contamination, thus assuring that some children would suffer the negative consequences of lead poisoning (Mielke, 2002). Should we evaluate the risk of the research by the relative standard of the incremental risk (or benefit) of the research when compared to the child's everyday life living in a lead-affected environment, or the absolute standard of the risk (or benefit) when compared to a healthy child presumably living in a lead free environment? Clearly remaining in contact with environmental lead involves some degree of risk to children. There may also be benefit to children from reducing the level of environmental lead exposure even if that reduction is not carried to the level of a complete abatement. However, whether or not the fact that a child may already be exposed to environmental lead should serve as a justification for continued exposure to environmental lead, even in the presence of partial abatement and monitoring procedures, is far from clear. On the one hand, the fact that limited socioeconomic resources create the child's condition of living in a lead-affected environment, then justifies an increased risk exposure, and limits the locally available interventions to only partial rather than full lead abatement seems unfair. On the other hand, partial abatement may be better than no abatement. If the ideal of complete lead abatement cannot be achieved, does research on partial abatement grounded in the socioeconomic realities of the local context offer more hope of helping children?

Reframing the Research Question

The question of whether partial lead abatement is effective in the primary prevention of childhood lead poisoning can be reframed as the question of how much environmental lead can be left behind before a young child develops an elevated blood lead concentration. Blood lead concentration is a well-established surrogate marker for the adverse event of cognitive impairment. Thus, the Baltimore lead abatement study sought to establish the level of environmental lead at which there is no observable adverse effect on young children as measured by blood lead concentration (defined as an absolute level of < 20 µg/dL, or a rise from baseline of > 5 µg/dL; Kennedy Krieger Institute, 2001). Using lead as a paradigm of an environmental neurotoxin, does the Baltimore lead abatement study provide any guidance for the ethical design of research to reduce environmental health hazards? How should we approach research into the neurodevelopmental effects of toxins that have been or will be introduced into the environment, such as pesticides? Should research designed to establish the neurotoxin level at which there is no observed adverse effect be conducted in humans? Under what conditions, if any? Should children be included or excluded? Low-income families and people of color are more likely to be exposed to environmental neurotoxins either in the workplace or in substandard housing (Ryan & Farr, 2002). Some question whether individuals living in these circumstances are capable of making informed and voluntary choices to participate in such research. To what extent should the affected community be involved in the design or conduct of such research?

Human Testing of Pesticides

The role of human testing in determining the "safe" dose of an environmental toxin such as pesticides has been the subject of recent debate (Anonymous, 2003; CropLife America, 2003b; Environmental Working Group, 1998; Phibbs, 2003a, 2003b). Usually the "no observable adverse effect level" (NOAEL) of a pesticide is calculated by applying a series of uncertainty factors to the most sensitive animal results. A 10-fold uncertainty factor is applied to account for the variability between animals and humans. A second 10-fold uncertainty factor is used to account for intrahuman variability, and a third 10-fold uncertainty factor is applied for an additional margin of safety to protect children. Following passage of the 1996 Food Quality Protection Act (1996), the Office of Pesticide Programs of the U.S. Environmental Protection Agency (EPA) has received a number of studies designed to establish the NOAEL in humans so that the initial 10-fold uncertainty factor can be eliminated. A Joint Subcommittee of the Science Advisory Board and the Federal Insecticide, Fungicide and Rodenticide Act Scientific Advisory Panel issued a report in September 2000 that supported "the intentional administration of pesticides to human subjects" under limited conditions. However, a strongly worded minority report argued that the final report did not reflect the "strong doubts about both the ethics and scientific validity of exposing humans to organophosphate pesticides" expressed by most members of the joint subcommittee (EPA, 2000). In a press release on December 14, 2001, the EPA announced an interim policy whereby it would not use data from third-party research in which human subjects were intentionally dosed with pesticides (EPA, 2001). The EPA also requested that the National Academy of Sciences review "the complex scientific and ethical issues" and "furnish recommendations" about the potential acceptability of such studies (EPA, 2001; National Research Council Committee on the Use of Third Party Toxicity Research with Human Research Participants, 2004). This interim policy was vacated on procedural grounds by a federal court on June 3, 2003, in response to a lawsuit filed by an association representing pesticide manufacturers (U.S. Court of Appeals, 2003). For the moment, the EPA will evaluate third-party human studies on a case-by-case basis pending initiation of the federal process of proposed rule making (EPA, 2003; Werner, 2003).

The American Crop Protection Association (now known as CropLife America) argued, in a statement submitted to the above mentioned Joint Subcommittee on November 30, 1999, that human testing of pesticides can be conducted using rigorous ethical, legal, and scientific standards. Drawing an analogy to phase I human volunteer testing of drugs, CropLife America argued that pesticide testing was less risky as the human "no observed effect level" was defined as that dose at which there was *any* side effect seen as opposed to the maximum tolerated dose based on an *unacceptable* side effect (CropLife America, 1999). However, the analogy to phase I drug testing breaks down at several points. First, phase I drug testing simply establishes the dose that is selected for phase II testing in which the safety profile of the drug is further defined. The number of individuals enrolled in a phase I drug study is simply insufficient to ascertain the true incidence of an adverse event. For rare adverse events, the Food and Drug Administration relies on post marketing experience when the medication is administered to hundreds of thousands of patients. As pointed out by the minority report, a prohibitively large number of human subjects (2,500 or more) would be required to detect a small effect (EPA, 2000). After phase I testing is complete, the wider exposure of subjects within the context of phase II testing is justified by the search for a potential benefit in treating a target disease or condition—a requirement that the administration of a pesticide cannot meet. Second, phase I drug testing is usually short-term and focused on acute toxicity. Phase I testing is ill-suited to study long-term neurodevelopmental or cognitive adverse effects. In addition, the negative impact of environmental lead on cognitive development, and the correlation with blood lead concentration, was established using epidemiological methods. Absent an appropriate surrogate marker such as a blood lead concentration, phase I testing of environmental neurotoxins in adults would provide little information applicable to the safety of children. The concern registered by the minority report was that "children will be placed at higher risk of exposure to neurotoxic pesticides" if the EPA allowed for limited adult testing in order to establish a human no observed effect level that eliminated a 10-fold uncertainty factor (EPA, 2000).

Third, the analogy to phase I testing breaks down as the initial testing of drugs in children is held to a different ethical and regulatory standard than such testing in adult volunteers. The administration of a drug, even if limited to a single dose, does not qualify as minimal risk and thus cannot be given to a child without a relevant condition. When administered to a child with an appropriate condition (i.e., a child who either has or would be at risk for the condition to be treated), the administration of a single dose of the drug must present only a minor increase over minimal risk. The administration of a known (i.e., lead) or unknown (i.e., a new pesticide) neurotoxic chemical clearly presents more than a minor increase over minimal risk (National Human Research Protections Advisory Committee, 2002). As such, the phase I administration of an experimental chemical must offer a prospect of direct benefit to the individual child that is comparable to the available alternatives and present risks that are justified or balanced by any anticipated benefit. The administration of a known neurotoxic chemical cannot meet this standard of providing a prospect of direct benefit, regardless of any socioeconomic benefits to society at large from the use of that chemical. To the extent that the Baltimore lead abatement study sought to establish the residual level of environmental lead at which there was no observable adverse effect, the study design is deeply problematic. The essential difference then between the intentional administration of escalating levels of a neurotoxic pesticide and the partial removal of differing amounts of a neurotoxic chemical such as lead appears to be the difference between an act of omission and commission. Are we any less culpable for failing to remove a known level of environmental lead as we would be for introducing that same level of lead into the environment?

Omission, Commission, and Environmental Justice

The simple comparison of the Baltimore lead abatement study with the human testing of pesticides on the grounds that both sought to determine the no observed adverse effect level of an environmental neurotoxin assumes symmetry between an act of omission and an act of commission. Based on this assumption, failing to remove differing levels of environmental lead from lead-affected housing containing young children should be judged no differently than introducing differing levels of lead into lead free housing containing young children. A young child may be left with an elevated blood lead concentration and the associated neurological injury in either case. However, this claim of symmetry based on simple causality assumes that there is no other morally relevant difference between the two types of research (Frankfurt, 1994; Smith, 2003).

All parties to the debate over the ethics of the Baltimore lead abatement study agree that the intentional exposure of young children to environmental lead is morally wrong. The disagreement arises in how to describe the Baltimore lead abatement study. Those who consider the study to be justified focus on the potential benefit of even partially reducing a young child's exposure to environmental lead; those who consider the study to be unjustified emphasize the cognitive damage from any residual level of environmental lead and the fact that some children were moved into lead-affected housing that had only been partially abated (i.e., the initially vacant housing in the intermediate group). This conflict is difficult to resolve because there are features of the study suggesting that both of these positions are accurate.

Regardless of whether the study is viewed as offering children a potential benefit or placing them at risk, one feature common to all descriptions of the Baltimore lead abatement study is the limited local housing conditions and the potential socioeconomic advantages of partial lead abatement. Lead-affected housing is often abandoned by landlords given the high costs of complete lead abatement, leading to a shortage of affordable and lead-free urban housing. Effective and less expensive methods of partial lead abatement might ameliorate this problem, yet would leave residual lead behind that places future children at some risk. In criticizing the study, some point out that "a conflict of interest existed between the residents and the interests of property owners who from the findings can now determine how little they need to invest in lead reduction in order to salvage their investments and keep their properties on the rental market" (Pinder, 2002). From this perspective, the risks of the research were borne by the child participants while the economic benefits accrued to the landlords.

This same trade-off between the risk of individual harm to human subjects and the benefits to pesticide companies and to society is seen in the debate over the human testing of pesticides. The EPA Scientific Advisory Board, in discussing whether human testing of pesticides should proceed, argued that "it is not enough to determine a risk/benefit ratio; it is important also to consider the distribution of risks and of benefits, and to ensure that risks are not imposed on one population for the sake of benefits to be enjoyed by another" (EPA, 2000). Generally, the research risks of ongoing exposure to neurotoxic chemicals falls disproportionately on low-income workers and/or families, with any socioeconomic benefits accruing to pesticide companies and potentially to society at large. Low-income families and people of color are more likely to live in substandard housing and to have limited housing options or a higher occupational exposure to pesticides (Ryan & Farr, 2002). From their perspective, the risks of ongoing exposure may not be balanced by the health benefit of partial lead abatement regardless of the socioeconomic benefit to others. Given this reality, how can we move forward in conducting interventional research on the reduction of health risks from environmental toxins?

Justice and the Baltimore Lead Abatement Study

One critique of the Baltimore lead abatement study emphasized the failure of the researchers to consider the principle of justice, and specifically environmental justice, in the design and implementation of the research (Pinder, 2002). Although apparently meeting the local legal standard that usually does not require complete lead abatement in the absence of a lead-poisoned child, the study did not conform to the moral standard of removing a young child from known lead hazards whenever possible. Participating families may not have had a clear understanding of the different levels of partial lead abatement nor the risks of exposure to remaining lead (Pinder, 2002; McNeilly, 2002). The study served the interests of property owners by determining the most economic way to keep a rental property on the market. An important presupposition of the study is the failure of either political or economic will to support complete lead abatement. Although most of the children in the study experienced a fall in their blood lead concentration, methods of partial lead abatement are only short-term strategies that reduce but not eliminate environmental contamination and thus simply delay "the inevitable—another lead-poisoned child" (Pinder, 2002). As Shepard notes: "The struggle for environmental justice by people of color, who bear the brunt of pollution in the United States

and around the world, has escalated with a growing awareness that this disproportionate burden contributes to egregious disparities in health by race/ethnicity
and social class" (Shepard, Northridge, Prakash, & Stover, 2002). Would the local
tenant community have accepted the risks of ongoing lead exposure as a necessary
trade-off to maintain adequate and affordable housing, or sought other avenues
to ameliorate the problem?

Community-Based Participatory Research

Community-based participatory research (CBPR) has been recommended as a
method to be used for the conduct of environmental research. CBPR is "a methodology that promotes active community involvement in the processes that shape
research and intervention strategies, as well as in the conduct of research studies."
Emphasizing a number of benefits for both researchers and community members,
O'Fallon and Dearry (2002) identify six principles or features of CBPR: (1) active
collaboration and participation, (2) co-learning, (3) community driven, (4) dis-
semination of results in useful terms, (5) culturally appropriate, and (6) the community as a unit of identity. The Baltimore lead abatement study apparently involved community organizations in the design of the three levels of intervention.
These organizations included a city program experienced in lead abatement, nonprofit housing organizations, and state and federal agencies (EPA, 1997c). Missing, however, were community advocacy groups and tenant organizations that
might represent the views of those living in the lead-affected housing. In effect,
the Baltimore lead abatement study did not involve the local community who
would be most affected by the results as collaborators in the design and implementation of the research. Another, albeit controversial, principle that has been
proposed as a guideline for environmental research and policy is the precautionary
principle (Myers, 2002). Faced with an uncertain threat of harm to human health
from an environmental contaminant, the precautionary principle argues for increased public participation in decision making (along with preventive action,
exploring alternatives, and shifting the burden of proof to demonstrating safety
rather than harm) (Kriebel et al., 2001). The importance of public participation
arises out of the policy implications of scientific research, and the observation
that scientists often make value judgments during the design, implementation, and
interpretation of research (Myers, 2002). Apart from the question of scientific
merit of the precautionary principle for guiding environmental policy, it provides
an ethical foundation for research by ensuring that the views of the broader community affected by the study are represented. Scientific uncertainty about the
threat of harm as a condition for using the precautionary principle does not readily
apply as lead is a known neurotoxin (Tickner, Raffensperger, & Myers, 1998).

Nevertheless, there was uncertainty about the level of *environmental* lead to which a young child can be exposed without adverse effect. The precautionary principle, as does the CBPR model, advocates for public involvement of those most affected by research and policy decisions about methods of lead abatement. If a CBPR model had been used, the design of the Baltimore lead abatement study may or may not have been different. However, the families living in (or moving into) the lead-affected housing may have been better informed given the higher visibility within and involvement of the local community fostered by such an approach.

CONCLUSION

The Baltimore lead abatement study offered the prospect of direct benefit to those children who were living in the lead-affected housing at the time of enrollment. Assuming the children were not lead-poisoned (i.e., blood lead concentration > 20 µg/dL), the potential benefit of partial lead abatement was comparable to the local legal standard that usually did not require complete lead abatement absent a lead-poisoned child. The study was designed so that a child with an elevated blood lead concentration at enrollment was likely to be placed in housing that had been abated to the same postabatement standards as required for complete lead abatement (i.e., the high-level intervention). A child who developed an elevated blood lead concentration during the study was to be treated according to the local standard of care, which presumably would involve closer monitoring and complete lead abatement (if available). Thus, with the possible exception of those children who were moved into the housing that had undergone the intermediate-level partial lead abatement, the Baltimore lead abatement study appeared to offer the enrolled children the prospect of direct benefit.

The risk of partial lead abatement should not be considered minimal under 45 CFR 46.404 (U.S. Department of Health and Human Services, 1983), because living in lead-affected housing is not "that level of risk associated with the daily activities of a normal, healthy, average child" (National Human Research Protections Advisory Committee, 2002). Although the risks of partial lead abatement may be commensurate with the risks of living in lead-affected housing, the category of a "minor increase over minimal risk" (45 CFR 46.406) should be limited to those "risks that are a little more than minimal and pose no significant threat to the child's health or well-being" thereby excluding any level of known lead exposure (National Human Research Protections Advisory Committee, 2002). For an intervention that offers the prospect of direct benefit to be approvable under 45 CFR 46.405, the risk must be justified by the anticipated benefit to the child and the relation of the anticipated benefit to the risk must be at least as favorable to the child as that presented by available alternative approaches. Thus, whether the study is approvable under 45 CFR 46.405 hinges on whether the available alternative approaches are limited to what is "locally available" or should include full lead abatement (U.S. Department of Health and Human Services, 1983).

From the start of the research, there was no expectation that the partial methods of lead abatement would be comparable to full lead abatement (EPA, 1997c). Should we be satisfied with methods of partial lead abatement that may meet the local legal standard in the absence of a lead poisoned child or advocate for complete lead abatement as a more universally accepted intervention? There are some who argue that the decision to study methods of partial lead abatement is morally suspect as it then aligns the research with those individuals that stand to gain financially from the continued failure to enforce existing lead abatement statutes. As Needleman (2002) observes, the vision of primary prevention through comprehensive lead abatement gave way to an "enfeebled pseudopragmatism" that sought to determine how little we could spend and still reduce blood lead concentrations in the short term. Alternatively, following the principle of justice, it is the community who are living in lead-affected housing that should decide whether methods of partial lead abatement offer a sufficient prospect of direct benefit to be approvable under 45 CFR 46.405. Framed within the context of CBPR, the Baltimore lead abatement study could have been approved within the existing regulatory framework perhaps with two modifications. First, absent an independent review of housing options, a child should not be moved into partially abated housing as one could not otherwise assume such a move offered that particular child potential direct benefit. Second, the question of whether environmental lead exposure could have been measured using skin contamination as opposed to blood lead concentrations should have been addressed (Mielke, 2002).

Interventional research designed to reduce exposure to environmental toxins can involve children and be conducted ethically under limited conditions. The most important condition is the involvement of the affected community in the design and implementation of the research, following the model of CBPR. Following existing federal regulations, the research must be designed to offer each child the prospect of direct benefit, combined with close monitoring and removal should the risk to an individual child become unacceptable. However, our ability to apply the lessons learned from the Baltimore lead abatement study to other environmental research may be hampered by an important scientific limitation—the lack of a surrogate marker of neurological damage (i.e., blood lead concentrations or skin contamination). Absent the capability of monitoring such a surrogate marker, the precautionary principle dictates the complete removal of a child from the environmental neurotoxin.

Questions for Discussion

1. Did the children enrolled in the Baltimore lead abatement study stand to benefit from the research?

2. Were these children healthy, or did they have a condition that warranted intervention?

3. Do you think that children who were either living in or moved into housing that was only partially abated (i.e., the low or intermediate intervention groups) were placed at an unacceptable risk?

4. How should we investigate the neurodevelopmental effects of toxins that have been or will be introduced into the environment, such as pesticides? Should research designed to establish the neurotoxin level at which there is no observed adverse effect be conducted in humans? Under what conditions, if any? Should children be included or excluded?

5. To what extent should the affected community be involved in the design or conduct of such research?

6. Which standard should we use to evaluate the risk of the research- the relative standard that compares the research risk to the child's everyday life living in a lead contaminated environment, or the absolute standard that compares the risk to that for a healthy child presumably living in a lead free environment?

7. What is the ethical difference between the intentional administration of escalating levels of a neurotoxic pesticide and the partial removal of differing amounts of a neurotoxic chemical such as lead?

8. Do you think it is reasonable to compare of the Baltimore lead abatement study with the human testing of pesticides? Why or why not?

9. The EPA Scientific Advisory Board, in discussing whether human testing of pesticides should proceed, argued that "it is not enough to determine a risk/benefit ratio; it is important also to consider the distribution of risks and of benefits, and to ensure that risks are not imposed on one population for the sake of benefits to be enjoyed by another" (EPA, 2000). How would you apply this argument to the research risks of ongoing exposure to neurotoxic chemicals?

10. What would be the criticism of the Baltimore lead abatement study with regard to the principle of environmental justice?

11. What are the two guideline models for environmental research presented by the writer? Do you think the Baltimore lead abatement study adheres to the principles of these models?

12. Do you agree with the writer that the risk of partial lead abatement should not be considered minimal under 45 CFR 46.404?

13. Can research designed to reduce but not eliminate the risks of environmental toxins be conducted using children under existing federal regulations?

14. Does the Baltimore lead abatement study provide any general guidance for the ethical design of research to reduce environmental health hazards?

▬

References

Anonymous. (2003). Human subject testing: EPA human testing notice seeks comment on broad range of issues for upcoming rule. *Medical Research Law & Policy Report, 2*(10), 375.

Centers for Disease Control and Prevention. (1991, October). *Preventing lead poisoning in young children: A statement by the centers for disease control.* Atlanta, GA: Department of Health and Human Services.

CropLife America. (1999). *Summary statement, testing pesticides in humans.* Retrieved July 27, 2004 from http://www.croplifeamerica.org/public/issues/medtest/11_99doc.html

CropLife America. (2003 June 3). *News release: CropLife America welcomes court ruling on consideration of clinical test data.* Retrieved July 27, 2004 from http://www.croplifeamerica.org/public/news/nrs/nr060303.html

Environmental Working Group. (1998). *The English patients: Human experiments and pesticide policy.* Retrieved July 27, 2004 from http://ww.ewg.org/reports/english/English.pdf

EPA. (1997a, August). *Executive summary: Lead-based paint abatement and repair and maintenance study in Baltimore: Findings based on the first year of follow-up.* EPA 747-R-97-001. Rev. October 31, 2003. Retrieved July 27, 2004 from http://www.epa.gov/lead/12mo-rpt.htm

EPA. (1997b, December). *Executive summary: Lead-based paint abatement and repair and maintenance study in Baltimore: Findings based on two years of follow-up.* EPA 747-R-97-005. Rev. October 31, 2003. Retrieved July 27, 2004 from http:/www.epa.gov/lead/24folup.pdf

EPA. (1997c, December). *Lead-based paint abatement and repair and maintenance study in Baltimore: Findings based on two years of follow-up.* EPA 747-R-97-005. NTIS PB99-101453. Retrieved July 27, 2004 from http://www.ntis.gov/search/product.asp?ABBR=PB99101453& starDB=GRAHIST

EPA. (1998, December). *Review of studies addressing lead abatement effectiveness: Updated edition.* EPA 747-B-98-001. Rev. October 31, 2003. Retrieved July 27, 2004 from http://www.epa.gov/lead/finalreport.pdf

EPA. (2000, September). *Comments on the use of data from the testing of human subjects. A report by the Science Advisory Board and the FIFRA Scientific Advisory Panel.* EPA-SAB-EC-00-017. Rev. October 31, 2003. Retrieved July 27, 2004 from http://epa.gov/sab/pdf/ec0017.pdf

EPA. (2001, December 14). *Press release: Agency requests national academy of sciences input on consideration of certain human toxicity studies; announces interim policy.* Rev. November 5, 2003. Retrieved July 27, 2004 from http://www.epa.gov/newsroom/

EPA. (2003). Human testing; Advance notice of proposed rulemaking. *Federal Register, 68*(88), 24410–24416.

Farfel, M. R., Rohde, C., Lees, P.S.J., Rooney, B., Bannon, D. I., & Derbyshire, W. (1996, August). *Lead-based paint abatement and repair and maintenance study in Baltimore: Pre-intervention findings.* EPA/747/R-95/012. NTIS PB97-115745. Washington, DC: U.S. Environmental Protection Agency. Retrieved July 27, 2004 from http:/www.ntis.gov/

Food Quality Protection Act of 1996. (1996, August 3). Public Law 104–170. Retrieved July 27, 2004 from http://www.epa.gov/oppfead1/fqpa/gpogate.pdf.

Frankfurt, H. (1994). An alleged asymmetry between actions and omissions. *Ethics, 104*(April), 620–623.

Kennedy Krieger Institute. (2001). *Lead-based paint study fact sheet.* Retrieved November 1, 2001 from (copy available from author).

Kriebel, D., Tickner, J., Epstein, P., Lemons, J., Levins, R., Loechler, E. L., et al. (2001). The precautionary principle in environmental science. *Environmental Health Perspectives, 109*(9), 871–876.

Maryland Court of Appeals. (2001a). *Ericka Grimes v. Kennedy Krieger Institute, Inc.* (No. 128); *Myron Higgins, a minor, etc., et al. v. Kennedy Krieger Institute, Inc.* (No. 129). Rev. October 31, 2003. Retrieved July 27, 2004 from http://www.courts.state.md.us/opinions/coa/2001/128a00.pdf

Maryland Court of Appeals. (2001b). *Ericka Grimes v. Kennedy Krieger Institute, Inc.* (No. 128); *Myron Higgins, a minor, etc., et al. v. Kennedy Krieger Institute, Inc.* (No. 129). *Reconsideration Denied.* Rev. November 1, 2003. Retrieved July 27, 2004 from http://www.law.uh .edu/healthlaw/law/StateMaterials/Marylandcases/grimesvkennedykriegar.pdf

McNeilly, P. J. (2002). *Office for human research protections to the Johns Hopkins University School of Medicine and the Kennedy Krieger Institute, 19 August.* Rev. October 31, 2003. Retrieved July 27, 2004 from http://www.hhs.gov/ohrp/detrm_letrs/YR02/aug02c.pdf

Mielke, H. W. (2002). Research ethics in pediatric environmental health: Lessons from lead. *Neurotoxicology and Teratology, 24*(4), 467–469.

Myers, N. (2002). The precautionary principle puts values first. *Bulletin of Science, Technology and Society, 22*(3), 210–219.

National Human Research Protections Advisory Committee. (2002). *Clarifying Specific Portion of 45 CFR 46 Subpart D that Governs Children's Research.* Rev. November 1, 2003. Retrieved July 27, 2004 from http://www.hhs.gov/ohrp/nhrpac/documents/nhrpac16.pdf.

National Research Council Committee on the Use of Third Party Toxicity Research with Human Research Participants. (2004). *Intentional Human Dosing Studies for EPA Regulatory Purposes: Scientific and Ethical Issues.* Washington, DC: The National Academics Press.

Needleman, H. L. (2002). What is not found in the spreadsheets. *Neurotoxicology and Teratology, 24*(4), 459–461.

Nelson, R. M.. (2002). Appropriate risk exposure in environmental health research: The Kennedy-Krieger lead abatement study. *Neurotoxicology and Teratology, 24*(4), 445449.

O'Fallon, L. R., & Dearry, A. (2002). Community-Based participatory research as a tool to advance environmental health sciences. *Environmental Health Perspectives, 110*(Suppl. 2), 155–159.

Phibbs, P. (2003a). Human subject testing: Court asked to vacate interim policy in which human data not considered. *Medical Research Law & Policy Report, 2*(2), 256.

Phibbs, P. (2003b). Human subject testing: Chemical, pesticide manufacturers oppose house amendment to ban human test data. *Medical Research Law & Policy Report, 2*(16), 600.

Pinder, L. (2002). Commentary on the Kennedy Krieger Institute lead paint repair and maintenance study. *Neurotoxicology and Teratology, 24*(4), 477–479.

Roig-Franzia, M. (2001, August 25). My kids were used as guinea pigs: Lead paint study adds to debate on research. *Washington Post*, p. A01.

Ryan, D. & Farr, N. (2002). Confronting the ethical challenges of environmental health research. *Neurotoxicology and Teratology, 24*(4), 471–473.

Shepard, P. M., Northridge, M. E., Prakash, S., & Stover, G. (2002). Preface: Advancing environmental justice through community-based participatory research. *Environmental Health Perspectives, 110*(Suppl. 2), 139–140.

Smith, P. (2003). Bad samaritans, acts, and omissions. In R.G. Frey & C. H. Wellman (Eds.), *A companion to applied ethics* (pp. 475–486). Malden, MA: Blackwell Publishing Ltd.

Tickner, J., Raffensperger, C., & Myers, N. (1998). *The precautionary principle in action: A handbook.* The Science and Environmental Health Network. Rev. November 1, 2003. Retrieved July 27, 2004 from http://www.sehn.org/rtfdocs/hardbook-rtf.rtf

U.S. Court of Appeals for the District of Columbia Circuit. (2003). *CropLife America, et al. v. Environmental Protection Agency.* No. 02-1057. Rev. October 31, 2003. Retrieved July 27, 2004 from http://pacer.cadc.uscourts.gov/docs/common/opinions/200306/02-1057a.pdf

U.S. Department of Health and Human Services. (1983). 45 CFR Part 46: Additional protections for children involved as subjects in research. *Federal Register, 48*(8 March), 9814.

Werner, K. L. (2003). Human subject testing: Federal court vacates EPA third-party policy; Human testing to be accepted case-by-case. *Medical Research Law & Policy Report, 2*(12), 450.

10

Behavioral Research With Children: The Fenfluramine Challenge

Gerald P. Koocher

CASE DESCRIPTION

Although psychosocial and behavioral science research rarely present serious medical hazards or threats to the physical well-being of participants, such studies can raise a wide range of ethical dilemmas and controversies. When children participate in such research some special concerns related to their unique developmental vulnerabilities, relative social and financial dependency on others, and status as minors under the law demand particular consideration. One recent set of studies based on a "fenfluramine challenge" protocol provides an interesting model for discussion in this context.

The research in question involved a behavioral science drug study, carried out at prestigious institutions. The studies had no therapeutic benefit or intent, used child participants from impoverished families, and employed a set of questionable recruitment practices. Many people in the lay and scientific communities saw the research as inappropriate or misguided. The investigators, well-intentioned and competent scientists, felt unfairly assailed by their critics. A government investigation of very limited scope determined that required regulatory oversight and informed consent procedures were followed. The study's authors (Wasserman & Pine, 2004) believe that description of the investigation of the Federal Office of Protection from Research Risk of their work as being of limited scope constitutes a mischaracterization. Their written rationale, in response to reading this chapter, rests on finding that IRB review attended to "the requirements of 45 CFR Part 46, Subpart D." Sadly, this response overlooks the fact that focusing almost exclusively on Subpart D precludes review of many of the issues raised in this chapter, such as distributive justice issues. Readers will have to decide the ethical appropriateness of the study and adequacy of regulatory oversight for themselves.

In the fall of 1997, a group known as Citizens for Responsible Care and Research, co-founded by Professor Adil Shamoo of the University of Maryland, began alerting advocacy groups and the public media regarding some published studies involving fenfluramine challenge research using children as participants (Shamoo & Tauer, 2002). The work originated at the New York State Psychiatric Institute and Columbia University's College of Physicians and Surgeons. A series of official complaints and media accounts of the study followed (Hilts, 1998; Montero, 1998).

The Study

Daniel S. Pine, a physician specializing in psychopharmacological research, and his colleagues believed that a relationship might exist among serotonin levels, aggressive behavior, and "a childhood history of socially adverse-rearing conditions" (Pine et al., 1996, 1997). They decided to study the biochemical responses of a group of young boys who showed "clinically significant" aggressive behavior *or* who were growing up in an environment "conducive to the development of chronic aggression." In particular, the investigators wanted to study the prolactin response of such boys who were administered a dose of fenfluramine hydrochloride (i.e., a fenfluramine challenge).

Pine et al. (1997) noted a cluster of research reports suggesting that a significant relationship may exist between chronic aggression with a childhood onset and abnormalities in the serotonergic nervous system. They describe an inverse correlation between indices of aggressive behavior and the prolactin response to a "fenfluramine hydrochloride challenge" in adults. Administration of fenfluramine increases synaptic serotonin levels by triggering release of serotonin from nerve terminals and inhibiting serotonin reuptake. Increased levels of synaptic serotonin stimulates a rise in prolactin levels, the magnitude of which indexes central serotonergic activity (Coccaro et al., 1989; Halperin, Newcorn, Kopestein, et al., 1997; Halperin, Newcorn, Schwartz, et al., 1997). The published studies generally provide detailed accounts of drug administration, sampling, and measurement techniques, for example, "double-antibody radioimmunoassay with intra-assay and interassay coefficients of variation" (Pine et al., 1997, p. 840). In an ironic contrast between expectations of biomedical versus ethical rigor in much of the scientific literature, this particular study and others of the same genre usually do not address the ethical issues involved in drug studies using healthy children as participants. Although any drugs will have both main and side effects, and despite the fact that fenfluramine has been linked to adverse side effects with some populations in some studies, Pine et al. did not address these issues in their published work. In fairness to Pine et al., such discussions of side effects and the risk-to-benefit ratios of conducting drug studies with healthy children, while generally well addressed by institutional review boards (IRBs), rarely accompany published research reports.

The research protocol in the 1997 study required all of the boys to follow low-monoamine diets for 4 days, fast the night before the challenge, and receive nothing by mouth during the challenge portion of the study. According to published accounts, an intravenous catheter was inserted by 8:30 a.m. and baseline blood samples were collected at 9:45 a.m. and 10:00 a.m. Oral fenfluramine hydrochloride (10 mg/kg) was given at 10:00 a.m. Blood was sampled hourly until 2:00 p.m. In addition to fasting and taking nothing by mouth from the evening before the study until after 2:00 p.m. the following day, the children were required to remain inactive from 8:30 a.m. to 2:00 p.m. on the day of the study.

The 34 boys who participated in this study were drawn from a subset of 126, all of whom were younger brothers of incarcerated "delinquents in New York, NY." Families were contacted after an older brother was identified through court records, with the help of juvenile authorities. Exclusion criteria included physical illness, abnormal blood chemistries or blood counts, current use of prescribed or illicit drugs, and needle phobias. After psychiatric examination, 56 nonexcluded boys were approached for this study, 36 children (with parental permission) agreed to participate and two were excluded for failing to follow the preparation protocol (i.e., fasting or diet limitations). Pine (2003) reported that assent was obtained from child participants, although details of the process and copies of actual forms used were unavailable.

All 34 boys lived in families described by the investigators as "impoverished." All of the participants were children of color, with 44% identified as African American and 56% as Hispanic. Most of the families had previously participated in research with the investigators. Age of the boys at original intake averaged 8.4 years ± 1.5 years, and age at time of challenge was 10.0 ± 1.5 years. A "trained interviewer" talked with caretakers of the child participants and completed ratings of aggression and other personality variables using the Child Behavior Checklist (Achenbach, 1991) and the Diagnostic Interview Schedule for Children–Revised (Shaffer et al., 1993).

Potential participants were selected because they had an incarcerated sibling and therefore were considered prospectively "at risk" for aggressive or violent behavior. Names from sealed court records had been provided to researchers, so that siblings of convicted juvenile offenders could be identified (Montero, 1998). The juvenile probation authorities did not seek or obtain court consent to unseal the records (Shamoo & Tauer, 2002).

The study found a positive correlation between aggression ratings, as measured by caregiver reports obtained using the Child Behavior Checklist and the Diagnostic Interview Schedule for Children–Revised, and the prolactin response to fenfluramine challenge in the participants. No evidence suggested a relationship between the psychiatric measures used by the investigators and the timing of peak prolactin response. Associations between disruptive psychiatric disorder diagnoses and prolactin levels appeared to occur at both 3 and 4 hours but not at 1 or 2 hours after oral fenfluramine ingestion. According to the investigators, data suggested that "adverse rearing circumstances" correlated with larger prolactin responses. The data also led the authors to conclude that aggressive behavior and social circumstances deemed conducive to developing aggressive behavior are positively correlated with a biomarker for central serotonergic activity.

The investigators noted four limitations to their study. First, it was not possible to study demographically matched comparison children without a family history of delinquency. Second, there were limitations to the assessment of serotonergic activity due to their inability to use placebo challenges in prepubertal children. Third, they focused on mother–son interactions and serotonin in boys, omitting consideration of paternal interactions. Finally, they noted that the two constructs studied (i.e., rearing environment and serotonergic activity) are dynamic systems studied at single points in time.

By the time of the study, fenfluramine had been withdrawn from the public marketplace due to evidence of heart valve damage in patients taking it as a component of "Fen-Phen" anti-obesity treatments (Connolly et al., 1997; Kolata, 1997). Although only a single does was administered in this nontherapeutic research, fenfluramine has caused adverse effects in adults after only a single dose, with as many as 90% of recipients in one study reporting side effects (Muldoon, Manuck, Jansma, Moore, & Mann, 1996).

Discussion With the Senior Investigators

Personal telephone and electronic mail conversations with two of the senior investigators provided the following additional information (Pine, 2003; Wasserman, 2003). The participants in this study were a subset of a larger sample of children used in many studies by the same team of investigators over several years. For the fenfluramine challenge study, Drs. Pine and Wasserman both recalled that inducement of approximately $150 in the form of "gift certificates to Toys R Us or a sneaker store" were provided to subjects. Neither Pine nor Wasserman could recall precise details of the inducement or consent forms, and neither had current access to original consent forms or IRB documents. After viewing an earlier draft of this chapter, Wasserman and Pine (2004) provided some previously unavailable documents, including IRB forms indicating that the actual compensation included a $25 gift certificate for the child, $100 paid to the parents, "for your child," and $25 to cover transportation costs.

When asked about any questions raised by the IRB regarding the nature of the study and consent process, Dr. Wasserman noted that she had no access to the records but believed that the key concerns expressed by IRB members at the time the proposed study was reviewed focused on the nature of compensation to participants. Dr. Wasserman recalled, "The only ethical concern of the IRB was whether the mothers would agree to anything in exchange for money. They (i.e., the IRB) wanted to give all the money to the kids in the form of gift certificates."

Both Drs. Pine and Wasserman reported that all child participants gave assent and were told about their right to withdraw at any time, but none did. Both also stated that cooperation with the research protocol (i.e., diet restrictions, fasting, blood drawing, and activity limitations) did not become problems because the children were kept company by research assistants during the procedure and had access to television, video tapes, and games that did not require significant physical activity.

When asked about recruitment issues and whether families may have felt some pressure to participate because of the nature of referral, Dr. Wasserman reported that, by the time of the fenfluramine challenge study, "[m]any parents had forgotten how they were recruited 2 years after the fact." She added, "The piece about which you inquire was one component in a longitudinal, multifaceted investigation, and we had extended relationships with the families over time. They provided us with access to information about themselves in multiple ways at many time points" (Wasserman, 2003). Notwithstanding Dr. Wasserman's sincere beliefs, at least one mother reportedly stated that she hoped her younger son's participation in the study might help her older, incarcerated son, a reasonable expectation given the involvement of the probation department (Guart, 1999).

When asked about the difficulty in maintaining compliance with food deprivation and inactivity during the procedure, Dr. Pine reported,

Staff were with the children at all times. Family were also encouraged to stay with the kids. Kids were provided with games and movies to watch. Second, the test occurred after we had already met the families on prior visits. As a result, families had considerable time to consider if they really wanted to participate. Some subjects initially thought they might want to participate, but upon reflection or discussion changed their mind and decided not to come in for the study. These subjects did not come to the center for this test at all. Therefore, families who ultimately came had considered alternatives before even coming to the center. We monitored how kids were doing throughout the procedure, both using standard rating forms completed regularly with children as well as through staff observations. These assessments revealed no signs of significant upset. Therefore, the procedure never had to be interrupted. Children and families were told that we could stop the procedure at any point that they so desired with no loss to them. (Pine, 2003).

Dr. Pine's comments seem reasonably supported by the 36% refusal rate reported in the published paper (Pine et al., 1997), suggesting that some potential participant families felt free to refuse despite any real or perceived connection of the study referral mechanism to the probation department and despite the offer of compensation, as described earlier.

—

ETHICAL ANALYSIS AND DISCUSSION

Exploration of the ethical hazards associated with this research can reasonably follow the order in which each occurred: access to potential participants, enrollment in the study, interventions during the data collection phase, the hazards of having an "at-risk" designation, and issues of distributive justice.

Was Access to the List of Potential Subjects a Breach of Confidentiality?

One significant concern raised by the study involves invasions of privacy in granting the investigators access to information about potential participants. The families of the juvenile offenders and the offenders themselves had a reasonable expectation of privacy, given the general operating standards of the juvenile courts and sealed nature of juvenile court records. Their confidentiality was breached by probation authorities, at the request of the researchers. This issue was not addressed in either the published papers or the investigation conducted by the federal Office of Protection from Research Risks (OPRR). One cannot totally blame the investigators for this significant violation of the families' privacy, since the decision to release the information was made by others. The researchers appear to have protected the identities of participants after the disclosure by authorities and any participation in the research.

Some interesting questions related to the ethical preservation of privacy rights remain unanswered in the context of this study. Did the participant families have a reasonable expectation of privacy that was violated by the juvenile court authorities? Should the investigators have sought access to these confidential and socially sensitive data, even if juvenile probation authorities seemed willing to provide it? Should the IRB have questioned such access? Do scientific interests ever justify the use of such access to confidential court records for purposes of research participant recruitment strategies?

Juvenile court records have historically been treated confidentially. The names of juvenile offenders do not appear in press accounts of arrests or legal proceedings except in the case of major crimes when the case is transferred for trial in adult court. The records of youthful offenders are generally expunged when offenders graduate from the authority of the juvenile justice system. The families of these offenders would have every reasonable expectation of privacy. We have no information about why the juvenile authorities agreed to assist the investigators by providing otherwise confidential identifying information and do not know who made the decision or how vetting of the request occurred. We do know that the investigators had a longstanding relationship with the juvenile authorities and the fenfluramine study represents a subset of the work done on a larger sample of the families of the juvenile offenders (Pine, 2003). In the aftermath of public criticism of the study in the media no juvenile authorities admitted responsibility for releasing the information. No IRB process took place under the auspices of juvenile authorities, and nothing suggests that the institutional review at the investigators' institutions addressed their access to the identities of potential participants. It seems reasonable to conclude that no independent body weighed the risks to participants against the potential scientific benefits of the study.

The investigators certainly believed that their work might ultimately answer significant questions about the heritability of potential to engage in violent behavior. Access to identities of families with adjudicated juvenile offenders and younger male siblings may have seemed an ideal opportunity to test important hypotheses. However, with no direct benefit apart from financial incentive, potential drug side effects, and psychosocial risks to the participating children, objective review of the access to the population should have been sought.

Subtle Coercion to Participate

Inadequacy of consent in this study presents major ethical problems. Original parental permission and child assent forms as approved by the IRB[1] were not available for review in the preparation of this chapter; however, the content of the forms hardly matters. By definition, informed consent must be knowing and voluntary. The fact that the child participants' parents knew the probation department had cooperated in making their names available constitutes a de facto coercive pressure of significant proportions. The mother who reported hoping that her incarcerated son might benefit because of his younger brother's cooperation in the drug study (Guart, 1999) clearly illustrates this point.

It matters little whether the IRB approved permission and assent forms contain traditional disclaimers asserting no connection between agreement to participate and the incarcerated siblings' circumstances. Ethnic minority families living below the poverty line may interpret a request or invitation from governmental authorities or investigators differently from their better situated fellow citizens, as carrying the weight of significant societal pressure. Even though the researchers had no formal authority in the lives of participants' families, they held high social status as medical professionals with prestigious academic appointments. In addition, they appeared to approach the families with the official imprimatur of the juvenile justice system and had longitudinal relationships with some of the families. For people of color living at the poverty level suspicions about obtaining fair treatment from civil authority figures, perception becomes reality, and the voluntariness essential to the informed consent process effectively vanishes.

Similarly, offers of financial incentives in the form of gift certificates ranging from $125 to $175 (Pine, 2003; Shamoo & Tauer, 2002; Wasserman, 2003) may have a powerful influence on the decision to participate. As Dr. Wasserman noted in her oral communications, the IRB recognized this fact to some extent when members expressed concern that all or most of the compensation should go to the participating children who experienced the stresses associated with the study (i.e., fasting, medication side effects, blood drawing, and inactivity), as opposed to their parents. The relatively significant compensation most likely brought some pleasure into the lives of the impoverished children who received the gift certificates.

Did the children realize that they could leave the study at any time they felt uncomfortable enough to do so, and still claim the compensation? We do not know. Would an 8- to 10-year-old African-American or Hispanic boy feel comfortable asserting a wish to terminate participation in the study to their parents or to the investigator doctor in the lab coat? Again, we do not know. We do know that 36% of those invited into the study either did not agree to enroll or dropped out prior to the drug challenge by virtue of noncooperation with the fasting or other prestudy requirements. This statistic tells us that 36% of potential participants were not coerced into the study, but tells us little of the motives or pressures experienced by the 64% who did complete their participation. We can reasonably assume that the perception of potential benefit to an incarcerated older brother, the relatively significant value of the gift certificate, and the social demand characteristics involved in wishing to please or satisfy the higher status researchers, aligned to create a powerful set of inducements to participate.

Treatment of Participants During the Study

Apart from the potential coercive forces described above, other social pressures may have operated during the course of the study. Parents of normal 8- to 10-year-old boys will most likely marvel at the prospect of their child sitting quietly, with an intravenous catheter in place for 5.5 hours, from 8:30 a.m. to 2:00 p.m., having had nothing to eat since dinner the night before. Dr. Pine's sincere account of attendance by caring assistants, nearby family members, and distractions such as television and games (Pine, 2003) affords a degree of reassurance regarding the boys' emotional support, but also implies a degree of coercion. How easy is it to say, "I'm tired of this and hungry, I want to quit now," in such a situation? We have no information on how often the child participants were subtlety dissuaded from exiting the study prior to completion of data collection. Situational factors of a social psychological nature (i.e., pressures toward group conformity, deference to individuals with perceived high social or economic status, and reluctance to question authority) often referred to by social psychologists as "demand characteristics" frequently influence people's behavior. Although we have no reason to believe that inappropriate overt pressures were applied, the social demand characteristics tending to promote full compliance in such circumstances seem quite clear.

Hazards of "At-Risk" Designation

A significant body of research attests to the potential adverse consequences of applying stigmatizing labels to children. This includes describing certain children as being "at-risk" for some social or behavioral consequence. In what has become a classic study in the sociology of education, Rosenthal and Jacobson (1968) gave an intelligence test to all of the students at an elementary school at the beginning of the school year. They then selected 20% of the students at random, without any regard to their intelligence test results, and advised the teachers that these students could be expected to "bloom" or "spurt" in their academic achievements that year. At the end of the year, they came back and retested all the students. The results described in Rosenthal & Jacobson (1968) demonstrated a positive shift in the children's achievement levels presumably linked chiefly to teachers' expectations.

A more ominous example of the potential research risks to those labeled as "at risk" for less desirable traits originates in the work of the nineteenth century Italian neurologist Cesare Lombroso. His classic *L'Uomo delinquente* (1896–97) described the concept of a criminal type or "born criminal" and led to eugenic suggestions of preventive incarceration based on physiological measurements. The work of Goffman (1986) and Hobbs (1978) also provide ample evidence that applying an "at-risk" label to a child may lead to significant adverse future consequences.

Pine, Wasserman, and their colleagues acknowledge their failure to study white delinquents as a limitation of their work. This limitation raises additional issues of distributive justice, described below. However, we do not know whether local juvenile justice authorities or the parents of the boys participating in the study came to view those children as prone to future problems. We have no way to know whether racial or social class stereotypes about youth violence in the minds of the families and authorities became heightened as a result of the "at-risk" designation applied in the course of the study. We also do not know whether the boys in the study came to view themselves as being like, hence as likely to emulate, their older incarcerated brothers as a result of the invitation they received to participate in the study.

Distributive Justice

OPRR investigated a total of four studies conducted in the New York City area using the fenfluramine challenge paradigm. Federal regulations currently allow some "greater-than-minimal-risk" research with children who may potentially benefit (45 CFR 46.101–124, 45 CFR 46.405) and with children who have a disorder or condition because of the need to develop knowledge about that disorder or condition (45 CFR 46.406). Some confusion exists about what constitutes "a condition." OPRR determined that in two of the four studies (not under Dr. Pine's direction), the consent forms were inadequate in describing reasonably foreseeable risks and discomforts (Halperin, Newcorn, Kopestein, 1997; Halperin, Newcorn, Schwartz, et al., 1997). The participants in those two studies (except for four normal controls) all had attention deficit hyperactivity disorder (ADHD) and their ethnicity and race were not specified.

As an aside, it seems worth noting that participants with ADHD in two of the studies had to abstain from taking the medication prescribed for the ADHD for up to 4 weeks prior to the study. Presumably, these children performed less well in school or became more likely to experience behavioral problems during the interval in which they abstained from taking the medication. Some might regard such abstention as incremental risk, beyond a normal month's experience in the lives of the children.

The application of these principles to competent adults is fairly straightforward, since adults generally have the ability to assess risks and benefits and advocate for themselves. In the case of children, the application of these principles becomes much more difficult. Special recommendations and federal regulations have been developed to govern the ethics of research with children (45 CFR 46.401–409). Generally accepted practice has dictated that when IRBs follow the federal regulations, and when parents have full information about risks and benefits of the research, then parents may grant permission for their children's participation.

A Maryland Court of Appeals decision recently stated that, regardless of parental permission, a child may not be allowed to participate in research unless it is in the child's best interests to do so (*Grimes v. Kennedy Krieger Institute, Inc.*, 2001). The Grimes decision seems to preclude involvement of a child in any research that does not promise benefit to that child. In a later clarification, the Court of Appeals acknowledged that nonbeneficial "minimal risk" research (i.e., involving risks comparable to those encountered in the everyday lives of ordinary children) might be allowable (*Grimes v. Kennedy Krieger Institute, Inc.*, 2001b; Kopelman, 2002).

Research involving healthy children clearly poses complex ethical and social dilemmas. In order to develop medical or behavioral treatments and practices that protect and benefit children as a group, it may be methodologically desirable to conduct some research using healthy children who will not directly benefit. At the same time, the health and well-being of individual child participants in research must be protected (for review, see Tauer, 1999; also Kopelman, 2000). Similar tensions occur in research with other populations where individuals' decisional capacity may be impaired, such as the severely mentally ill (Shamoo and Keay 1996; Shamoo and O'Sullivan, 1998).

The current American Psychological Association's ethical code (American Psychological Association, 2002) cautions psychologists to take note that special safeguards may be necessary to protect the rights and welfare of persons or communities whose vulnerabilities impair autonomous decision making. The code also calls for attempts to eliminate the effect of biases based on factors such as cultural, individual, and role differences, including those based on age, gender, gender identity, race, ethnicity, culture, national origin, religion, sexual orientation, disability, language, and socioeconomics when working with members of such groups. Psychologist are discouraged from knowingly participating in or condoning activities of others based upon such prejudices. These standards did not specifically apply to the fenfluramine challenge studies, as they were not adopted until 2002, but they do articulate a way of framing and thinking about distributive justice issues.

In each of the studies, young boys had the drug fenfluramine administered in order to investigate possible correlations between serotonergic activity and aggression. While some of the subjects had previously displayed aggressive behavior, others were identified only because of possible risk factors for aggression; for example, having a sibling who was incarcerated, or adverse rearing circumstances such as parental substance abuse or harsh rearing practices (Halperin, Newcorn, Kopestein, et al. 1997; Halperin, Newcorn, Schwartz, et al., 1997; Pine et al., 1996, 1997). In this context, the failure of investigators to study a racially, ethnically, and socioeconomically diverse group of children constitutes an ethical failure as well as a methodological limitation.

To the extent that population sampling inadequacies contribute to findings that support adverse social stereotypes or misleading attributions applicable to a particular group, distributive justice issues arise. Researchers who defend such limitations with answers such as, "These participants are typical of the neighborhood," or, "We could not get access to the younger siblings of white juvenile offenders in other communities," miss the point. For example, suppose that the same investigators given access to sealed case information from African-American and Hispanic youth in New York City had attempted to get access to similar data from suburban Long Island or affluent Westchester County where a greater percentage of the population and juvenile offenders are white. Would the juvenile authorities in those neighborhoods have furnished the same confidential data obtained on the children of color? If not, what does that fact tell us about the degree of fairness and justice afforded the less affluent minority families? Research of such limited scope may serve to magnify stereotypes by cloaking them behind a scientific aura rationalized by citing convenient access to potential participants and acknowledging limitations. Sadly, discussion of full implications of study limitations seldom appears in abstracts and subsequent citations of the work.

CONCLUSION

The investigators who conducted this study are serious behavioral and biomedical people with worthy research goals. They followed procedures specified by the research oversight authorities of their institution and did not cause known or measurable harm to any identifiable people. They did, however, gain access to data that should have remained confidential, offered substantial inducements to elicit participation by impoverished children, took advantage of power and social position to recruit participants, and put healthy child participants at some medical and psychosocial risk with no chance of direct benefit. They did all this to conduct a study with trivial statistical power, inadequate control participants, and highly questionable generalizability but significant potential to perpetuate social stereotypes. Nonetheless, the study survived peer review and attained publication. The reader is left to determine the ethical propriety of the fenfluramine challenge study.

Questions for Discussion

1. According to this chapter, one of the investigators in the study recalled, "The only ethical concern of the IRB was whether the mothers would agree to anything in exchange for money. They (i.e., the IRB) wanted to give all the money to the kids in the form of gift certificates." Can you identify ethical concerns beyond the issue of compensation? Had you

been the investigator, what strategy would you propose to assure that compensation did not distort parental decision making?

2. Do you think the right to privacy of the potential participants' siblings and their families was violated by probation authorities? Does the fact that the juvenile probation authorities provided the investigators with confidential and socially sensitive data mitigate the culpability of the investigators for the breach of confidentiality?

3. In terms of putting coercive pressure on the participants' families:
   a. How significant is the fact that the child participants' parents knew the probation department had cooperated in making their names available to the investigators?
   b. How significant is the fact that the investigators had long term relationship with the participants' families?
   c. Would these factors be more likely to contribute to or ameliorate coercive pressure?

4. According to the author of this chapter, how did the following effect the decision to participate in the study:
   a. The way in which the participants' parents were approached?
   b. The social status of the investigators who approached the families?
   c. The type of incentive offered to the participants?
   Do you support the author's opinion?

5. How does the fact that 36% of those invited into the study either did not agree to enroll or dropped out prior to the drug challenge impact your opinion of the quality of the informed consent process that took place? Does this prove that the 64% who did complete their participation made a free and voluntary consent decision?

6. Do you think the attendance of caring assistants, nearby family members, and distractions such as television and games supports the assertion that investigators' provided for the boys' emotional support, or do these collateral benefits make you concerned about some degree of coercion?

7. How significant is the concern about stigmatization that may be associated with describing certain children as being "at risk" and therefore eligible for the fenfluramine challenge study? Did the investigators do anything to address that concern in this case?

8. What is the appropriate balance between the need to develop medical or behavioral treatments that benefit children as a group and the need to protect the health and well-being of individual child research participants? How does your ethical analysis of the fenfluramine challenge study influence your answer?

9. Had the current American Psychological Association's ethical code been adopted prior to the fenfluramine challenge studies, would you determine

that the studies were conducted in violation of the code? Why or why not?

10. Do you think the investigators in the fenfluramine challenge studies acted in accordance with the principle of distributive justice?

11. Do you agree with the author's conclusion? How would you modify the study so that it meet the investigators' goals and yet be considered ethically permissible?

▬

Note

1. Informed consent can only be granted for oneself. Thus, when a parent or guardian is asked to authorize participation of a child in research the proper term is permission, rather than consent.

References

Achenbach, T. M. (1991). *Manual for the child behavior checklist/4–18 and 1991 profile*. Burlington, VT: University of Vermont.

American Psychological Association. (2002). Ethical principles of psychologists and code of conduct. *American Psychologist, 57*(12), 1060–1073.

Coccaro, E. F., Siever, L. J., Klar, H. M., Maurer, G., Cochrane, K., Cooper, T. B., Mohs R. C., & Davis, K. L. (1989). Serotonergic studies in patients with affective and personality disorders. Correlates with suicidal and impulsive aggressive behavior.

Connolly, H. M., Crary, J. L., McGoon, M. D., Henrud, D. D., Edwards, B. S., Edwards, W. D., et al. (1997). Valvular heart disease associated with fenfluramine-phentermine. *New England Journal of Medicine, 337*, 581–588.

Goffman, E. (1986). *Stigma: Notes on the Management of Spoiled Identity* (Re-issued Edition). New York: Touchstone Books.

Grimes v. Kennedy Krieger Institute, Inc., Circuit Court for Baltimore City. Case numbers 24-C-99-000925 (2001).

Guart, A. (1999, May 30). Mom: I was duped when son became "drug guinea pig." *New York Post,* p. 6.

Halperin, J. M., Newcorn, J. H., Kopestein, I., McKay, K. E., Schwartz, S. T., Siever, L. J., et al. (1997a). Serotonin, aggression, and parental psychopathology in children with attention-deficit hyperactivity disorder (ADHD). *Journal of the American Academy of Child and Adolescent Psychiatry, 56,* 1395–1398.

Halperin, J. M., Newcorn, J. H., Schwartz, S. T. Sharma, V., Siever, L. J., Koda, V. H., et al. (1997b). Age-related changes in the association between serotonergic function and aggression in boys with ADHD. *Biological Psychiatry, 41,* 682–689.

Hilts, J. (1998, April 15). Experiments on children are reviewed: Research involved now-banned drug. *New York Times,* p. B3.

Hobbs, N. (1978). The Future of Children: Categories, Labels, and Their Consequences. San Francisco: Jossey-Bass.

Kolata, G. (1997, September 16). Two popular diet pills are withdrawn from market. *New York Times,* p. A1.

Kopelman, L. M. (2000). Moral problems in assessing research risk. *IRB: A Review of Human Subjects Research, 22,* 7–10.

Kopelman, L. M. (2002). Group benefit and protection of pediatric research subjects: Grimes v. Kennedy Krieger and the lead abatement study. *Accountability in Research, 9,* 177–192.

Lombroso, C. (1896–97). *L'uomo delinquente.* (Transl. as *Criminal Man,* 5th ed., 1911,)

Montero, D. (1998, April 18). City aide aided recruit of drug-experiment kids. *New York Post,* p. 2.

Muldoon, M., Manuck, S. B., Jansma, C. L., Moore, A. L., & Mann, J. J. (1996). D,L-Fenfluramine challenge test: Experience in nonpatient sample. *Biological Psychiatry, 39,* 761–768.

Pine, D. S. (2003, July). Personal communication: Information on conduct of fenfluramine study.

Pine, D. S., Coplan, J. D., Wasserman, G. A., Miller, L. S., Fried, J. E., Davies, M., et al. (1997). Neuroendocrine response to fenfluramine challenge in boys. Associations with aggressive behavior and adverse rearing [Comment]. [Erratum appears in *Archives of General Psychiatry,* 1998, *55*(7), 625.] *Archives of General Psychiatry, 54*(9), 839–846.

Pine, D. S., Wasserman, G., Coplan, J., Fried, J. A., Huang, Y. Y., Kassir, S., et al. (1996). Platelet serotonin 2A (5-H T_{2A}) receptor characteristics and parenting factors for boys at risk for delinquency: A preliminary report. *American Journal of Psychiatry, 153,* 538–544.

Rosenthal, R., & Jacobson, L. (1968). *Pygmalion in the classroom.* New York: Rinehart and Winston.

Shaffer, D., Schwab-Stone, M., Fisher, P., Cohen, P. Piacentini, J., Davies, M., et al. (1993). The Diagnostic Interview Schedule for Children Revised Version (DISC-R): Preparation, field testing, inter-rater reliability, and acceptability. *Journal of the American Academy of Child and Adolescent Psychiatry, 32,* 643–650.

Shamoo, A. E., & Tauer, C. A. (2002). Ethically questionable research with children: The fenfluramine study. *Accountability in Research, 9,* 143–166.

Shamoo, A. E. and Keay, T. (1996). "Ethical Concerns about Relapse Studies. *Cambridge Quarterly of Health Care Ethics, 5,* 373–386.

Shamoo, A. E., and O'Sullivan, J. O. (1998). The Ethics of Research on the Mentally Disabled. In *Health Care Ethics: Critical Issues for the 21st Century,* Edited by Thomasma, D. C. and Monagle, J. Gaithersburg, Maryland: Aspen Publishers, 239–250.

Tauer, C. A. (1999). Testing drugs in pediatric populations: The FDA mandate. *Accountability in Research, 7,* 37–58.

Wasserman, G. A. (2003, July). Personal communication: Information on conduct of fenfluramine study.

Wasserman, G. A., & Pine, D. (2004. Letter to the author, dated May 27, 2004.

11

The Ethics of Predictive Genetic Testing in Prevention Trials Involving Adolescents

Gail Geller

CASE DESCRIPTION

You are an institutional review board (IRB) member at an academic medical center known for its advances in genetic research. You are asked to review two prevention protocols in which at-risk children/adolescents between the ages of 10 and 17 undergo predictive genetic testing.

One protocol focuses on minors with a family history of familial adenomatous polyposis of the colon (FAP), ascertained through their affected or at-risk parent. All adult patients at the cancer prevention clinic who are found to carry the risk-conferring APC (adenomatous polyposis coli) mutations would be invited to enroll their children in the study. Participants would first undergo APC testing (on a saliva sample) and learn their results. Then all mutation carriers would be assigned to a chemopreventive intervention with a drug that has been shown to reduce the risk of FAP in adults. The purpose of this study would be to determine if the risk:benefit ratio of the drug is as favorable in adolescents as it is in adults, and to assess the impact of the genotype information itself on the adolescents' psychological health and compliance with risk-reducing regimens.

The second protocol focuses on adolescents in the general population who might have an increased susceptibility to smoking-related behaviors (e.g., initiating, continuing, quitting smoking) and nicotine addiction. This protocol involves community-based recruitment strategies such as distributing leaflets in middle and high schools or posting advertisements in newspapers. Adolescents would be recruited before they start to smoke, and their saliva would be tested for genetic polymorphisms that increase their risk of initiating smoking and becoming addicted to nicotine. They would be told their test results and then participate in an intensive smoking prevention program. The purpose of the research would be to see if the genotype information, itself, has an impact on their compliance with and the success of the intervention. You realize that there are different ethical implications of each, but seek guidance about how to frame these differences. You are uncertain about whether the IRB should approve either of the protocols.

———

ETHICAL ANALYSIS AND DISCUSSION

Predictive genetic testing of children and adolescents for adult-onset disease or complex behavioral traits is likely to become an integral part of many types of intervention studies, including prevention trials. The existence of a preventive or therapeutic intervention is widely considered to be a necessary precondition of predictive genetic testing in children (American Academy of Pediatrics, 2001; ASHG Social Issues Committees, 1995) and, in the case of newborn screening, has provided moral justification for the disclosure of genetic results to families (Ross, 2003). However, it is not clear whether the inclusion of a prevention strategy in predictive genetics research involving older children and adolescents is sufficient to justify disclosure of genetic results to them. The existence of a preventive intervention may lead those reviewing the ethics of such studies to single-mindedly focus on the physical risks and benefits of the intervention itself, obscuring the risks and benefits of the genetic testing component of the research. The disclosure of genetic information is itself an intervention, accompanied by its own set of psychosocial and economic risks and potential benefits. This chapter considers the ethical implications of disclosing the results of predictive genetic testing as a part of prevention trials involving minor adolescents. The case of *newborn* genetic screening *in the absence of an intervention* is covered elsewhere in this book (Ross, 2003).

The chapter begins with a brief justification for the relevance and timeliness of this topic. Then it addresses the moral acceptability of the smoking prevention study described above. Next it compares the morally relevant characteristics of genetic susceptibility research that focuses on complex behaviors as compared to genetic studies of adult onset diseases. The chapter concludes with a discussion of threats to voluntary and informed decision making likely to arise in the conduct of adolescent prevention trials involving predictive genetic testing as well as strategies for dealing with those threats.

This chapter focuses on children older than 10 years, for several reasons. First, this is the age at which many children enter puberty. Changes in physical development and body image can be associated with changes in perceptions of vulnerability, risk, and health. Second, this is the age at which environmental exposures such as hormonal changes begin to interact with inherited predispositions (Ziegler, 1998), making this population a desirable target for those interested in genetic epidemiologic research. Third, this is the age at which parents seem to feel that children should be included in decisions about research participation, or should be told their genetic test results (Michie et al., 1996; Patenaude et al., 1996). Finally, empirical evidence indicates that children older than 10 have increasing capacity to engage in informed and voluntary decision making regarding research participation (Bruzzese & Fisher, 2003; Geller et al., 2003; Ondrusek et al., 1998; Petersen & Leffert, 1995; Santelli et al., 1995; Weithorn & Scherer, 1994).

The Timeliness of Gene-Based Pediatric Prevention Trials

The discovery of new genes and their functions can allow doctors to identify individual response to medications and will result in new disease management and prevention strategies. The tantalizing potential of pharmacogenetics represents a major medical breakthrough that will bring great benefits to patients in the 21st century. Careful research must be conducted before these benefits can be realized. Although the focus of genome research is currently on adults, these genetic discoveries will certainly affect children (Williams, 2000). There is general agreement that genetic tests should be evaluated in the context of clinical research before they are used routinely in clinical practice in order to establish efficacy and to avoid harm to the population (Holtzman & Watson, 1997). Therefore, children and adolescents who are at high risk of future disease because of their family history or who are at increased risk of developing potentially harmful behaviors or traits are increasingly likely to be considered for participation in genetic susceptibility research (Toriello, 2002). This trend will be promoted by the identification of greater numbers of susceptibility-conferring mutations (Collins, 1999), evidence that risk factors during childhood are related to the development of several adult-onset diseases (Berenson et al., 1998; Berkey, Frazier, Gardner, & Colditz 1999; Ziegler, 1998), the federal mandate to include children in clinical research (National Institutes of Health, 1998), and the American Academy of Pediatrics (2001) call for additional research on testing for late-onset conditions in the pediatric population.

To date, there has been a paucity of empirical research involving children from high-risk families (Geller et al., 2003). Most of these studies have explored the psychological effect on children of testing family members for susceptibility to adult-onset disease (Fanos, 1997; Michie, Bobrow, & Marteau, 2001; Petersen & Leffert, 1995; Tercyak et al., 2001a; Tercyak, Peshken, Streisand, & Lerman, 2001b) or of being tested themselves (Codori, Petersen, Boyd, Brandt, & Grardello, 1996; Codori et al., 2003). One study explored at-risk children's perceptions of the benefits and harms of participating in genetic susceptibility research (Bernhardt, Tambor, Fraser, Wissow, & Geller, 2003; Geller, Tambor, Bernhardt, Wissow, & Fraser, 2000) and the role that at-risk children would play in making decisions about research participation (Geller et al., 2003).

Now, and for years to come, research involving genetic testing, followed by preventive or therapeutic interventions, is likely to be proposed for genetically susceptible children to reduce future morbidity. A chemoprevention study of the efficacy of sulindac (a nonsteroidal anti-inflammatory) in reducing risk of FAP, a condition that invariably leads to colon cancer, has already been conducted among children who carry mutations on the risk-conferring APC gene (Giardiello et al., 2002). Similar studies using COX-2 inhibitors are likely to follow based on promising results in studies of adults (Steinbach et al., 2000). It is easy to imagine several other examples of this kind of research. For example, children with elevated lipid levels, who are often misclassified based on cholesterol levels alone (Humphries, Galton, & Nicholls, 1997), could be enrolled in prevention research in which they would be tested for mutations in the low-density lipoprotein receptor gene and randomized to various interventions such as dietary and lifestyle modifications (Obarzanek et al., 2001; Shamir & Fisher, 2000) or lipid-lowering medications (Humphries et al., 1997). Similarly, adolescent girls from families with BRCA1 or BRCA2 mutations could be recruited into a study in which they undergo BRCA1/2 testing themselves, and mutation carriers would then be randomized to a dietary or lifestyle intervention or a tamoxifen-like drug (Bernhardt et al., 2003; Geller et al., 2000).

Recent developments in human behavioral genetics (ASHG Statement, 1997) could lead to research scenarios involving several common complex traits that are highly prevalent in children and have potentially significant health consequences. For example, there is ample evidence that attention deficit hyperactivity disorder (ADHD) has a strong genetic component (Biederman &Faraone, 2002) and that dopamine transporter and receptor genes are implicated in its pathogenesis (Anderson & Cook, 2000; DiMaio, Gruzenko, & Joober, 2003). One can easily imagine a study that assesses the impact of population-based testing of children for susceptibility to ADHD followed by preventive interventions that are tailored to children with the risk-conferring genotype. Obesity is another behavioral trait that is increasingly prevalent among adolescents, associated with type II diabetes and other adult-onset diseases and partially attributable to mutations in the leptin (O'Rahilly, 2002), melanocortin 4 receptor (Farooqi et al., 2003), APOE4 (Feigenbaum & Hutz, 2003), and UPC3 (Kimm et al., 2002) genes. Early identification of certain genetic polymorphisms in children at risk of obesity may influence their responsiveness to dietary interventions (Vincent et al., 2002) or to pharmacologic treatments (Bickerdike, 2003).

The ethics of enrolling adolescents in prevention research involving genetic susceptibility testing are described below, beginning with the smoking case (Wilfond, Geller, Lerman, Audrain-McGovern, & Shields, 2002).

Background on Smoking Prevalence and Genetic Influences

Decades of clinical research and intensive public health efforts have failed to dislodge smoking from its position as the lead cause of preventable death in the United States (McGinnis & Foege, 1993). Most adult smokers begin smoking before the age of 18 (Office of Smoking and Health, 1994), and two-thirds of adolescents try smoking, continue to smoke, or attempt to quit (or some combination thereof; Johnston, O'Malley, & Bachman, 2001; CDC, 2002). A substantial number of these adolescents have shown symptoms of nicotine addiction (Colby, Tiffany, Shiffman, & Niaura, 2000; Stanton, 1995). Despite considerable knowledge about the psychological, social, and environmental components of adolescent smoking, studies such as that of Sussman, Lichtman, Ritt, and Pallonen, (1999) show that efforts thus far to prevent adolescents from smoking and to help them quit have not been very successful.

Researchers are now turning their attention to genetic factors, a stance consistent with the large-scale public health goal of understanding gene-gene and gene-environment interactions and their impact on health and disease (Sternberg, Gwinn, & Khoury, 2001). In the specific case of smoking, genes related to dopaminergic and serotonin pathways, as well as genes related to nicotine metabolism, contribute to the tendency to smoke and the ability to quit; ongoing studies will further our understanding of genotype-phenotype relationships for smoking behavior (Lerman & Berrettini, 2002). Studies are also being proposed to test adolescents for genetic susceptibility to smoking-related health consequences (Thelin, Sveger, & McNeil, 1996). Although adolescents have been enrolled in studies addressing the role of genetics in smoking behavior, these studies have not revealed information on genetic status to participants (Audrain & Tercyak, 2002). The involvement of adolescents in research on smoking has received some support on ethical grounds (Moolchan & Mermelstein, 2002), but the moral justifiability of targeting adolescents for smoking prevention research in which genetic information is disclosed to them requires more attention and further analysis.

The Ethics of Including Adolescents in Gene-Based Smoking Prevention Trials

There is little controversy about whether it is morally acceptable to enroll adolescents in smoking prevention trials that are not based on genotype. That the vast majority of smokers begin smoking in adolescence supports the wisdom of including adolescents in such trials, both in terms of efficient use of resources and potential to reduce the public health burden. Furthermore, the physiological, psychological, and social characteristics of adolescents differ from adults to a degree that can make findings from adult studies meaningless for the adolescent population (Cohn, Macfarlane, & Yanez, 1995; Murray, 2000; Skinner, Chapman, & Baltes, 1988). For example, differences in vulnerability to peer pressure and social acceptability of a particular behavior may make it impossible to predict adolescents' compliance with a preventive intervention from studies of adults' compliance with that intervention.

More debatable, however, is whether including genetic susceptibility testing as part of a smoking prevention trial for adolescents *and* disclosing the results to participants changes the moral analysis. One argument against conducting gene-based smoking prevention studies of adolescents is that only those identified as having certain genetic traits would have access to the intervention (Wilfond et al., 2002). A greater percentage of adolescents would benefit from efforts aimed at modifying their social environment, regardless of their genotype. Moreover, environmental approaches would not pose the same social risks as those associated with genetic testing for complex behaviors, such as stigmatization and/or discrimination against teens identified with specific smoking-associated genetic variants. My colleagues and I have argued elsewhere (Wilfond et al., 2002) that adolescents should be excluded from genotype-based smoking prevention trials, at least until studies of adults have provided sufficient information about the likelihood or magnitude of benefits and risks of disclosing genetic information to participants. Our arguments are based on a determination that the social risks to individuals currently outweigh the public health or individual benefits.

Assessment of Risks to Adolescents of Genotype-Based Smoking Prevention Trials

In the case of research on inherited susceptibility to disease or complex traits, characterization of risk is more complicated than the physical risks of drawing blood, which would be considered "minimal risk." The risks of genetic information are primarily psychosocial; some of them may be ordinarily encountered in the daily life of minor adolescents (e.g., changes in self-image), and some may not (e.g., fear of future disease, potential loss of insurance coverage). Most of these risks center around stigma and discrimination.

The major social risks of information regarding one's genetic susceptibility to complex behaviors such as smoking stem from the socially sensitive nature of the behavior, the extent to which it pits personal responsibility (O'Brien & McLellan, 1996; McLellan, Lewis, O'Brien, & Kleber, 2000) against determinism (Arnold et al., 1995; Mann, 1994), and the degree to which the genetic polymorphisms are associated with other stigmatizing conditions or behaviors. This phenomenon of pleiotropy, in which a single gene has multiple phenotypic effects, has received little attention in the ethics literature (Wachbroit, 1998). Although the best-known example is the association of APOE4 mutations with both premature heart disease and Alzheimer's disease, pleiotropy also has relevance in the context of behavioral genetics.

Genes involved in dopamine and serotonin regulation, which have been a primary focus of the research on the genetics of smoking, have also been associated with risk for substance abuse more generally, including addiction to cocaine and alcohol use (Blum et al., 1990; Comings et al., 1999; Lichtermann et al., 2000; Matsushita et al., 2001; Noble, 2000), as well as a number of psychiatric conditions, for example, Tourette's syndrome (Comings et al., 1997), anxiety (Lesch et al., 1996), ADHD (Comings, Muhlcman, & Gysin, 1996; Muglia, Jain, Macciardi, & Kennedy, 2000), posttraumatic stress disorder (Comings et al., 1997), obsessive-compulsive disorder (Blum et al., 1995; Rowe et al., 1998), depression and suicide (Bellivier et al., 1998; Nielsen et al., 1998; Ogilvie et al., 1996). Genetic information relating to behaviors such as substance abuse and psychiatric disorders may be far more stigmatizing than genetic susceptibility to smoking (Davies, 2000; Link, Struening, Rahav, Phelan, & Nuttbrock, 1997; Link, Phelan, Bresnahan, Stueve, & Pescosolido, 1999; Phelan, Bromet, & Link, 1998; Ritson, 1999). Concerns about the stigma of psychiatric disorders led a National Institute of Mental Health workshop to conclude that prevention research on "at-risk" individuals was ethically questionable (Heinssen, Perkins, Applebaum, & Fenton, 2001).

Adult smokers already face possible discrimination in insurance, employment, and social acceptability (Burris, 2002). Could identification of smoking-related genes with pleiotropic effects lead to greater discrimination in these areas in the future (Garnick, Hendricks, Comstock, & Horgan, 1997; Hudson, Rothenberg, Andrews, Kahn, & Collins, 1995)? Or could genetic information become a mitigating factor in the explanation of and attitudes toward nicotine addiction? Given the current, relatively primitive understanding of pleiotropy and genotype-phenotype relationships in complex behaviors, the former scenario seems more likely: Compared with participants in smoking studies that yield information only about the risk for health consequences, participants in studies that reveal genetic information with potentially stigmatizing pleiotropic associations incur additional risks (Wilfond et al., 2002).

Further complicating these concerns is the possibility of racial variation in some of these polymorphisms. For example, preliminary evidence suggests that variants of two particular genes that are protective against nicotine addiction are more prevalent among Caucasians (Lerman et al., 1997). As a result, racial minorities may be at higher genetic risk for the development of nicotine addiction. Racial variation has also been observed in genes associated with increased susceptibility to obesity, with African-American women being at greater risk (Cooper

& Luke, 2003; Kimm et al., 2002). Although scientific evidence is mounting against the use of race to distinguish between certain groups (Collins & Mansoura, 2001), studies of human genetic variation in common polymorphisms may continue to categorize people by race. With the laudable intention of reducing racial disparities in health outcomes, African-American adolescents, who are already marginalized and stigmatized, may become targets of genotype-based prevention research.

Adolescents in our culture face the twin tasks of developing a positive self-image and a belief in their ability to shape the future. Telling them (and others) that they are at risk for addiction and/or health complications of smoking may harm them in both respects (Cohn et al., 1995; Davis, 1997; Murray, 2000; Skinner et al., 1988). "At-risk" children and adolescents may perceive themselves differently from counterparts who have no known inherited susceptibility to diseases or to complex traits, or from those who are already ill. How these differences in perception manifest themselves is likely to affect "at-risk" adolescents' willingness to participate in research on susceptibility to future disease as well as the impact of such participation on their well-being.

Senior, Marteau, and Peters (1999) express concern that the "geneticization" of society may lead to increased fatalism, adversely affecting motivation to change behavior in order to reduce health risks. In the case of adolescents and smoking, such fatalism could lead to two undesirable outcomes: On the one hand, teens who are told they have a genetic risk of nicotine addiction may become deterministic and abandon attempts to quit; on the other, those who are told they are not at genetic risk may mistakenly assume that they can smoke without ever developing a serious habit. The very information intended to promote healthy behavior could therefore have the exact opposite effect (Wilfond et al., 2002).

In light of the paucity of available evidence about the nature and degree of risk to adolescents of participating in genotype-based smoking prevention trials, it is difficult to determine whether this research represents a minor increase over minimal risk or more than minimal risk. The guidelines of the National Institutes of Health NIH 45 CFR 46 (2001) stipulate that children should be excluded from research if "insufficient data are available in adults to judge potential risk in children." Assigning the appropriate regulatory category under 45 CFR 46 subpart D (2001) is made even more difficult by all that is unknown about the prospect of direct benefit. Therefore, proposals to enroll adolescents in genotype-based smoking prevention trials should not be approved under subpart D 405 or 406 until we have more information about the nature and degree of potential risks and benefits.

Assessment of Benefits to Adolescents of Genotype-Based Smoking Prevention Trials

In order for adolescents who participate in gene-based prevention trials to benefit from disclosure of their genotype, two conditions would have to be met. First, the genotype–phenotype relationships would have to be fairly strong. This ability to predict particular behaviors given the presence of certain genes is known as clinical validity. Second, there would have to be persuasive evidence that relaying information about one's genotype leads to significant behavioral change. The positive impact of the information on one's behavior is known as clinical utility. In the case of gene based prevention trials involving adolescents, there is insufficient evidence of clinical validity or clinical utility.

Studies of twins suggest that heritable factors may account for about 50% of the variance in the initiation of smoking and about 70% in the progression to nicotine dependence. Some studies have linked smoking behavior to genetic variation in the dopamine pathway (Lerman et al., 1999; Sabol et al., 1999), but such findings have been inconsistent (Bierut et al., 2000; Jorm et al., 2000). Other studies have focused on the serotonin pathway and found some associations there with likelihood of starting to smoke and with the age at which smoking begins (Sullivan & Kendler, 1999; Lerman et al., 2001). Nevertheless, taken together these and other studies provide only tentative understanding of the complex genotype-phenotype associations involved in smoking and do not meet the criterion of robustness for the utility of genetic information in clinical research (Lerman & Berrettini, 2002). Even in the case of a robust genotype–phenotype relationship, data from other contexts indicate that a person's knowledge of such a relationship does not necessarily alter smoking behaviors. Piitulainen and Sveger (1998) found that informing children and their parents of the robust link between alpha-1 antitrypsin deficiency (ATD) and early-onset emphysema in smokers did not reduce smoking behaviors. Yet proposals have been made to screen preadolescents for ATD to prevent adolescent smoking (Sveger, Piitulainen, & Arborelius,1995; Thelin et al., 1996). (It should be noted that studies of adults have failed to show much evidence of a positive impact of genetic information about smoking-related disease susceptibility on the rate of quitting [Audrain et al., 1997; Lerman et al., 1997; McBride et al., 2002].)

In contexts other than that of smoking, genetic information has been shown to have limited impact on behavior in children. In the case of phenylketonuria, while dietary interventions are effective in maintaining phenylalanine levels within an acceptable range to avoid neurocognitive effects, adolescents do not always stay on the diet. In a recent study from the United Kingdom, approximately 70% of children younger than 10 years were able to keep their phenylalanine levels in the acceptable range, but this decreased to approximately 20% for adolescents older than 15 years age (Walter et al., 2002). Thus, even when a clearly genetic disorder is manifest *and* an effective intervention exists, adolescents may not comply. Adolescents may be even less likely to comply with a smoking prevention intervention when the evidence of increased genetic risk of smoking is less clear.

Balancing Benefits and Risks

Regulations promulgated by the U.S. Department of Health and Human Services prohibit research that exposes children to more than a minor increase over minimal risk unless there is a "prospect of direct benefit" to the subject that justifies the risk (U.S. Department of Health and Human Services, 1991). However, it is quite difficult to weigh risks and benefits when one is trying to prevent a disease of indeterminate likelihood (Roth, 2001). The attraction of using genetic information in prevention studies of adolescent smoking lies in its potential to ease this seemingly intractable problem. However, in accordance with the letter and spirit of the regulations as well as with common sense, there is no justification for exposing adolescents to more than minimal risk by including them in genetically based prevention trials that have not yet been shown to be effective in improving the public health of adult smokers. My colleagues and I have argued elsewhere (Wilfond et al., 2002) that initial gene-based smoking intervention research should target adult smokers because of a more favorable risk:benefit ratio. Since smokers are already engaged in a behavior with significant health risks, the potential direct benefit to them is likely to be greater. Moreover, the harms stemming from discrimination may be less of a concern for smokers who already face significant discrimination. Only after adult studies have provided greater clarity about risk:benefit ratios should prevention trials involving adolescents be initiated. These prevention trials should first be conducted in young adults between the ages of 18 and 25 before enrolling minor adolescents. As we have previously stated (Wilfond et al., 2002), members of this age group are old enough to make their own decisions, but young enough to still be at risk of beginning to smoke.

Ethical Differences Between Predictive Genetic Testing for Complex Traits Versus Diseases

The smoking case described above stands in stark contrast to the scenario of enrolling minors at increased risk of FAP in gene-based disease prevention trials. A comparison of these two cases highlights the ethical differences between predictive genetic testing for complex traits or behaviors more generally and predictive genetic testing for susceptibility to disease. Table 1 provides examples of some of the morally relevant characteristics associated with susceptibility tests for three diseases (FAP, common adult-onset cancers such as those of the breast, and heart disease) and two complex traits (obesity and smoking). These differences influence our judgments about whether it is justified to include or even target children and adolescents in prevention research involving genetic susceptibility testing.

One of the most notable differences is the prevalence and penetrance of the risk-conferring mutations. The prevalence of mutations associated with an increased susceptibility to complex traits is high. However, although these single-nucleotide polymorphisms (SNPs) are, by definition, common in the general population, the degree to which they express themselves phenotypically (e.g., their penetrance) is small. By contrast, disease-susceptibility mutations are rare, but when present have a relatively high likelihood of causing disease. These differences in prevalence and penetrance influence the clinical validity (sensitivity, specificity, and predictive value) and utility of the genetic test (Holtzman & Watson, 1997), as well as the moral acceptability of targeting certain populations for

TABLE 11.1 Morally Relevant Characteristics
of Genetic Susceptibility Tests in Minor Adolescents

	FAP	Breast cancer	Heart disease	Smoking or obesity
Prevalence of mutation?	Low	Low	High	High
Penetrance of mutation?	High	High-moderate	Low	Low
Does disease/trait occur in adolescence?	Yes	No	No	Yes
Fear of mortality/ severity	High	High	Moderate	Low
Is there an effective preventative intervention?	Yes	Unknown or risky	Exists but ? efficacy	Exists but ? efficacy
Pleiotrophy?	No	No	Yes	Yes
Variable prevalence of particular mutations?	I1307K[a] > in Jews	Higher in Jews?	Higher in African Americans?	Higher in African Americans?

[a] Unlike most mutations on the APC gene that are associated with the development of FAP, this is a polymorphism of low penetrance that does not lead to FAP. Nevertheless, it is associated with an increased risk of other forms of familial colorectal cancer, and is more prevalent among Jews (Lynch & de la Chapelle, 1999).

research. For example, screening the general population of adolescents for susceptibility to FAP would never be justified because APC mutations are extremely rare. Thus, even though APC mutations are virtually 100% penetrant (e.g., all carriers will develop the disease), the likelihood of identifying carriers in the general population would be very low. By contrast, population-based screening of adolescents for SNPs associated with complex behaviors may identify large numbers of young people at increased risk, but the poor predictive value of positive test results would render the risk:benefit ratio unfavorable.

In determining the moral acceptability of gene-based prevention trials involving children and adolescents, other considerations include the age at which the condition actually manifests itself, how prospective participants are likely to view the severity and preventability of these conditions, and how effective risk-reducing interventions are. Although FAP and smoking often occur during adolescence, these phenotypes have very different effects on lifespan and quality of life. Given the variability in adolescents' perceptions about the heritability, seriousness, and preventability of disease in general (Michielutte & Diseker, 1982; Ponder, Lee, Green, & Richards, 1996), it is likely that such variation exists in adolescents' perceptions of FAP and of smoking.

Moreover, in the case of FAP, interventions can be offered to participants *while they are teenagers* that will alter their chances of developing the disease. Even in the context of providing clinical care, there is general consensus that testing children and adolescents for FAP is morally justified, based on a determination that the benefits of testing outweigh the harms. Because the polyps actually develop during adolescence, colonoscopies, if started early, can identify the polyps in enough time to intervene and forestall the development of the disease. Moreover, children who are found *not* to carry the risk-conferring mutations are spared the burden and risk of frequent and uncomfortable screening (ASHG Social Issues Committees, 1995; Clayton, 1995; Kodish, 1999; Marteau, 1994; Wertz, Fanos, & Reilly, 1994). In light of the moral acceptability of *clinical* genetic testing of children for FAP susceptibility, it is ethically acceptable to enroll at-risk children in gene-based chemoprevention *research,* particularly if evidence exists from studies of adults that the chemopreventive agent is effective in reducing the risk of developing FAP. This was the case for the sulindac trial (Giardiello et al., 2002).

With respect to the more common adult-onset diseases, evidence of available and effective risk-reducing interventions in adults does not provide moral justification for enrolling at-risk minors in gene-based chemoprevention trials. These diseases, by definition, do not manifest themselves during adolescence. Since there may be significant physical risks associated with the interventions themselves, and psychosocial risks associated with disclosure of genetic information, enrolling young people in such trials would mean subjecting them to greater than minimal risk without the prospect of direct or immediate benefit. In contrast to common adult-onset diseases, complex behaviors do often become manifest early in life and low-risk behavioral interventions do exist. However, it is not clear whether these interventions are effective or whether their efficacy is influenced by knowledge of one's genotype.

Additional factors to consider in determining the moral acceptability of enrolling adolescents in gene-based prevention trials are the extent to which pleiotropy exists and whether there is racial or ethnic variation in the prevalence of the mutation or polymorphism. In the case of FAP testing, there is little if any evidence of pleiotropy. Genes associated with smoking or obesity, on the other hand, are known to have pleiotropic associations. In addition, racial variation in some of the polymorphisms associated with an increased susceptibility to complex traits may exacerbate the risks of stigma and discrimination already experienced among minority subgroups of the adolescent population.

There are considerable parallels between the criteria listed above and several of the principles of population screening (Burke, Coughlin, Lee, Weed, & Khoury, 2001). For example, the "condition" (e.g., disease or trait) should be an important one in the particular population (e.g., adolescents), a suitable (e.g., clinically valid) test should be available, and an accepted treatment (e.g., intervention) should be available for people with the recognized condition. Application of these stringent criteria to assessments of gene-based prevention research involving adolescents will facilitate the determination of their moral acceptability.

Once it is determined to be ethically acceptable to include minor adolescents in gene-based prevention studies, ethical questions and concerns will arise about adolescents' ability to engage in a valid and meaningful informed consent process. The main threats to informed and voluntary decision making by adolescents are their capacity to understand the risks of the research and their vulnerability to undue influences to enroll in research (Levine, 1995; Nelson, 1998; Santelli et al., 1995; Weithorn & Scherer, 1994). Although these threats apply when children and adolescents are enrolled in any kind of research, there are some unique aspects of these concerns in the specific case of studies that employ genetic testing (Knoppers, Avard, Cardinal, & Glass, 2002; Weir & Horton, 1995).

Factors That Influence Informed and Voluntary Decision Making by At-Risk Adolescents

Research in which at-risk adolescents undergo predictive genetic testing may present particular challenges to the informed consent process because of the adolescent's incomplete or inaccurate understanding of heredity and disease, the probabilistic nature of genetic information, and that information's potential value for and impact on the entire family (Bernhardt et al., 2003; Geller et al., 1997; Ponder et al., 1996; Richards, 1998). Moreover, studies of parental perceptions of informed consent for research involving children suggest that adults are relatively poor judges of children's ability to understand explanations of an illness or event (Harth & Thong, 1995). This tendency is worrisome in the context of recruiting adolescents to participate in research (Scherer & Reppucci, 1988). The vulnerability of minors is particularly important in research that provides genetic information because of the potential for psychological harm (Codori et al., 1996, 2003) and the unknown likelihood of social harm associated with being labeled "at risk."

Another concern is the extent to which adolescents will be subjected to undue influences from others. Although the potential for undue influence is a risk in any research involving minors, there may be added risk of undue influence by parents and other family members in genetics research precisely because genetics is a "family affair." However, the degree of added risk of undue influence in genetics research turns on two issues: whether genetic test results will be disclosed to the participant as part of the research, and how involved the minor would be in deciding to participate in a given study.

Adolescents are more likely to be involved in informed consent discussions than younger children and their opinions given more weight because they are farther along in cognitive and emotional development (Miller, 2000; Rich et al., 2000). However, most studies involving minors have been limited to populations of *un*healthy children participating in clinical/therapeutic research (Broome, 1999; Broome, 2003; Broome et al., 2001; Michie et al., 2001; Susman, Dorn, & Fletcher, 1992) or psychosocial research (Miller, 2000; Rich, Lamola, Gordon, & Chalfen, 2000) as opposed to populations of genetically at risk but currently healthy older children and adolescents (e.g., those between 10 and 17 years of age). It is important to understand how they would assess the benefits and risks of participating in studies that disclose information to them about their genetic susceptibility to diseases and/or complex traits.

Evidence from families at increased risk of breast cancer or premature heart disease suggest that at-risk children older than 10 years are capable of thinking about the implications of receiving genetic test results, and are able to apply their own assessment of the relative balance of risks and benefits to making a decision about participating in a hypothetical study involving predictive genetic testing (Bernhardt et al., 2003; Geller et al., 2000). Some children think positive genetic test results would make them worry, while others think they would benefit in the long run by knowing. Many children would only want to know their test results if there was something that could be done to prevent the condition from occurring. Children are also able to consider the ramifications of disclosing their test results to others. While some children think that being labeled as genetically at-risk could lead to stigmatization, others believe the sharing of test results could increase intimacy and support from family and friends. Such assessments of risks and benefits take time and often require some probing. If the assent of the minor to participate in gene-based prevention research is accepted without encouraging him/her to think about test implications, it is unlikely that the assent would be truly informed (Bernhardt et al., 2003).

Evidence also suggests that parents from at-risk families are interested in involving their older children in decision making about research participation. However, the degree to which parents include their adolescents in decision making varies, in part, according to the whether the research is therapeutic or nontherapeutic. The more ambiguous the benefit, as is the case in prevention research generally and genetic testing research in particular, the more decision-making authority the minor adolescent would have. Parents are likely to defer to their adolescent children regarding decisions about participation in "nontherapeutic" genetic susceptibility research (Geller et al., 2003). By contrast, gene-based studies that offer adolescents the opportunity to participate in a preventive intervention might be perceived by parents as having potential benefits for their adolescents. Parents are thus more likely to encourage their children to participate in such studies or to override their children's refusal (Bernhardt et al., 2003; Geller et al., 2000, 2003).

Even in studies that offer preventive interventions, there may be differences in the degree of adolescents' "veto" power depending on the nature of the targeted disease or trait. The more severe or the less preventable the condition, the more parents might want to enroll their children in research that is thought to provide benefit. For example, parents from families with a high incidence of breast cancer, who perceive few effective preventive or therapeutic options, would be more willing to subject their daughters to research-related risks if the child's own risk of developing the disease was high and a preventive intervention was being offered. By contrast, parents from so-called heart disease families, who tend to think there are several effective preventive and therapeutic options outside of research participation, would be less willing to subject their children to research-related risks even if the child's own risk of developing the disease was high (Geller et al., 2003).

Two other aspects of the familial nature of genetic information render the informed consent process for enrolling minors in gene-based prevention research more challenging. First, at-risk minors are often concerned about the disease that runs in their family and might perceive research participation as a way to benefit their relatives. Indeed, a substantial minority of at-risk minors would be motivated to participate in gene-based research for altruistic reasons (Bernhardt et al., 2003). This motivation may be even stronger among children whose parents are actually affected with the condition than among those whose parents are at higher risk (Geller et al., 2000).

Second, genetic information about adolescents has potential relevance for the parents themselves. In the case of gene-based smoking prevention trials, parents might derive some personal benefit from knowing more about their family's susceptibility to nicotine addiction or risk of lung cancer. In the case of gene-based disease prevention trials, parents might want to know if the disease-conferring mutation that runs in the family has been transmitted to the child, and might be relieved to enroll their at-risk children in prevention research. Thus, parents' perception of personal benefit might lead them to coerce their adolescents into participating in gene-based prevention research (Bernhardt et al., 2003; Geller et al., 2003).

The risk of parental coercion is exacerbated in families where communication between parents and children is already strained (Geller et al., 2003). Communication difficulties are particularly worrisome in the context of recruiting adolescents to participate in research that discloses genetic information (Geller et al., 2003), which carries with it the risk of disrupting familial relationships even further (Knoppers et al., 2002). Additional safeguards may be necessary in families where the parents are eager to enroll the child(ren) and the interpersonal dynamics require the minor adolescents to comply (Gordon & Bonkovsky, 1996). Use of facilitators in the decision-making process may provide such a safeguard in families at increased genetic risk, where there are biologic as well as emotional ties that may exert unique influences on the communication between parents and adolescent children (Geller et al., 2003).

Several strategies are recommended to reduce the threats to informed and voluntary decision making by adolescent participants in gene-based prevention research. First, genetic counseling should be part of the informed consent process (Knoppers et al., 2002). Such counseling would maximize prospective participants' understanding of heredity, the probability of developing the disease or trait, the clinical validity of the genetic test including pleiotropy, and the potential for adverse social and psychological consequences arising from disclosure of genetic test results. Genetic counseling should be offered to parents as well as adolescents because parents' decisions about enrolling their children are influenced by their knowledge about testing (Hamann et al., 2000).

Second, when enrolling adolescents from high-risk families in disease-prevention research, long-term psychological support should be made available to participants and their parents and siblings, because test results can affect entire families, and some adolescents show clinically significant anxiety symptoms in response to predictive genetic testing (Codori et al., 2003; Roth, 2001). Some have argued for the inclusion of psychological screening of minors prior to participation in research that is potentially anxiety-provoking (McCarthy et al., 2001). However, psychological screening or support may not be necessary when enrolling adolescents in population-based prevention trials of complex traits involving lower-penetrance gene variants, because such studies are associated with a different set of risks (Beskow, 2001).

Third, the decision-making process should take place in two stages. In the first stage, the parents and the adolescent would be given an opportunity to discuss the prospect of research participation as a family, with or without a member of the research team present to answer questions and resolve disagreements. In the second stage, the consent of the adolescent would be sought in a setting away from the influential adults, one that provides them with respect, privacy and time to think and ask questions (Broome et al., in press; Geller et al., 2003).

Providing adolescents with the opportunity to discuss a proposed study with a researcher separately from the parent does not imply a disregard for the importance of parental involvement in decision making. On the contrary, evidence suggests that many adolescents want parental input into their decisions about research participation, even those who think the final decision should be theirs (Geller et al., 2003), and perceive a greater need for parental consent when the protocols involve more invasive procedures (Sikand, Schubiner, & Simpson, 1997). Recent theoretical literature on adolescent development and decision making (Gilligan, 1988) reminds us of the reality of interdependence between children and parents and the possibilities for cooperation, particularly when it comes to decisions that could potentially harm the child or affect the entire family. Thinking about families in terms of conflicting interests is misguided, and stems from a narrow notion of informed consent (Kuczewski, 1966). In fact, where families are concerned, viewing informed consent as a process of shared decision making, whereby adolescents are involved in decisions about research participation, can actually enhance their autonomy within the family (Weithorn & Scherer, 1994). The shared decision-making process, whose primary goal is to help the adolescent clarify his or her values and preferences, should be tailored to the adolescent's level of maturity (Dorn, Susman, & Fletcher, 1995) and the family's communication style.

CONCLUSION

The desire to prevent early-onset disease and the progress in genetics research are combining to produce a growing interest in conducting clinical research that uses genetic information in conjunction with other strategies to motivate behavior, or to select the optimal treatment and/or preventive interventions for adolescents based on their genetic profiles (Lerman et al., 2002; Lerman & Niaura, 2002). However, such research raises several ethical concerns about the clinical validity and utility of the genetic information and the potential psychosocial harms that result from being labeled "at risk." Consideration must be given to the morally relevant differences between predictive genetic testing for complex traits or be-haviors as compared to adult-onset diseases. These differences influence our judg-ments about whether it is justified to include or even target adolescents in research involving genetic susceptibility testing.

Once a determination has been made that it is morally defensible to enroll or target adolescents for gene-based prevention trials, special care must be taken to overcome threats to their informed and voluntary decision making. The in-formed consent process should give adolescents sufficient opportunity to explore the meaning, benefits and risks associated with the disclosure of genetic test results, and to exercise their right to refuse participation without parental influence that might result from the parent's own health status, their desire for information about familial risk, or their faith in prevention.

Pediatric researchers and IRBs should not underestimate the awareness and maturity that many minor adolescents possess when addressing the prospect of enrolling in gene-based research. However, the obligation of investigators and reviewers to protect participants from research risks (Kodish, 2003) also requires them to be mindful of the potential for adverse psychological and social harm that could result from adolescent participation in such research. Guidelines on the communication of genetic results to minors should be developed. In addition, members of ethics boards need continuing education to keep them abreast of the areas of genetic research, such as pharmacogenomics, that are developing at a rapid pace (Knoppers et al., 2002).

Questions for Discussion

1. What distinguishes gene-based studies of adolescents (such as the smok-ing prevention trial) from studies that do not involve subjects' genetic information?

2. How might the disclosure of results of a gene-based study to an adoles-cent participant improve her situation? How might disclosure worsen it?

3. What is the central ethical dilemma involved in the disclosure of genetic information obtained in the course of research? How does is differ from clinical genetic testing?

4. How would you address Senior et al.'s (1999) concerns regarding the "geneticization" of society? Answer the question in terms of policy and in practice.

5. In your view, how would clear evidence of increased genetic risk of smok-ing, discovered by participation in research, effect adolescents' compli-ance with a smoking prevention intervention?

6. Do you agree with the author's position that the first stage of initial gene-based smoking intervention research should target adult smokers rather than adolescents because of a more favorable risk:benefit ratio?
7. According to the author, in determining the moral acceptability of gene-based prevention trials involving children and adolescents, what are the factors that should be taken into consideration? Had you been policy maker, would you suggest other factors?
8. What are the particular challenges to the informed consent process presented by a research in which at-risk adolescents undergo predictive genetic testing?
9. According to the author of this chapter, which factors effect the degree to which parents involve their adolescents in decision making about genetic based research participation? Which of the factors do you find desirable? Would you engage other factors?
10. Do you find the strategies recommended by the author to reduce the threats to informed and voluntary decision making by adolescent participants in gene-based prevention research persuasive? Why/why not?

Acknowledgments

This chapter is drawn from my experience with three distinct projects. The first was a grant (R01 HD36189-01) entitled "Minors at-risk of future disease: Their role in research," which I received from the National Institute of Child Health and Development (NICHD), with an administrative supplement from the National Human Genome Research Institute (NHGRI). I am indebted to my colleagues Barbara Bernhardt, Ellen Tambor, Gertrude Fraser, and Larry Wissow, as well as the parents and children who participated in that study. Second, I was a member of the NIH Cancer Genetics Studies Consortium and Co-Chair of its Informed Consent Task Force. Third, I participated in the consensus panel on "Emerging Issues in Smoking and Genetics" which was supported by the Robert Wood Johnson Foundation (A. Shields, P.I.) and a Transdisciplinary Tobacco Use Research Center grant from the National Cancer Institute, the National Institute on Drug Abuse (P5084718; C. Lerman, P.I.). I thank my collaborators and co-authors Ben Wilfond, Caryn Lerman, Janet Audrain-McGovern, and Alexandra Shields, as well as Ruth Faden and Pat King for advancing our thinking on these issues. This chapter is dedicated to the memory of Dorothy Wertz, Ph.D. and John Fletcher, Ph.D.

References

American Academy of Pediatrics Committee on Bioethics. (2001). Ethical issues with genetic testing in pediatrics. *Pediatrics, 107,* 1451–1455.

Anderson G. M., & Cook, E. H. (2000). Pharmacogenetics: Promise and potential in child and adolescent psychiatry. *Child & Adolescent Psychiatric Clinics of North America, 9,* 23–42.

Arnold, L. E., Stoff, D. M., Cook, E. Jr., Cohen, D. J., Kruesi, M., Wright, C., et al. (1995). Ethical issues in biological psychiatric research with children and adolescents. *Journal of the American Academy of Child & Adolescent Psychiatry, 34,* 929–939.

ASHG Social Issues Committees. (1995). ASHG/ACMG Report. Points to consider: Ethical, legal and psychosocial implications of genetic testing in children and adolescents. *American Journal of Human Genetics, 57,* 1233–1240.

ASHG Statement. (1997). Behavioral genetics '97: Recent developments in human behavioral genetics: Past accomplishments and future directions. *American Journal of Human Genetics, 60,* 1265–1275.

Audrain, J., & Tercyak, K. P. (2002). Recruiting adolescents into genetic studies of smoking behavior. *Cancer Epidemiology, Biomarkers & Prevention, 11,* 249–252.

Audrain, J., Boyd, N. R., Roth, J., Main, D., Caporaso, N. F., Lerman, C. (1997). Genetic susceptibility testing in smoking cessation treatment: One year outcomes of a randomized trial. *Addiction Behavior, 22,* 741–742.

Bellivier, F., Henry, C., Szoke, A., Schurhoff, F., Nostand-Bertrand, M., Feingold, J., et al. (1998). Serotonin transporter gene polymorphisms in patients with unipolar or bipolar depression. *Neuroscience Letters, 255,* 143–146.

Berenson G. S., Srinivasan, S. R., Bao, W., Newman, W. P. 3rd, Tracy, R. E., Wattigney, W. A. (1998). Association between multiple cardiovascular risk factors and atherosclerosis in children and young adults: The Bogalusa Heart Study. *New England Journal of Medicine, 338,* 1650–1656.

Berkey, C. S., Frazier, A. L., Gardner, J. D., Colditz, G. A. (1999). Adolescence and breast carcinoma risk. *Cancer, 85,* 2400–2409.

Bernhardt, B. A., Tambor, E. S. Fraser, G., Wissow, L. S., Geller, G. (2003). Parents' and children's attitudes toward the enrollment of minors in genetic susceptibility research: Implications for informed consent. *American Journal of Medical Genetics, 116A,* 315–323.

Beskow, L. M., Burke, W., Merz, J. F., Barr, P. A., Terry, S., Penchaszadeh, V. B., et. al. (2001). Informed consent for population-based research involving genetics. *Journal of the American Medical Association, 286,* 2315–2321.

Bickerdike, M. J. (2003). 5-HT2C receptor agonists as potential drugs for the treatment of obesity. *Current Topics in Medical Chemistry, 3,* 885–897.

Biederman, J., & Faraone, S. V. (2002). Current concepts on the neurobiology of attention deficit hyperactivity disorder. *Journal of Attention Disorders, 6*(Suppl. 1), S7–16.

Bierut, L. J., Rice, J. P., Edenburg, H. J., Goate, A., Foroud, T., Cloninger, C. R., et al. (2000). Family-based study of the association of the dopamine D2 receptor gene (DRD2) with habitual smoking. *American Journal of Medical Genetics, 90,* 299–302.

Blum, K., Sheridan, P. J., Wood, R. C., Braverman, E. R., Chen, T. J., Comings, D. E. (1995). Dopamine D2 receptor gene variant s: Association and linkage studies in impulsive, addictive and compulsive disorders. *Pharmacogenetics, 5,* 121–141.

Blum, K., Noble, E. P., Sheridan, P. J., Montgomery, A., Ritchie, T., Jagadeeswaran, P., et al. (1990). Allelic association of human dopamine D2 receptor gene in alcoholism. *Journal of the American Medical Association, 236,* 2055–2060.

Broome, M. E. (1999). Consent (assent) for research with pediatric patients. *Seminars in Oncology Nursing, 15,* 96–102.

Broome, M. E., Kodish, E., Geller, G., Siminoff, L. A. (2003). Children in research: New perspectives and practices for informed consent. *IRB: Ethics & Human Research.* 2003 Sep-Oct; Suppl 25(5):S20-S23.

Broome, M. E., Richards, D., Hall, J. (2001). Children in research: The experience of ill children and adolescents. *Journal of Family Nursing, 7,* 32–49.

Bruzzese, J.-M., & Fisher, C. B. (2003). Assessing and enhancing the research consent capacity of children and youth. *Applied Developmental Science, 7,* 13–26.

Burke, W., Coughlin, S. S., Lee, N. C., Weed, D. L., Khoury, M. J. (2001). Application of population screening principles to genetic screening for adult-onset conditions. *Genetic Testing, 5,* 201–211.

Burris, S. (2002). Disease stigma in US public health law. *Journal of Law, Medicine & Ethics, 30,* 179–190.

CDC. (2002, May 17). *Trends in cigarette smoking among high school students—United States (1991–2001).* Retrieved MMWR 2002;51:409–412 from http://www.cdc.gov/mmwr/preview/mmwrhtml/mm5119a1.htm

Clayton, E. W. (1995). Removing the shadow of the law from the debate about genetic testing of children. *American Journal of Medical Genetics, 57,* 630–634.

Codori, A.M., Petersen, G. M., Boyd, P. A., Brandt, J., Giardiello, F. M. (1996). Genetic testing for cancer in children: Short-term psychological effects. *Archives of Pediatrics & Adolescent Medicine, 150,* 1131–1138.

Codori, A.-M., Zawacki, K. L., Petersen, G. M., Miglioretti, D. L., Bacon, J. A., Trimbath, J. D., et al. (2003). Genetic testing for hereditary colorectal cancer in children: Long-term psychological effects. *American Journal of Medical Genetics, 116A,* 117–128.

Cohn, L. D., Macfarlane, S., & Yanez, C. (1995). Risk perception: Differences between adolescents and adults. *Health Psychology, 14,* 217–222.

Colby, S. M., Tiffany, S. T., Shiffman, S., Niaura, R. S. (2000). Measuring nicotine dependence among youth: A review of available approaches and instruments. *Drug & Alcohol Dependence, 59*(Suppl. 1), S23–24.

Collins, F. S. (1999). Shattuck lecture: Medical and societal consequences of the human genome project. *New England Journal of Medicine, 341,* 28–37.

Collins, F. S., & Mansoura, M. K. (2001). The Human Genome Project: Revealing the shared inheritance of all humankind. *Cancer, 91,* 221–225.

Comings, D. E., Gonzalez, N., Wu, S., Saucier, G., Johnson, P., Verde, R., et al. (1999). Homozygosity at the dopamine DRD3 receptor gene in cocaine dependence. *Molecular Psychiatry, 4,* 484–487.

Comings, D. E., Gade, R., Wu, S., Chiu, C., Dietz, G., Muhleman, D., et al. (1997). Studies of the potential role of the dopamine D1 receptor gene in addictive behaviors. *Molecular Psychiatry, 2,* 44–56.

Comings, D. E., Muhleman, D., Gysin, R. (1996). Dopamine D2 receptor (DRD2) gene and susceptibility to posttraumatic stress disorder: A study and replication. *Biological Psychiatry, 40,* 368–372.

Cooper, R., & Luke, A. (2003). Racial differences in susceptibility to obesity. *American Journal of Clinical Nutrition, 77,* 751–753.

Davies, M. R. (2000). The stigma of anxiety disorders. *International Journal of Clinical Practice, 54,* 44–47.

Davis, D. S. (1997). Genetic dilemmas and the child's right to an open future. *Rutgers Law Journal, 28,* 549–592.

DiMaio S., Gruzenko, N., & Joober, R. (2003). Dopamine genes and attention-deficit hyperactivity disorder: A review. *Journal of Psychiatry & Neuroscience, 28,* 27–38.

Dorn, L. D., Susman, E. J., & Fletcher, J. C. (1995). Informed consent in children and adolescents: Age, maturation and psychological state. *Journal of Adolescent Health, 16,* 185–190.

Fanos, J. H. (1997). Developmental tasks of childhood and adolescence: Implications for genetic testing. *American Journal of Medical Genetics, 71,* 22–28.

Farooqi, I. S., Keogh, J. M., Yeo, G. S., Lank, E. J., Cheetham, T., O'Rahilly, S. (2003). Clinical spectrum of obesity and mutations in the melanocortin 4 receptor gene. *New England Journal of Medicine, 348,* 1085–1095.

Feigenbaum, M., & Hutz, M. H. (2003). Further evidence for the association between obesity-related traits and the apolipoprotein A-IV gene. *International Journal of Obesity & Related Metabolic Disorders, 27,* 484–490.

Garnick, D. W., Hendricks, A. M., Comstock, C., Horgan, C. (1997). Do individuals with substance abuse diagnoses incur higher charges than individuals with other chronic conditions? *Journal of Substance Abuse, 14,* 457–465.

Geller, G., Botkin, J. R., Green, M. J., Press, N., Biesecker, B. B., Wilfond, B., et al. (1997). Genetic testing for susceptibility to adult-onset cancer: The process and content of informed consent. *Journal of the American Medical Association, 277,* 1467–1474.

Geller, G., Tambor, E. S., Bernhardt, B. A., Fraser, G., Wissow, L. S. (2003). Informed consent for enrolling minors in genetic susceptibility research: A qualitative study of at-risk children's and parents' views about children's role in decision making. *Journal of Adolescent Health, 32,* 260–271.

Geller, G., Tambor, E. S., Bernhardt, B. A., Wissow, L. S., Fraser, G. (2000). Mothers and daughters from breast cancer families: A qualitative study of their perceptions of the risks and benefits associated with minors' participation in genetic susceptibility research. *Journal of the American Medical Association, 55,* 280–284.

Giardiello, F. M., Yang, V. W., Hylind, L. M., Krush, A. J., Petersen, G. M., Trimbath, J. D., et al. (2002). Primary chemoprevention of familial adenomatous polyposis with sulindac. *New England Journal of Medicine, 346,* 1054–1059.

Gilligan, C. (1988). Exit-Voice dilemmas in adolescent development. In Carol Gilligan, Janie Victoria Ward, Jill McLean Taylor (Eds.), *Mapping the moral domain: A contribution of women's thinking to psychological theory and education* (pp. 141–158). Cambridge, MA: Harvard University Press.

Gordon, V. M., & Bonkovsky, F. O. (1996). Family dynamics and children in medical research. *Journal of Clinical Ethics, 7,* 349–354.

Hamann, H. A., Croyle, R. T., Venne, V. L., Baty, B. J., Smith, K. R., Botkin, J. R. (2000). Attitudes toward the genetic testing of children among adults in a Utah-based kindred tested for a BRCA1 mutation. *American Journal of Medical Genetics, 92,* 25–32.

Harth, S. C., & Thong, Y. H. (1995). Parental perceptions and attitudes about informed consent in clinical research involving children. *Social Science & Medicine, 40,* 1573–1577.

Heath, A. C., & Martin, N. G. (1993). Genetic models for the natural history of smoking: Evidence for a genetic influence on smoking persistence. *Addiction Behavior, 18,* 19–34.

Heinssen, R. K., Perkins, D. O., Appelbaum, P. S., Fenton, W. S. (2001). Informed consent in early psychosis research. National Institute of Mental Health Workshop, November 15, 2000. *Schizophrenia Bulletin, 27,* 571–583.

Holtzman, N. A., & Watson, M. S. (1997). *Promoting safe and effective genetic testing in the U.S.: Final report of the task force on genetic testing. NIH-DOE working group on ethical, legal, and social implications of human genome research* (pp. 26–28). Baltimore, MD: The Johns Hopkins University Press.

Hudson, K. L., Rothenberg, K. H., Andrews, L. B., Kahn, M. J., Collins, F. S. (1995). Genetics discrimination and health insurance: An urgent need for reform. *Science, 270,* 391–393.

Humphries, S. E., Galton, D., & Nicholls, P. (1997). Genetic testing for familial hypercholesterolaemia: Practical and ethical issues. *Quarterly Journal of Medicine, 90,* 169–181.

Johnston, L. D., O'Malley, P. M., Bachman, J. G. (2002). *Monitoring the future. National results on adolescent drug use: Overview of key findings, 2001.* NIH 02-5105. Bethesda, MD: National Institute on Drug Abuse 32, 1–61.

Jorm, A. F., Henderson, A. S., Jacomb, P. A., Christensen, H., Korten A. E., Rodgers, B., et al. (2000). Association of smoking and personality with a polymorphism of the dopamine transporter gene. Results from a community survey. *American Journal of Medical Genetics, 96,* 331–334.

Kendler, K. S., Neale, M. C., Sullivan, P., Corey, L. A., Gardner, C. O., Prescott, C. A. (1999). A population-based twin study in women of smoking initiation and nicotine dependence. *Psychological Medicine, 29,* 299–308.

Kimm, S. Y., Glynn, N. W., Aston, C. E., Damcott, C. M., Poehlman, E. T., Daniels, S. R., et al. (2002). Racial differences in the relation between uncoupling protein genes and resting energy expenditure. *American Journal of Clinical Nutrition 75,* 714–719.

Knoppers, B. M., Avard, D., Cardinal, G., Glass, K. C. (2002). Science and Society: Children and incompetent adults in genetic research: Consent and safeguards. *Nature Reviews Genetics, 3,* 221–225.

Kodish, E. (1999). Testing children for cancer genes: The rule of earliest onset. *Journal of Pediatrics, 135,* 390–395.

Kodish, E. (2003). Informed consent for pediatric research: Is it really possible? *Journal of Pediatrics, 142,* 89–90.

Kuczewski, M. G. (1996). Reconceiving the family: The process of consent in medical decision-making. *Hastings Center Report, 26*(2), 30–37.

Lerman, C., & Berrettini, W. (2002). Elucidating the role of genetic factors in smoking behavior and nicotine dependence. *American Journal of Medical Genetics,* 2003 Apr 1;118B(1):48–54. Review.

Lerman, C., Shields, P. G., Wileyto, E. P., Audrain, J., Pinot, A., Hawk, L., et al. (2002). Pharmacogenetic investigation of smoking cessation treatment. *Pharmacogenetics, 12,* 627–634.

Lerman, C., & Niaura, R. (2002). Applying genetic approaches to the treatment of nicotine dependence. *Oncogene, 21,* 7412–7420.

Lerman, C., Caporaso, N. E., Bush, A., Zheng, Y. L., Audrain, J., Main, D., et al. (2001). Tryptophan hydroxylase gene variant & smoking behavior. *American Journal of Medical Genetics, 105,* 518–520.

Lerman, C., Caporaso, N. E., Audrain, J., Main, D., Bowman, E. D., Lockshin, B., et al. (1999). Evidence suggesting the role of specific genetic factors in cigarette smoking. *Health Psychology, 18,* 14–20.

Lerman, C., Gold, K., Audrain, J., Lin, T. H., Boyd, N. R., Orleans, C. T., et al. (1997). Incorporating biomarkers of exposure and genetics susceptibility into smoking cessation treatment: Effects on smoking-related cognitions, emotions, and behavior change. *Health Psychology, 16,* 87–99.

Lesch, K. P., Bengel, D., Heils, A., Sabol, S. Z., Greenberg B. D., Petri, S., et al. (1996). Association of anxiety-related traits with a polymorphism in the serotonin transporter gene regulatory region. *Science, 274,* 1527–1531.

Levine, R J. (1995). Adolescents as research participants without permission of their parents or guardians: Ethical considerations. *Journal of Adolescent Health, 17,* 287–288.

Lichtermann, D., Hranilovic, D., Trixler, M., Franke, P., Jernej, B., Delmo, C. D., et al. (2000). Support for allelic association of a polymorphic site in the promoter region of the serotonin transporter gene with risk for alcohol dependence. *American Journal of Psychiatry, 157,* 2045–2047.

Link, B. G., Phelan, J. C., Bresnahan, M., Stueve, A., Pescosolido, B. A. (1999). Public conceptions of mental illness: Labels, causes, dangerousness, and social distance. *American Journal of Public Health, 89,* 1328–1333.

Link, B. G., Struening, E. L., Rahav, M., Phelan, J. C., Nuttbrock, L. (1997). On stigma and its consequences: Evidence from a longitudinal study of men with dual diagnoses of mental illness and substance abuse. *Journal of Health & Social Behavior, 38,* 177–190.

Lynch, H. T., & de la Chapelle, A. (1999). Genetic susceptibility to non-polyposis colorectal cancer. *Journal of Medical Genetics 36,* 801–818.

Mann, C. C. (1994). Behavioral genetics in transition. *Science, 264,* 1687–1689.

Marteau, T. M. (1994). The genetic testing of children. *Journal of Medical Genetics 31,* 743.

Matsushita, S., Yoshino, A., Murayama, M., Kimura, M., Muramatsu, T., Higuchi, S. (2001). Association study of serotonin transporter gene regulatory region polymorphism and alcoholism. *American Journal of Medical Genetics, 105,* 446–450.

McBride, C. M., Bepler, G., Lipkus, I. M., Lyna, P., Samsa, G., Albright, J., et al. (2002). Incorporating genetic susceptibility feedback into a smoking cessation program for African-American smokers with low income. *Cancer Epidemiology, Biomarkers & Prevention, 11,* 521–522.

McCarthy, A. M., Richman, L. C., Hoffman, R. P., Rubenstein, L. (2001). Psychological screening of children for participation in nontherapeutic invasive research. *Archives of Pediatrics & Adolescent Medicine, 155,* 1197–1203.

McGinnis, J. M., & Foege, W. H. (1993). Actual causes of death in the United States. *Journal of the American Medical Association, 270,* 2207–2212.

McLellan, A. T., Lewis, D. C., O'Brien, C. P., Kleber, H. D. (2000). Drug dependence, a chronic medical illness: Implications for treatment, insurance, and outcomes evaluation. *Journal of the American Medical Association, 284,* 1689–1690.

Michie, S., Bobrow, M. Marteau, T. M., & the FAP Collaborative Research Group. (2001). Predictive genetic testing in children and adults: A study of emotional impact. *Journal of Medical Genetics, 38,* 519–526.

Michie, S., McDonald, V., Bobrow, M., McKeown, C., Marteau, T. (1996). Parents' responses to predictive genetic testing in their children: Report of a single case study. *Journal of Medical Genetics, 33,* 313–318.

Michielutte, R., & Diseker, R. A. (1982). Children's perceptions of cancer in comparison to other chronic illnesses. *Journal of Chronic Diseases, 35,* 843–852.

Miller, S. (2000). Researching children: Issues arising from a phenomenological study with children who have diabetes mellitus. *Journal of Advanced Nursing, 31,* 1228–1234.

Moolchan, E. T., & Mermelstein, R. (2002). Research on tobacco use among teenagers: Ethical challenges. *Journal of Adolescent Health, 30,* 409–417.

Muglia, P., Jain, U., Macciardi, F., Kennedy, J. L., et al. (2000). Adult attention deficit hyperactivity disorder and the dopamine D4 receptor gene. *American Journal of Medical Genetics, 96,* 273–274.

Murray, J. S. (2000). Conducting psychosocial research with children and adolescents: A developmental perspective *Applied Nursing Research, 13,* 151–156.

National Institutes of Health. (2002, November). *Policy and guidelines on the inclusion of children as participants in research involving human participants. NIH Guide.* National Institutes of Health. Retrieved [–*–] from http://ohsr.od.nih.gov/guidelines/45cfr46.html#SubpartD

Nelson, R. M. (1998). Children as research participants. In Kahn, J. P., Mastroianni, A. C., Sugarman, J. (Eds.), *Beyond consent: Seeking justice in research* (pp. 47–66). New York: Oxford University Press.

Nielsen, D. A., Virkkunen, M., Lappalainen, J., Eggert, M., Brown, G. L., Long, J. C., et al. (1998). A tryptohan hydroxylase gene marker for suicidiality and alcoholism. *Archives of General Psychiatry, 5,* 593–595.

Noble, E. (2000). The DRD2 gene in psychiatric and neurological disorders and its phenotypes. *Pharmacogenomics, 1,* 309–333.

Obarzanek, E., Kimm, S. Y., Barton, B. A., Van Horn, L. L., Kwiterovich, P. O., Jr., Simons-Morton, D. G., et. al. (2001). Long-term safety and efficacy of a cholesterol-lowering diet in children with elevated low-density lipoprotein cholesterol: Seven-year results of the dietary intervention study (DISC). *Pediatrics, 107,* 256–264.

O'Brien, C. P., &McLellan, A. T. (1996). Myths about the treatment of addiction. *Lancet, 347,* 237–240.

Office of Smoking and Health. (1994). *Preventing tobacco use among young people: A report of the surgeon general.* Atlanta, Georgia: CDC National Center for Chronic Disease Prevention and Health Promotion, U.S. Department of Health and Human Services.

Ogilvie, A. D., Battersby, S., Bubb, V. J., Fink, G., Harmar, A. J., Goodwim, G. M., et al. (1996). Polymorphism in serotonin transporter gene associated with susceptibility to major depression. *Lancet, 347,* 731–733.

Ondrusek, N., Abramovitch, R., Pencharz, P., Koren, G. (1998). Empirical examination of the ability of children to consent to clinical research. *Journal of Medical Ethics, 24,* 158–165.

O'Rahilly, S. (2002). Leptin: Defining its role in humans by the clinical study of genetic disorders. *Nutrition Reviews, 60,* S30–34.

Patenaude, A. F., Basili, L., Fairclough, D. L., Li, F. P. (1996). Attitudes of 47 mothers of pediatric oncology patients toward genetic testing for cancer predisposition. *Journal of Clinical Oncology, 14,* 415–421.

Petersen, A. C., & Leffert, N. (1995). Developmental issues influencing guidelines for adolescent health research: A review. *Journal of Adolescent Health, 17,* 298–305.

Phelan, J. C., Bromet, E. J., Link, B. G. (1998). Psychiatric illness and family stigma. *Schizophrenia Bulletin, 24,* 115–126.

Piitulainen, E., & Sveger, T. (1998). Effect of environmental and clinical factors on lung function and respiratory symptoms in adolescents with alpha$_1$-antitrypsin deficiency. *Acta Paediatrica, 87,* 1120–1124.

Ponder, M., Lee, J., Green, J., Richards, M. (1996). Family history and perceived vulnerability to some common diseases: A study of young people and their parents. *Journal of Medical Genetics, 33,* 485–492.

Rich, M., Lamola, S., Gordon, J., Chalfen, R. (2000). Video intervention/prevention assessment: A patient-centered methodology for understanding the adolescent illness experience. *Journal of Adolescent Health, 27,* 155–165.

Richards, M. (1998). The genetic testing of children: Adult attitudes and children's understanding. In A. J. Clarke (Ed.), *The genetic testing of children* (pp. 157–168). Oxford: BIOS Scientific Publishers Ltd.

Ritson, E. B. (1999). Alcohol, drugs and stigma. *International Journal of Clinical Practice, 53,* 549–551.

Ross, L. F. (2003). Minimizing risks: The ethics of predictive diabetes screening research in newborns. *Archives of Pediatric & Adolescent Medicine, 157,* 89–95.

Roth, R. (2001). Psychological and ethical aspects of prevention trials. *Journal of Pediatric & Endocrinologic Metabolism, 14*(Suppl. 1), 669–674.

Rowe, D. C., Stever, C., Gard, J. M., Cleveland, H. H., Sanders, M. L., Abramowitz, A., et. al. (1998). The relation of the dopamine transporter gene (DAT1) to symptoms of internalizing disorders in children. *Behavioral Genetics, 28,* 215–225.

Sabol, S. Z., Nelson, M. L., Fisher, C., Gunzerath, L., Brody, C. L., Hu, S., et al. (1999). A genetic association for cigarette smoking behavior. *Health Psychology, 18,* 7–13.

Santelli, J. S., Smith Rogers, A., Rosenfeld, W. D., DuRant, R. H., Dubler, N., Morreale, M., et al. (1995). Guidelines for adolescent health research: A position paper of the society for adolescent medicine. *Journal of Adolescent Health, 17,* 270–272.

Scherer, D. G., & Reppucci, N. D. (1988). Adolescents' capacities to provide voluntary informed consent. *Law & Human Behavior, 12,* 123–141.

Senior, V., Marteau, T. M., & Peters, T. J. (1999). Will genetic testing for predisposition for disease result in fatalism? A qualitative study of parents' responses to neonatal screening for familial hypercholesterolemia. *Social Science & Medicine, 48,* 1857–1860.

Shamir, R., & Fisher, E. A. (2000). Dietary therapy for children with hypercholesterolemia. *American Family Physician, 61,* 675–682.

Sikand A, Schubiner, H., & Simpson, P. M. (1997). Parent and adolescent perceived need for parental consent involving research with minors. *Archives of Pediatric & Adolescent Medicine, 151,* 603–607.

Skinner, E. A., Chapman, M., & Baltes, P. B. (1988). Children's beliefs about control, means–ends, and agency: Developmental differences during middle childhood. *International Journal of Behavioral Development, 11,* 369–388.

Stanton, W. R. (1995). DSM-III-R tobacco dependence and quitting during late adolescence. *Addiction Behavior, 20,* 595–598.

Steinbach, G., Lynch, P. M., Phillips, R. K., Wallace, M. H., Hawk, E., Gordon, G. B., et al. (2000). The effect of celecoxib, a cyclooxygenase-2 inhibitor, in familial adenomatous polyposis. *New England Journal of Medicine, 342,* 1946–1952.

Steinberg, K. K., Gwinn, M., & Khoury, M. J. (2001). The role of genomics in public health and disease prevention. *Journal of the American Medical Association, 286,* 1635.

Sullivan, P., & Kendler, K. S. (1999). The genetic epidemiology of smoking. *Nicotine & Tobacco Research, 1,* S51–57.

Susman, E. J., Dorn, L. D., & Fletcher, J. C. (1992). Participation in biomedical research: The consent process as viewed by children, adolescents, young adults, and physicians. *Journal of Pediatrics, 121,* 547–552.

Sussman, S., Lichtman, K., Ritt, A., Pallonen, U. E. (1999). Effects of thirty-four adolescent tobacco use cessation and prevention trials on regular users of tobacco products. *Substance Use & Misuse, 34,* 1469.

Sveger, T., Piitulainen, E., Aborelius, M., Jr. (1995). Clinical features and lung function in 18-year-old adolescents with alpha$_1$–antitrypsin deficiency. *Acta Paediatrica, 84,* 815–816.

Tercyak, K. P., Hughes, C., Main, D., Snyder, C., Lynch, J. F., Lynch H. T., et al. (2001a). Parental communication of BRCA1/2 genetic test results to children. *Patient Education & Counseling, 42*(3), 213–24.

Tercyak, K. P., Peshkin, B. N., Streisand, R., Lerman, C. (2001b). Psychological issues among children of hereditary breast cancer gene (BRCA1/2) testing participants. *Psychooncology, 10*(4), 336–46.

Thelin, T., Sveger, T., McNeil, T. F., (1996). Primary prevention in a high-risk group: Smoking habits in adolescents with homozygous alpha₁-antitrypsin deficiency (ATD) *Acta Paediatrica, 85,* 1207.

Toriello, H. V. (2002). Effect of the human genome project on the practice of adolescent medicine. *Adolescent Medicine, 13,* 201–212.

U.S. Department of Health and Human Services. (1991). Additional protections for children involved as subjects in research [Revised]. 45 CFR 46 subpart D. *Federal Register, 56.* 56 FR 28032 p. 120 (Original published 1983, *Federal Register, 48,* 9814–9820)

Vincent, S., Planells, R., Defoort, C., Bernard, M. C., Gerber, M., Prudhomme, J., et al. (2002). Genetic polymorphisms and lipoprotein responses to diets. *Proceedings of the Nutrition Society, 61,* 427–434.

Wachbroit, R.. (1998). The question not asked: The challenge of pleiotropic genetic tests. *Kennedy Institute of Ethics Journal, 8,* 131–144.

Walter, J. H., White, F. J., Hall, S. K., MacDonald, A., Rylance, G., Boneh, A., et al. (2002). How practical are recommendations for dietary control in phenylketonuria? *Lancet, 360,* 55–57.

Weir, R. F., & Horton, J. R. (1995). Genetic research, adolescents and informed consent. *Theoretical Medicine, 16,* 347–373.

Weithorn, L. A., & Scherer, D. G. (1994). Children's involvement in research participation decisions: Psychological considerations. In M. A. Grodin & L. H. Glanz (Eds.), *Children as research participants: Science, ethics and law* (pp. 133–179). New York: Oxford University Press.

Wertz, D. C., Fanos, J. H., & Reilly, P. R. (1994). Genetic testing for children and adolescents: Who decides? *Journal of the American Medical Association, 272,* 875–881.

Wilfond, B. S., Geller, G., Lerman, C., Audrain-McGovern, J., Shields, A. E. (2002). Ethical issues in conducting behavioral genetics research: The case of smoking prevention trials among adolescents. *Journal of Health Care, Law & Policy, 6,* 73–88.

Williams, J. K. (2000). Impact of genome research on children and their families. *Journal of Pediatric Nursing, 15,* 207–211.

Ziegler, J. (1998). Exposure and habits early in life may influence breast cancer risk. *Journal of National Cancer Institute, 90,* 187–188.

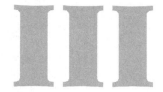

III

Research Involving Children With Serious Illness

12

Research Ethics and Maternal–Fetal Surgery

Rebecca Dresser

CASE DESCRIPTION

In April 1999, the *Wall Street Journal* reported on a new surgical procedure designed to reduce the damage done by spina bifida (also known as myelo-meningocele), a relatively common birth defect that can cause developmental delay, learning disabilities, impaired ability to walk, and bladder and bowel incontinence (Winslow, 1999). Although the precise causes of the disabilities are not fully understood, they are triggered in early embryonic development when bone and skin tissue fails to enclose the spinal cord.

Spina bifida can be diagnosed in the second trimester of pregnancy. Some women elect to terminate their pregnancies to avoid having an affected child, but others do not. Standard therapy for infants born with spina bifida is surgery to enclose the spinal cord. In most cases, physicians also insert a shunt to drain excess fluid in the brain (hydrocephalus) that can lead to further neurological impairment. The infants often are delivered by cesarean section to avoid added damage to the spinal cord (Olutoye & Adzick, 1999).

In an effort to improve the children's health, physicians devised a surgical intervention that is performed on pregnant women and fetuses at between 22 and 30 weeks of gestation. In the surgery, the woman's uterus is lifted out of her body, the fetus is exposed (in a process referred to as "open" surgery), and the abnormal opening in the fetal spinal cord is closed. The uterus is then replaced and the pregnancy is continued. The basis for this procedure is the hope that earlier repair will reduce damage to the spinal cord during the remainder of fetal development.

The *Wall Street Journal* reported that two centers, Vanderbilt University Medical Center and Children's Hospital of Philadelphia (CHOP), were offering the surgery. Indeed, the news report suggested that the two centers were competing with each other for patients and positive publicity from the innovation. The journal story focused on the entrepreneurial dimensions of the hospitals' actions and the surgery's potential economic consequences. But the story also revealed numerous ethical issues raised by the surgery. These issues concern (1) the appropriate availability and evaluation of new surgical procedures, (2) the assessment of potential benefits and harms when novel interventions affect both pregnant women and the infants they hope to deliver, (3) the justification for exposing women and infants to significant risks to reduce mild-to-moderate disabilities, and (4) decision making by women and their partners considering unproven interventions aimed at enhancing the health of their future children.

—

ETHICAL ANALYSIS AND DISCUSSION

Historical Context

The procedure described in the *Wall Street Journal* was not the first in utero intervention performed for the sake of a future child. Such interventions were initially attempted in the 1960s, when physicians transfused blood to fetuses whose lives were jeopardized by Rh factor incompatibility between the pregnant woman and fetus (Casper, 1998). Although open surgery was attempted at that time, most of the attempts were unsuccessful, and open surgery was replaced by alternative forms of intervention (Fauza, 1999).

The development of ultrasound revitalized interest in open surgery. Ultrasound improved physicians' ability to diagnose fetal abnormalities and to monitor surgical procedures (Casper, 1998). In the early 1980s, Dr. Michael Harrison and his colleagues at the University of California–San Francisco (UCSF) began performing open surgery to correct life-threatening fetal abnormalities, such as urinary tract obstructions and holes in the diaphragm. Many of these efforts fell short of expectations. A major problem is that open surgery usually causes preterm labor. Although drugs can delay birth for a while, nearly all the infants are born prematurely (Fauza, 1999). Physicians also found that children with many conditions had better outcomes if surgery was postponed until after birth (Marwick, 1993). Consequently, by the late 1990s, in utero surgery was regarded as a successful treatment method for only a few conditions (Simpson, 1999).

Despite these less-than-stellar results, physicians at Vanderbilt and CHOP believed there were good reasons to move forward with in utero surgery for spina bifida. Researchers reported positive outcomes in studies of sheep and monkey fetuses whose spinal cord defects were surgically repaired (Olutoye & Adzick, 1999). There was also some evidence that the disabilities associated with spina bifida were exacerbated by lengthy exposure of the spinal cord to amniotic fluid in the uterus. If this were true, covering the cord as soon as possible could reduce the severity of the impairments. Accordingly, in the late 1990s, the Vanderbilt and CHOP teams began performing the surgery on humans.

Pediatric Research Ethics and Parental Decisions

Most pediatric research intimately involves parents, but nowhere is the involvement more direct than in research on in utero surgery. In this context, both the pregnant woman and her fetus are research subjects. This duality significantly complicates the research ethics analysis. Risks and possible benefits to both subjects must be assessed and justified. Moreover, women and physicians may downplay risks to both subjects out of a strong desire to "rescue" at-risk infants.

The development of new surgical procedures can also raise complex ethical issues. Surgery has a history of innovation unaccompanied by formal research. In the absence of research, patients may undergo novel surgical procedures without a clear understanding of the procedures' unproven status. Innovative procedures may also be performed without the systematic data collection that is necessary to evaluate whether the procedures are safe and effective.

Both sources of ethical complexity exist in the case of in utero surgery for spina bifida. Women whose fetuses are diagnosed with spina bifida must decide whether to undergo novel surgery that presents risks to them and their future children. And they must do so in the absence of rigorous studies assessing the surgery's potential harms and benefits. The remainder of this chapter provides a discussion of research ethics and in utero surgery for spina bifida.

Innovation in Surgery and the Need for Systematic Research

The field of surgery lacks a strong research tradition. As a result, novel surgical procedures may become clinically available without receiving the close scrutiny given to other forms of medical innovation. The situation arose partly because surgeons often adjust their techniques based on the characteristics of individual patients. If an alteration appears to work well in one patient, the surgeon may try it in another. Eventually, this process can develop into a substantially novel approach that warrants formal study, but this may not be obvious because the changes occurred incrementally (Frader & Caniano, 1998).

The structure of the U.S. regulatory system also contributes to the lack of research in surgery compared with other medical fields. The Food and Drug Administration requires medical product manufacturers to submit research data showing that new drugs and devices are safe and effective before the products may be released for clinical use (Kessler, 1989; Kessler, Pape, & Sundwall, 1987).

The agency lacks jurisdiction over surgical procedures, however. As a result, the agency's research requirements do not apply to surgical innovations.

Novel surgical procedures are sometimes covered by a second U.S. oversight system, the Federal Policy for the Protection of Human Subjects (1991; also known as the Common Rule). Because this system applies to all human studies conducted in medical schools and hospitals that receive federal funds for research, it covers a great deal of surgical research. The Common Rule requires investigators to put into place many safeguards designed to protect the interests of early recipients of novel interventions, including ethics review by the institutional review board (IRB). Yet the Common Rule's provisions become effective only after an innovation is defined as the object of systematic study. For the Common Rule to apply, a team must first decide to conduct formal research to evaluate how well an innovation performs in humans (Federal Policy for the Protection of Human Subjects, 1991).[1]

Thus, the regulatory system aimed at protecting the recipients of novel surgical interventions applies solely to formal research projects. Innovators can be reluctant to undertake formal research, however. Launching a well-designed study is a formidable task. Innovators must obtain funding for the extra costs of data collection. To obtain funds, they usually must submit their proposals for peer review by experts in the field. As we have seen, IRB review can be required as well.

Surgical innovators have financial and other personal interests that could be jeopardized by research. A rigorous study could find that an innovation is not as beneficial as it initially appeared. Developers of a new procedure may not want to take the professional and economic risks of discovering that their innovation performed poorly in rigorous testing.

Serious ethical problems arise, however, when physicians make new interventions available without conducting research. Offering a surgical innovation as simply another medical option jeopardizes the interests of patients. Physicians owe information to patients asked to undergo novel procedures, whether or not patients are part of a formal research study. Adults capable of exercising self-determination—including pregnant women asked to undergo surgery for the sake of their future children—should receive information describing the intervention's unproven status, what is known about its potential harms and benefits, and the available alternatives to the intervention. Women need this information to make decisions that are consistent with their personal values and preferences. As prospective parents, they and their partners need this information to make decisions that are consistent with their responsibilities to future children (American Academy of Pediatrics Committee on Bioethics, 1999).

Physicians also owe patients protection from unacceptable risks. Novel procedures present unknown risks and uncertain benefits. In this sense, novel procedures are experimental even when they are not part of a formal study (McNeill, 1993). But because the medical system fails to demand formal peer or ethics review of novel procedures, such procedures may be made available even when they lack a defensible scientific foundation. A physician's intention or hope to benefit patients is not enough to protect patients from harm. There must also be an objective basis for the physician's belief, and that basis exists only when others in the field agree that a new procedure has a reasonable chance of helping patients (King, 1995).

If novel procedures are offered as simply another therapeutic alternative, the earliest human recipients may not obtain the information and protection they are owed. Patients can "become de facto research subjects without their knowledge or consent" (Gates, 1999, p. 208). They can also be exposed to undue risk, for risks can be greater when new procedures are performed in "haphazard and scientifically invalid experiments [rather] than in properly conducted scientific experimentation" (McNeill, 1993, p. 12).

Early recipients of new surgical procedures are not the only patients whose interests are threatened when innovations are offered in the pure clinical setting. The failure to conduct research on novel procedures can also be detrimental to later recipients. Without research, patients in general may be denied the information and protection they are owed.

According to widely accepted ethical and legal standards, patients have a right to receive information about the procedures their physicians propose. But if innovators fail to conduct formal research, physicians remain unable to give patients reasonably accurate information about a procedure's possible benefits and harms. Instead, patients must rely on physicians' subjective impressions, impressions that may be colored by the physicians' personal interests in encouraging or discouraging the procedure's use. When physicians fail to conduct well-designed studies, they deny patients the opportunity to make informed choices.

The failure to conduct research may also expose patients to risky and ineffective procedures. History is replete with cases in which physicians mistakenly assumed that an innovation was superior to existing therapy. In these cases, it took formal research to identify the mistakes. Research allows innovations to be evaluated using methods that produce a much more accurate picture of the intervention's quality. Research also allows others in the field to review the data and consider whether the investigators' conclusions are scientifically warranted.

Research advances the interests of the broader society, as well. Research data are needed to determine the appropriate allocation of health care resources. Different interventions must be compared so that limited funds can be devoted to the most effective therapies. In light of the need to control health care costs, resources should be reserved for new procedures that perform successfully in well-designed studies. For all these reasons, "surgeons who engage in the pioneering field of prenatal surgery have an enormous responsibility to conduct clinical trials that are scientifically sound and consistent with current regulations for research involving humans" (Caniano & Baylis, 1999, p. 307).

Initial Evaluation of In Utero Surgery for Spina Bifida

Unlike some other surgical innovations, in utero surgery for spina bifida drastically departs from the standard approach of performing surgery after the child's birth. Thus, its developers could not (and did not) seek to be excused from systematic evaluation on grounds that the surgery was simply an incremental deviation from ordinary care. The physicians who developed in utero surgery for spina bifida did collect and publish early data on the procedure.

In 1999, the *Journal of the American Medical Association* (*JAMA*) published accounts by the Vanderbilt and CHOP teams. The Vanderbilt team reported on an observational study in which infants receiving in utero surgery were compared to a historical control group of infants with similar medical characteristics who received surgery after birth (Bruner et al., 1999). The CHOP team presented a case series of patients who underwent in utero surgery (Sutton et al., 1999).

For their outcome measures, the Vanderbilt and CHOP teams evaluated the incidence of hindbrain herniation, which is a brain malformation associated with the hydrocephalus and other problems infants with spina bifida experience. The teams also collected data on the infants' need for a shunt, their birth weight and gestational age, and problems women experienced during pregnancy and childbirth.

Both teams concluded that infants undergoing in utero surgery had decreased levels of hindbrain herniation and as a result, were less likely to have hydrocephalus and require placement of a shunt. As in the earlier attempts at in utero surgery, however, premature birth was a major risk. Infants are classified as premature if they are born before 37 weeks' gestation. The 29 infants who underwent in utero surgery at Vanderbilt were delivered at a significantly earlier age than infants in the control group (mean gestational age of 33.2 weeks vs. 37 weeks). Five infants in the in utero surgery group were born before 30 weeks' gestation; one of them was born during the in utero surgery. At CHOP, 4 of the 10 infants receiving in utero surgery were born at 31 weeks' gestation or earlier, and one of them died. The rest were delivered by cesarean section at 36 weeks' gestation.

Even though prematurity is associated with numerous health problems, the Vanderbilt and CHOP physicians reported no significant morbidity in infants who underwent in utero surgery. As the Vanderbilt team acknowledged, however, the children might later demonstrate impaired cognitive abilities: "Open fetal surgery, followed by weeks of tocolysis [measures to halt premature labor], culminating in preterm labor and delivery of a premature infant are all risk factors for a poor neurologic outcome" (Bruner et al., 1999, p. 1824).

The Vanderbilt team identified risks to women, as well. The team compared maternal complications among women who did and did not undergo in utero surgery. Women in the surgery group experienced several complications. Forty-eight percent, compared to 4% in the control group, had some loss of amniotic fluid. This condition can create fetal risks, although the physicians reported that no infants in the in utero surgery group had to be delivered early because of this condition. Women who underwent surgery were also more likely to be hospitalized for premature labor (50% vs. 9%). They had a higher incidence of premature rupture of the membranes, too, an event that poses both immediate health risks and long-term risks to reproductive health (Lyerly & Mahowald, 2001). Finally, the surgery caused a small bowel obstruction in one woman that necessitated additional surgery during the pregnancy. The CHOP team reported no maternal complications in the 10 cases they described.

The two teams recognized certain ethical responsibilities to patients receiving the innovative surgical procedure. Before in utero surgery, CHOP patients met with clinicians to discuss risks and potential benefits, and their cases were reviewed by the "Institutional Fetal Therapy Advisory Committee." At Vanderbilt, patients considering in utero surgery spent 2–3 days in "comprehensive multidisciplinary counseling" designed to promote their understanding of the procedure. According to the *Wall Street Journal,* the process involved "grueling discussions with doctors, nurses, a social worker, and ethicists," and a visit to the neonatal intensive care unit to view the effects of premature birth. Patients in the Vanderbilt study were considered research subjects and the study was reviewed by the IRB.

Thus, physicians performing in utero surgery for spina bifida attempted to supply prospective parents with extensive information about the procedure. Physicians also submitted their plans to institutional review committees before proceeding. It is unclear whether these measures ensured that prospective parents understood the surgery's risks and unproven benefit, however. According to the *JAMA* articles, only one woman offered the surgery declined it. The CHOP physicians reported, "Women who were offered the procedure invariably chose to proceed with it." In an editorial commenting on the reports, another physician called the low refusal rate "troublesome" and an indication of "investigator exuberance" in describing the possible harms and benefits of the surgery (Simpson, 1999, p. 1874).

The same editorial addressed the quality of the scientific information presented in the reports. Among different types of studies, the "case series is generally the weakest of the research designs; other designs in order of increasing strength, are the case-controlled study . . . and the randomized clinical trial"

(Schaffner, 1995, p. 2270–2278). Neither of the in utero surgery teams conducted a randomized clinical trial (RCT) incorporating rigorous research methods designed to minimize biased results. Another problem was that neither team measured the children's functional abilities, such as walking and bladder and bowel control. [In another 1999 article comparing the infants receiving in utero surgery with two groups of historical controls, the Vanderbilt team found no differences in the infants' leg function at 8 months of age (Tulipan et al. 1999).]

As the *JAMA* editorial noted, the absence of functional outcome measures and rigorous research methods made it difficult to evaluate whether in utero surgery produced outcomes superior, equivalent, or inferior to the standard approach of operating on infants after they are born. According to the editorial, "the surgery remains unproved" and "certainly must be considered experimental" (Simpson, 1999, p. 1874). Thus, the developers of in utero surgery for spina bifida had not presented the information and results that would justify its widespread clinical use.

The newness of the surgical procedure partly explains the shortcomings of the two reports. When the data were gathered, children who had received in utero surgery were not old enough to walk or be toilet-trained. Furthermore, a pilot phase to evaluate a procedure's feasibility through less rigorous data gathering may be justified. But as Frader and Caniano (1998) caution, when this pilot phase is concluded, "surgeons should conduct an appropriately designed controlled clinical trial with sufficient patients (i.e., statistical power) to reach generalizable results about the efficacy of the new treatment" (p. 235).

By 2000, the medical community was urging the Vanderbilt and CHOP physicians to conduct such a study. That summer, the National Institutes of Health (NIH) sponsored a workshop on maternal-fetal surgery. Experts at the workshop highlighted the need for rigorous research on in utero surgery for spina bifida. After the workshop, physicians decided to seek NIH funding for an RCT evaluating the procedure.

The NIH agreed to support the proposed trial, which began in 2003. The RCT evaluating in utero surgery for spina bifida is being conducted at Vanderbilt, CHOP, and UCSF. In the trial, 200 pregnant women whose fetuses have been diagnosed with spina bifida will be randomly assigned to an experimental or control group. Women in the experimental group will undergo in utero surgery when their fetuses are between 19 and 25 weeks' gestational age. Women in the control group will not undergo the surgery, and their infants will receive standard treatment after birth. Women and infants will be followed for 2.5 years so that investigators can collect data on the children's functional abilities, as well as the women's physical and psychological health (National Institute of Child Health and Human Development, 2003).

The trial presents distinct ethical challenges because it involves both pregnant women and fetuses expected to develop into children. The surgical intervention's impact on two individuals complicates assessment of risks and expected benefits, including judgments about clinical equipoise. Promoting informed and voluntary decision making in this situation is also a challenge. These challenges are explored in greater detail below.

Evaluating Potential Harms and Benefits in Research Involving Pregnant Women and Fetuses

Like all human research, an RCT evaluating in utero surgery should be consistent with the ethical principle of beneficence. As articulated in the *Belmont Report* (National Commission, 1979) and Common Rule, this principle requires investigators to minimize and justify risks to study subjects. The beneficence principle is also incorporated in a second set of federal regulations relevant to the RCT evaluating in utero surgery for spina bifida, the Department of Health and Human Services regulations governing research involving pregnant women and fetuses (U.S. Department of Health and Human Services, 2001). These regulations require that interventions presenting greater than minimal risk offer a prospect of direct benefit to either the fetus or pregnant woman (National Commission, 1976–1977).[2]

When the RCT addressing in utero surgery for spina bifida was under consideration, what was known about potential benefits to children born after the procedure? Information on the potential benefits was limited. It appeared that surgery might reduce the children's need for a shunt, but this was uncertain. The children had not been followed long enough to determine the magnitude or duration of any other possible benefits. Meanwhile, it was clear that in utero surgery presented risks to children.

The surgery's primary risk to infants was premature birth, which can itself cause serious harm. The greatest risks are to infants born at 25 weeks' gestation or earlier. A study of 811 infants in this group admitted to an intensive care unit found that over half died in the hospital. The researchers were able to assess 283 of the surviving children at 2.5 years of age. Twenty-three percent were classified as severely disabled and 49% as disabled (Wood, Marlow, Costeloe, Gibson & Wilkinson, 2000). The prognosis improves for infants born later than 25 weeks, but serious medical problems remain a possibility (Lee et al., 2000). Only one infant reported in the Vanderbilt and CHOP series was born at 25 weeks or earlier, but extreme prematurity remains a risk of in utero surgery.

Although spina bifida at times produces serious disabilities, its effects range in severity. For example, the Vanderbilt team's *JAMA* article cited a study reporting an average IQ of 86 in a group of 285 children with spina bifida. Yet the

IQs in this group ranged from 24 to 141 (Bruner et al., 1999). In another article, CHOP physicians cited studies finding that the majority of children with spina bifida have normal intelligence (Olutoye & Adzick, 1999). The degree of physical disability also varies among children with the condition. And physicians have limited ability to predict how well individual fetuses and infants with spina bifida will function when they are older.

Some people question whether a possible decrease in disabilities justifies performing in utero surgery, since the operation itself could have lethal or disabling consequences. For example, the *Wall Street Journal* quoted the reaction a man with spina bifida had to the surgery: "I wouldn't have wanted my mother to risk my life in an effort to make me 'perfect.' My life has been and continues to be VERY rewarding" (Winslow, 1999, pp. A1, A10). From a disability rights perspective, physicians' and parents' willingness to expose future children with spina bifida to the risk of death and additional disability rests on the mistaken assumption that life with this condition is not worth living. To the contrary, because the condition typically causes only mild-to-moderate disability, people with spina bifida "can live good lives" if they have access to adequate medical care and support services (Saxton, 2000). The ethical question is whether it is appropriate to expose such infants to a risk of death or additional disability from in utero surgery to obtain a possible improvement in physical or neurologic functioning (Lyerly, Gates, Cefalo, & Sugarman, 2001).

Another controversial issue concerns the proper weight to assign to the surgery's impact on women. Lyerly and Mahowald (2001) argue that physicians performing in utero surgery tend to see the fetus as their sole patient. This attitude is evident in the language used to describe the practitioners—fetal surgeons—and the centers in which they operate. For example, Vanderbilt operates the Center for Fetal Diagnosis and Therapy and CHOP the Center for Fetal Diagnosis and Treatment. Lyerly and Mahowald contend that this attitude led physicians to give cursory attention to the effects of in utero surgery for spina bifida on pregnant women. For example, they say, the Vanderbilt and CHOP teams did not consider whether the women would be able to have other children and how risky any additional pregnancies would be (Farrell et al., 1999).[3] Another problem is that neither team assessed the procedure's psychosocial effects on women.

In summary, the plan to conduct an RCT was based on limited information about in utero surgery's effect on children with spina bifida. The information that existed failed to clarify whether the surgery produced a net benefit in children. At the same time, most of the infants survived, and animal data suggested that they might have improved function. It also seemed possible that they might avoid some of the burdens of standard therapy, including surgery for placement of a shunt and treatment for shunt-related infections (Bruner et al., 1999).

There was also some information about how the surgery affected women. Women faced the risks associated with the surgery itself, as well as increased rates of preterm labor, which in turn produced higher rates of hospitalization and use of drugs to maintain the pregnancy. Some obstetric complications had been documented, too. No data had been collected on the surgery's long-term physical or psychosocial effects on women; thus, it was unclear whether the procedure offered a psychological or other direct benefit to women. In these circumstances, was it appropriate to evaluate the surgery in an RCT? This question requires us to examine the concept of equipoise.

Equipoise in Research

Physicians conducting RCTs may encounter a conflict of professional responsibilities. Physicians have a duty to advance the patient's best interests. In practice, this means that physicians should offer the therapy they believe will be most effective for the individual patient. In an RCT, however, the physician-researcher asks the patient to consent to the chance of receiving an intervention that is less than optimal for that individual. The ethical conflict arises if a physician personally believes that one of the interventions being studied would be better for an individual patient. By enrolling in an RCT, the patient takes the risk of receiving what the physician believes is an inferior intervention. Thus, the physician allows the patient's care to be compromised so that research data can be generated. In effect, the physician puts the interests of the future patients who will benefit from the information the trial produces above the individual patient's interests.

As discussed above, however, the failure to conduct rigorous research raises ethical concerns, as well. Without an RCT evaluating in utero surgery for spina bifida, there would be continued uncertainty about whether the surgery's benefits outweighed its harms. The failure to conduct an RCT could thus lead to ongoing exposure of pregnant women and their future children to an ineffective or damaging surgical intervention.

Moreover, RCT defenders say there is a satisfactory response to the physician's apparent conflict of interest. They argue that physicians personally favoring one study intervention can ethically cooperate with an RCT, as long as the general medical community is uncertain about which intervention is best. These writers argue that when the medical community is uncertain—a situation called "clinical equipoise"—properly open-minded physicians will admit that they could be wrong about which intervention would be best for a patient. Thus, the physician may ethically permit patients to receive an intervention that other reputable physicians believe may be superior (Freedman, 1987).[4]

When the RCT on in utero surgery for spina bifida was proposed, physicians disagreed about whether the intervention was better for children than standard care. Some physicians contended that its risks outweighed any possible benefit to infants. On the other side, the teams performing the surgery thought there was strong evidence that the surgery had at least a short-term benefit to children and that long-term benefits were a definite possibility. Indeed, in its *JAMA* report, the Vanderbilt team expressed its belief "that the maternal and neonatal morbidity associated with in utero repair for myelomeningocele is outweighed by the apparent benefits of early closure" (Bruner et al., 1999, p. 1825).

But was the expert community's uncertainty about net benefits to children enough to establish equipoise? Commentators Lyerly and Mahowald believe it was not. Instead, they argue that "[t]o achieve the equipoise necessary for ethical research on [maternal-fetal surgery], investigators would have to determine a balance between risks and benefits for the woman" (Lyerly & Mahowald, 2001, p. 13). Because "there is really only one patient—the pregnant woman," potential harms and benefits of in utero surgery for spina bifida should be assessed solely from her perspective. The effect the surgery could have on a future child could be counted, they write, but this is a psychosocial benefit to the woman that remains undocumented. For Lyerly and Mahowald, then, insufficient data existed to establish equipoise.

Individuals in favor of conducting the RCT did not explicitly address this point. They probably thought it was reasonable to assume that surgery offered a benefit to women. They could make two claims to support this assumption. First, they could claim that a possible psychosocial benefit to women was adequately established by evidence that in utero surgery could give children improved functioning and freedom from the burdens of a shunt. Second, advocates could claim that this possible benefit to women was demonstrated by women's eagerness to undergo the procedure. Nearly all women offered the procedure consented to it, and this could be interpreted as evidence that women saw the possibility of reduced burdens to their children as a benefit they would experience, too.

The women's positive attitudes about the surgery could strengthen the case for conducting the RCT. Ordinarily, prospective recipients of an investigational procedure are not consulted when judgments about clinical equipoise are made. A newer concept called "community equipoise" departs from the traditional approach, however, by incorporating the views of patient representatives into decisions about equipoise (Karlawish & Lantos, 1997). Accordingly, if patient representatives believed that most women would experience a benefit to a future child as a benefit to themselves, that belief should count in evaluating possible benefits of in utero surgery.

The community equipoise concept might support the judgment that there was sufficient uncertainty to justify an RCT comparing in utero surgery and standard therapy. At the same time, however, if the views of pregnant women should be considered in determining whether equipoise existed, then the views of people with spina bifida should be considered, too. As noted above, at least some members of this group think in utero surgery presents unwarranted risks.

Community equipoise is a new idea and there is uncertainty about how to incorporate the views of different affected groups into equipoise determinations (Dresser, 2001). Another source of difficulty is the approach's reliance on patient representatives to have a reasonable understanding of a novel procedure's potential harms and benefits. As discussed in the next section, such an understanding may be lacking among pregnant women considering in utero surgery for spina bifida.

Informed and Voluntary Decisions About In Utero Surgery

Promoting informed and voluntary decision-making in the context of research on in utero surgery for spina bifida presents several challenges. Pregnant women and their partners must understand that it is uncertain whether the surgery actually benefits children. They must understand that the surgery carries a risk of premature birth, which could lead to additional disability and even death for a child. They must understand that surgery presents risks to pregnant women. They must also be aware that postbirth surgery is an option, and that children receiving standard therapy experience a range of outcomes. They must realize that many individuals with spina bifida have a good quality of life.

The psychological states of physicians and prospective parents possibly compromised the quality of initial decisions to undergo in utero surgery for spina bifida. The CHOP and Vanderbilt reports suggest that physicians might have presented the intervention in an unduly positive light. According to the reports, only 1 woman in 40 decided against in utero surgery. One signal of the adequacy of an information disclosure process is the rate at which people refuse an intervention (Shimm & Spece, 1992). The low refusal rate at the two institutions thus creates a basis for concern.

Moreover, the formal disclosure process is just one information source for patients. People develop beliefs about interventions outside the medical setting. Publicity about a novel intervention shapes expectations that may persist in the face of more detailed and accurate information (Lyerly et al., 2001). Thus, innovators and institutions should be accurate and balanced in all public statements about an unproven procedure.

Some of the initial publicity regarding in utero surgery for spina bifida fell short of this standard. The Vanderbilt and CHOP teams both posted material on Web sites implying that the surgery was proven therapy. (By the time the RCT began, the questionable claims had been removed.) Pregnant women and their partners may have been especially sensitive to language suggesting that in utero surgery was established therapy. Reports in the popular media described couples seeking to do everything possible for a future child. For example, a reporter described one woman's response as follows: "When Kelly saw Vanderbilt's Web site one night, a few days after her ultrasound, she knew that she wanted the surgery. 'Just knowing it would help—or the possibility that it would help—made me decide,' she says. 'It's *doing* something for [my child]' " (Jones, 2001, p. 42).

The prospective parents' state of mind only heightens the physician-investigators' responsibility to avoid presenting in utero surgery in an unduly positive light. Physicians performing in utero surgery should "temper their possible enthusiasm . . . with some sensitivity to the fact that the pregnant woman may be desperate to save her fetus and thus be vulnerable to the lure of the spectacular achievements in prenatal therapy" (Caniano & Baylis, 1999, p. 307). Physicians performing in utero surgery for spina bifida should also give prospective parents an opportunity to meet people with the condition "to gain a more balanced understanding of living with a disability" (Lyerly et al., 2001, p. 696).

Besides raising questions about their communications with prospective parents considering in utero surgery, physicians' enthusiasm could complicate the effort to conduct an RCT evaluating the procedure. When members of the medical community present an unproven procedure as beneficial therapy, it can be difficult to recruit people to participate in an RCT. People actively seeking novel interventions often do so because they are dissatisfied with standard therapy. In turn, they may be unwilling to enroll in an RCT because they might be assigned to receive an existing treatment, rather than the experimental approach. As long as the experimental intervention is available as a clinical option, such individuals are likely to decline RCT participation.

To avoid this problem, the Vanderbilt, CHOP, and UCSF teams agreed to refrain from providing the surgery outside the trial. The procedure will be available solely to trial participants, who will have a 50% chance of being assigned to the in utero surgery group (Lyerly et al., 2001, p. 695). People who assume the surgery is beneficial may be dissatisfied at having their access restricted. Yet physicians are not obligated to perform experimental interventions; rather, performing such interventions outside research raises serious ethical concerns:

> Once the professional community has agreed that a procedure requires formal investigation, off-protocol use of an intervention in an effort to benefit a particular patient undermines the discipline's obligation both to develop treatments that are safe and effective and to not cause unintended harm (Lyerly et al., 2001, p. 694)

In this situation, it is ethically defensible to limit the surgery's availability. The appropriate response to those criticizing the restrictions on access is to stress that the surgery may be ineffective or even harmful and that the trial is necessary to determine whether the surgery actually helps children and families.

CONCLUSION

This analysis of in utero surgery points to two overriding ethical responsibilities for clinicians and researchers. One is the duty to conduct rigorous research to discover whether an innovative procedure is actually better than currently available treatments. In the absence of rigorous research, patients may continue to be exposed to procedures whose overall outcome could be the same or worse than standard care.

The second responsibility is to communicate honestly about the unproven status of novel procedures. The optimistic publicity about in utero surgery is just one illustration of a common tendency to portray innovations in an unduly positive light. In many cases, experimental interventions fall short of initial expectations. Whether to advance their own economic and professional interests, or out of a genuine desire to help children with spina bifida, physicians might have promoted unwarranted hope in novel approaches. The case of in utero surgery demonstrates the need for physicians and researchers to strive for accuracy whenever they discuss experimental interventions with patients and the public.

——

Questions for Discussion

1. What are the unique characteristics of maternal-fetal surgery that make the ethical dilemmas more complicated than the dilemmas raised by pediatric research ethics in general?

2. What are the historical, legal, and contextual reasons that explain the lack of a research tradition the field of surgery compared with other medical fields? What are the implications of this situation?

3. According to the author, innovators can be reluctant to undertake formal research because of the added costs and review requirements. Do the requirements present an unjustified obstacle to the development of innovative new procedures?

4. This chapter asserts that physicians sometimes make new interventions available without conducting rigorous research to assess them. What principles should be considered in analyzing the ethics of this practice?

5. Whose interests are threatened when innovations are offered in the clinical setting, without being accompanied by a formal research? What are those interests?

6. Ethically speaking, what are the shortcomings of the Vanderbilt and CHOP reports on in utero surgery for spina bifida?

7. The *JAMA* editorial noted the absence of functional outcome measures and rigorous research methods in the in utero surgical report. Was there an acceptable reason for those omissions?

8. What are the ethical challenges presented by the randomized clinical trial (RCT) that was scheduled to begin in 2003?

9. Are there moral justifications for the RCT from a disability rights perspective? Does this perspective support the RCT?

10. How should the surgery's impact on women be applied to the case presented in the chapter? Can a feminist ethics perspective contribute to the moral analysis of the issues raised by maternal-fetal surgery?

11. What is the conflict of professional responsibilities physicians face in the case of in utero surgery? What are the reasons for and against conducting the RCT?

12. What is the main ethical violation in portraying in utero surgery for spina bifida in an "unduly positive light"? Can you think of circumstance where this sort of violation is justified?

━━━

Notes

1. The Common Rule covers human research, which is defined as "a systematic investigation, including research development, testing and evaluation, designed to develop or contribute to generalizable knowledge" (Federal Policy for the Protection of Human Subjects, 1991, p. 28,013).

2. Minimal research risks in this context are interpreted as risks comparable to those present in normal fetal development and routine obstetric care (National Commission, 1976–1977).

3. One study found little impact on subsequent fertility among women who had undergone surgery to address other fetal problems (Farrell et al. 1999). Lyerly and Mahowald (2001) question these findings, however, due to methodological problems with the study.

4. Freedman (1987). This chapter's description of RCTs is based on my discussion of the topic in Shapiro M., Spece, R., & Clayton, E., (2003).

References

American Academy of Pediatrics Committee on Bioethics. (1999). Fetal therapy—ethical considerations. *Pediatrics, 103,* 1061–1063.

Bruner, J. P., Tulipan, N., Paschall, R., Boehm, F., Walsh, W., Silva, S., et al. (1999). Fetal surgery for myelomeningocele and the incidence of shunt-dependent hydrocephalus. *Journal of the American Medical Association, 282,* 1819–1825.

Caniano, D. A., & Baylis, F. (1999). Ethical considerations in prenatal surgical consultation. *Pediatric Surgery International, 15,* 303–309.

Casper, M. J. (1998). *The making of the unborn patient: A social anatomy of fetal surgery.* Brunswick, NJ: Rutgers University Press.

Dresser, R. (2001). *When science offers salvation: Patient advocacy and research ethics.* New York, Oxford University Press.

Farrell, J. A., Albanese, C. T., Jennings, R., Kilpatrick, S., Bratton, B., Harrison, M. (1999). Maternal fertility is not affected by fetal surgery. *Fetal Diagnosis and Therapy, 14,* 190–192.

Fauza, D. O. (1999, July/August). The littlest patient. *The Sciences,* pp. 34–38.

Federal Policy for the Protection of Human Subjects. (1991). *Federal Register, 56,* 28012–28018.

Frader, J. E., & Caniano, D. A. (1998). Research and innovation in surgery. In L. B. McCullough, J. W. Jones, & B. A. Brody (Eds.), *Surgical ethics* (p. 216). New York: Oxford University Press.

Freedman, B. (1987). Equipoise and the ethics of clinical research. *New England Journal of Medicine, 317,* 141–145.

Gates, E. (1999, July/August). Two challenges for research ethics: Innovative treatment and fetal therapy. *Women's Health Issues, 9,* 208–210.

Jones, M. (2001, July 15). A miracle, and yet. *New York Times Magazine,* p. 42.

Karlawish, J. H., & Lantos, J. (1997). Community equipoise and the architecture of clinical research. *Cambridge Quarterly of Healthcare Ethics, 6,* 385–396.

Kessler, D. A. (1989). The regulation of investigational drugs. *New England Journal of Medicine, 320,* 281–288.

Kessler, D. A., Pape, S. M., & Sundwall, D. N. (1987). The federal regulation of medical devices. *New England Journal of Medicine, 317,* 357–366.

King, N. M. P. (1995, July/August). Experimental treatment: Oxymoron or aspiration? *Hastings Center Report, 25,* 6–15.

Lee, S. K., McMillan, M., Ohlsson, A., Pendray, M., Synnes, A., Whyte, R., et al. (2000). Variations in practice and outcome in the Canadian NICU network (1996–97). *Pediatrics, 106,* 1070–1079.

Lyerly, A. D., & Mahowald, M. B. (2001). Maternal-fetal surgery: The fallacy of abstraction and the problem of equipoise. *Health Care Analysis, 9,* 1–15.

Lyerly, A. D., Gates, E., Cefalo, R., Sugarman, J. (2001). Toward the ethical evaluation and use of maternal-fetal surgery. *Obstetrics & Gynecology, 98,* 689–697.

Marwick, C. (1993). Coming to terms with indications for fetal surgery. *Journal of the American Medical Association, 270,* 2025, 2029.

McNeill, P. M. (1993) *The ethics and politics of human experimentation.* New York: Cambridge University Press.

National Commission for the Protection of Human Subjects of Biomedical and Behavioral Research. (1979). The Belmont Report: Ethical Principles and Guidelines for the Protection of Human Subjects of Research. Washington, D.C.: Government Printing Office.

National Commission for the Protection of Human Subjects of Biomedical and Behavioral Research. (1976–1977). Research on the fetus: Deliberations and conclusions. *Villanova Law Review, 22,* 300–324.

National Institute of Child Health and Human Development.(2003, September 22). Overview of management of myelomeningocele study. Retrieved July 22, 2004 from http://www.spinabifidamoms.com/english/overview.html

Olutoye, O. O., & Adzick, N. S. (1999). Fetal surgery for myelomeningocele. *Seminars in Perinatology, 23,* 462–473.

Saxton, M. (2000). Why members of the disability community oppose prenatal diagnosis and selective abortion. In E. Parens & A. Asch (Eds.), *Prenatal testing and disability rights* (pp. 147–164). Washington, DC: Georgetown University Press.

Schaffner, K. F. (1995). Research methodology: Conceptual issues. In W. T. Reich (Ed.), *Encyclopedia of bioethics* (pp. 2270–2278). New York: Macmillan.

Shapiro, M. H., Spece, R., Dresser, R., Clayton, E. (2003). *Bioethics and law: Cases, materials and problems* (2nd ed.). St. Paul, MN: West Group.

Shimm, D. S., & Spece, R. G. (1992, March/April). Rates of refusal to participate in clinical trials. *IRB: A Review of Human Subjects Research, 14,* 7–9.

Simpson, J. L. (1999). Fetal surgery for myelomeningocele. *Journal of the American Medical Association, 282,* 1873–1874.

Sutton, L. N., Adzick, N., Bilaniuk, L., Johnson, M., Crombleholme, T., Flake, A. (1999). Improvement in hindbrain herniation demonstrated by serial fetal magnetic resonance imaging following fetal surgery for myelomeningocele. *Journal of the American Medical Association, 282,* 1826–1831.

Tulipan, N., Bruner, J., Hernanz-Schulman, M., Lowe, L., Walsh, W., Nickolaus, D., et al. (1999). Effect of intrauterine myelomeningocele repair on central nervous system structure and function. *Pediatric Neurosurgery, 31,* 183–188.

U.S. Department of Health and Human Services. (2001). Additional protections for pregnant women, human fetuses, and neonates involved in research. *Federal Register, 66,* 56778–56780.

Winslow, R. (1999, April). Fetal operation raises hope for some parents but lots of questions. *Wall Street Journal, 20,* pp. A1, A10.

Wood, N. S., Marlow, N., Costeloe, K., Gibson, A., Wilkinson, A. (2000). Neurologic and developmental disability after extremely preterm birth. *New England Journal of Medicine, 343,* 378–384.

13

Testing Drugs in Developing Countries: Pediatric Research Ethics in an International Context

Michelle Eder

CASE DESCRIPTION

In 2001, a pharmaceutical company submitted a proposal to the Food and Drug Administration to study a new surfactant drug, Surfaxin, in premature infants with respiratory distress syndrome (RDS). The proposed trial design included three arms or treatment groups with 325 subjects in each arm: (1) a group receiving the new, experimental surfactant drug, Surfaxin; (2) a group receiving an established, approved surfactant drug; and (3) a placebo group. The company requested approval to conduct the study in four Latin American countries (Bolivia, Ecuador, Peru, and Mexico). Upon learning of the proposed trial, the directors of Public Citizen, a nonprofit consumer watchdog group, wrote a letter to the secretary of the U.S. Department of Health and Human Services labeling the study as unethical and urging that approval for the study be denied (Lurie, Wolfe, & Klaus, 2001). In the letter, they pointed out that this trial would not be permissible in the United States because a proven effective treatment exists and thus the use of a placebo arm would not be ethical. They also questioned the acceptability of testing the drug in a population that would not be able to afford it if it is proven effective.

The company justified their use of a placebo group in this study because the established drug is not available to the majority of people in the resource-poor Latin American countries where they plan to conduct the study (Flaherty & Stephens, 2001; National Bioethics Advisory Commission, 2001). Because they don't have access to the proven effective treatment, those in the placebo group would not be left any worse off than if they had not participated in the research. Also, the director of the company agreed to provide training, equipment, and Surfaxin, if proven effective, at a discounted cost for 10 years throughout the countries in which the study would be conducted (Charatan, 2001; Flaherty &

Stephens, 2001; National Bioethics Advisory Commission, 2001,). Lurie et al. (2001) maintained that conducting research in a developing country that would not pass ethical muster in the United States constitutes exploitation of a vulnerable population.

RDS *and Surfactant Therapy*

RDS is the most common cause of respiratory failure in neonates (Verma, 1995). It is the fourth largest cause of infant mortality in the United States, constituting about 20% of all neonatal deaths (Verma, 1995). Between 60,000 and 70,000 infants born each year in the United States have RDS, and 5,000 of these infants dic (Wiswell & Mendiola, 1993). RDS is especially prevalent in premature newborns, and its incidence is inversely related to gestational age due to lack of lung development. Surfactant is a phospholipid substance in the lungs that prevents the alveoli from collapsing during expiration (Miller & Armstrong, 1990). Surfactant production occurs primarily in the third trimester so many premature infants are born without sufficient surfactant, and this surfactant deficiency results in RDS (Ishisaka, 1996).

The administration of exogenous surfactant is now considered the standard of care for premature newborns with RDS (Curley & Halliday, 2001; Ishisaka, 1996; Jobe, 1993; Kresch, Lin, & Thrall, 1996; Wiswell & Mendiola, 1993,). RDS-related deaths have decreased significantly with the use of this surfactant replacement therapy. More than 35 randomized controlled trials (RCTs) of exogenous surfactants, both animal and synthetic, were conducted between 1985 and 1992, and four of these surfactants have been approved and are now available for use in the United States (Jobe, 1993; Lurieet al., 2001). A meta-analysis of these RCTs showed a 30–40% decrease in mortality with surfactant therapy (Jobe, 1993). A later report showed a 40–60% decrease in morbidity and mortality from RDS with the use of exogenous surfactant therapy (Ishisaka, 1996).

———

ETHICAL ANALYSIS AND DISCUSSION

This case provides a good example of the complex set of issues involved in the conduct of pediatric research in developing countries. When investigators from the United States are conducting research in another country, they must adhere to federal ethical, legal, and regulatory requirements such as those in the Code of Federal Regulations. These regulations apply to "research conducted, supported or otherwise subject to regulation by the Federal Government outside the United States" (U.S. Department of Health and Human Services, 1991). In addition to these federal regulations, there are several documents that serve as guidelines for conducting research in the international context. These include (1) the Nuremberg

Code (Trials of War Criminals, 1949), (2) the *Declaration of Helsinki* (World Medical Association, 2000), (3) the Council for International Organizations of Medical Sciences (CIOMS) *International Ethical Guidelines for Biomedical Research Involving Human Subjects* (CIOMS/WHO, 2002), (4) the National Bioethics Advisory Commission (NBAC) *Report and Recommendations on Ethical and Policy Issues in International Research* (National Bioethics Advisory Commission, 2001), and (5) the International Conference on Harmonisation *Guideline on the Choice of Control Group and Related Issues in Clinical Trials* (International Conference on Harmonisation 2000). Many writers have raised questions regarding discrepancies in the recommendations given by these various international guidelines (e.g., Weijer & Anderson, 2001). While recognizing that it is a problem, I will not attempt to answer these regulatory questions in this chapter but rather focus on how the guidelines can aid an analysis of the ethical issues raised by the Surfaxin case.

The principles laid out by the National Commission for the Protection of Human Subjects of Biomedical and Behavioral Research in the *Belmont Report* (National Commission, 1978) provide a useful structure for the ethical discussion of the Surfaxin case because all human subjects research should be consistent with its three fundamental ethical principles of beneficence, respect for persons, and justice.

Beneficence

Research that is in accord with the principle of beneficence must be designed to minimize risks to the subject and balance these risks with benefits to the subject, the larger community or group to which the subject belongs, and other patients with the disorder or condition that is being studied (45 CFR 46.111). Children are generally considered to be a vulnerable population that requires extra protection from research risk due to their lack of capacity to provide valid informed consent to participation in research. In pediatric research, parents act as surrogate decision-makers. Because the child-subjects are not making decisions about research participation for themselves, closer scrutiny of the risks involved in research is necessary to protect them from harm. When conducting research with children in developing countries, an additional level of vulnerability is present because the children and their families are socioeconomically disadvantaged. In these populations, increased attention to the minimizing of risks in relation to benefits is warranted to avoid exploitation by investigators from wealthier countries. This is recognized in Article 8 of the *Declaration of Helsinki*: "Medical research is subject to ethical standards that promote respect for all human beings and protect their health and rights. Some research populations are vulnerable and need special protection. The particular needs of the economically and medically disadvantaged must be recognized."

Subpart D of the Code of Federal Regulations (45 CFR 46.401–46.409) provides additional protections for children involved as subjects in research. These additional protections stipulate that research conducted on children is only permissible if the research involves less than minimal risk or, if it involves greater than minimal risk, has the prospect of direct benefit to individual subjects or is likely to yield generalizable knowledge about the subject's disorder or condition (U.S. Department of Health and Human Services, 1991).

Application of these federal regulations fails to clarify the ethical acceptability of the Surfaxin trial. In this case, the primary risks to be considered are the risks to the placebo group who will not receive any active treatment. Public Citizen based their risk analysis on the results of previous surfactant trials and concluded that placing 325 infants in a placebo group would result in the preventable deaths of 17 infants (Lurie et al., 2001). Therefore, the Surfaxin case would certainly fall under the greater than minimal risk category because those infants in the placebo control group are at an increased risk of severe morbidity and mortality. As discussed below, however, standard effective treatment is not available to these infants so the subjects in the placebo group would not be any worse off than if they had not participated in the research. The guidelines are unclear on how to factor this into the risk evaluation.

The question of whether the study offers the prospect of direct benefit is more complicated. Those infants who are randomized to one of the treatment groups will benefit from receiving therapy for RDS. However, those infants who are randomized to the placebo group will not receive the benefit of treatment. If the analysis of benefits takes place prior to randomization, then it could be argued that all children in the study have some chance for benefit because they might be randomized to one of the active treatment groups. A prerandomization analysis of benefits seems inappropriate in these circumstances, though, because it would allow for research that provides a less than favorable risk:benefit ratio to a significant number of subjects. Some contend that those on the placebo arm do receive some benefits, such as ventilation, more intensive health care monitoring, and access to health care professionals trained in neonatology, and that these types of benefits should be considered in the ethical evaluation of the trial (Barry, 1991; Lurie et al., 2001).

Choice of Control Group

The main objection to the design of the Surfaxin study is the inclusion of a placebo control group when a standard proven therapy exists. Many of the ethical issues relating to placebo use in pediatric research are covered elsewhere (see chapter 16 in this volume), so this discussion focuses primarily on the issues that are specific to the international context. Debate about placebo trials has increased markedly in the past 10 years with the proliferation of HIV studies being conducted in developing countries by investigators from the United States. For example, several trials in Africa that tested the effectiveness of a short course treatment for the prevention of maternal–fetal transmission of HIV raised concerns regarding the use of a placebo arm (Angell, 1998, 1999; Annas, 2003; Guay et al., 1999; Lallemant et al., 1998; Lurie & Wolfe, 1999; Schuklenk, 1998; Thomas, 1998; Varmus & Satcher, 1999). These trials have many characteristics in common with the Surfaxin case, but some key differences between them lead to a very different ethical analysis.

Regarding the choice of control group, Article 29 of the *Declaration of Helsinki* states: "The benefits, risks, burdens and effectiveness of a new method should be tested against those of the best current prophylactic, diagnostic, and therapeutic methods. This does not exclude the use of placebo, or no treatment, in studies where no proven prophylactic, diagnostic or therapeutic method exists." A note of clarification on article 29 issued in 2001 added:

> a placebo-controlled trial may be ethically acceptable, even if proven therapy is available, under the following circumstances:
>
> - Where for compelling and scientifically sound methodological reasons its use is necessary to determine the efficacy or safety of a prophylactic, diagnostic or therapeutic method; or
> - Where a prophylactic, diagnostic or therapeutic method is being investigated for a minor condition and the patients who receive placebo will not be subject to any additional risk of serious or irreversible harm."

In a section devoted to ethical issues surrounding the use of a placebo control, International Conference on Harmonisation (2000) guideline E10 reads: "In cases where an available treatment is known to prevent serious harm, such as death or irreversible morbidity in the study population, it is generally inappropriate to use a placebo control."

There is general agreement in these regulations and in the scientific community that placebos shouldn't be used when proven therapy exists and withholding that proven therapy could result in death or serious harm (Emanuel & Miller, 2001; Temple & Ellenberg, 2000). According to this reasoning, the Surfaxin study would not be ethically permissible because withholding proven therapy would result in an increased chance of death.

Many of the arguments made in favor of the Surfaxin study refer to the scientific advantages of placebo use. These arguments regarding the scientific necessity of placebo use will not be discussed at length here because many of them are covered in chapter 16 in this volume. Briefly, proponents of the Surfaxin study point to the decreased time and sample size needed to get results regarding the effectiveness of the treatment under study when a placebo is used (Charatan, 2001; Flaherty & Stephens, 2001; Lurie et al., 2001; National Bioethics Advisory Commission, 2001). However, the argument for speed of results doesn't apply in this case because four surfactant drugs are already approved and available for use in the United States, but are not available to most infants in the Latin American countries where the trial will be conducted due to cost and other considerations. Nor is there any reason to believe that Surfaxin, if proven effective, will be available to these infants (National Bioethics Advisory Commission, 2001). Placebo controlled studies are generally less expensive to carry out because they require fewer subjects to answer the research question, but as Rothman and Michels (1994) stress, "the costs saved by the drug company are borne by patients, who receive placebos instead of effective treatments" (p. 396).

Those in favor of the Surfaxin study's trial design also suggest that the need for assay sensitivity (the ability to determine how a new treatment performs in comparison to another) demands the use of placebo. While it is true that studies must be methodologically sound in order to be considered ethical, the ethical requirement to test new treatments against proven therapy if it exists takes precedence over these scientific considerations (Rothman & Michels, 1994; Weijer & Anderson, 2001). Put another way, Emanuel and Miller (2001) propose that scientific validity *is* an ethical reason to use placebo controls, but it would not constitute a *sufficient* reason because research must be scientifically valid *and* minimize risks to subjects in order to be ethical.

Proponents of this Surfaxin trial also cite the need for a placebo control because there is a lack of information about the effectiveness of the standard proven surfactant therapy in the Latin American context. Because there is uncertainty regarding whether the standard therapy would be effective in Latin America, it is necessary to compare the standard therapy to placebo. There is a concern that a different epidemiological setting, such as in Latin America where infant mortality is 2–3 times higher than in developed countries, might affect the success of surfactant therapy (Freedman, Weijer, & Glass, 1996; Rossello et al., 1997). There is also the possibility that differences in the health care infrastructure, such as the quality of neonatal care available, may influence the outcome of surfactant therapy.

These arguments overlook a key study (Rossello et al., 1997) describing the effects of surfactant therapy in Latin America that used a nonconcurrent untreated control because the researchers considered a placebo control to be unethical due to the existence of effective surfactant therapy. Rossello et al. compared infants with RDS who were treated with surfactant to those who were not treated in the

2 years prior to the availability of surfactant in 19 Neonatal intensive care units (NICUs) from five Latin American countries. Their results showed that surfactant significantly improved outcomes for infant morbidity and mortality. Specifically, use of surfactant therapy resulted in a 50% decrease in early mortality and an 18% decrease in global mortality at discharge for infants weighing between 700 g and 999 g at birth.

Although advocates of placebo-controlled trials would argue that historical controls are inadequate because of their inability to ensure the comparability of the treatment and control groups, the limitations related to the use of a historical control were minimized by Rossello et al. (1997). The infants in the historical control group met the same inclusion criteria as those in the surfactant group, were taken from the same 19 NICUs, and had similar clinical features, such as Apgar scores. In addition, Rossello et al. contend that "[d]uring the two years prior to surfactant use, no major changes occurred in the NICUs that could affect neonatal outcomes" (p. 281). The group treated with surfactant did have a lower mean birth weight and gestational age, but this bias in group composition was corrected for by performing comparisons stratified by birth weight. This study provides evidence that the surfactant therapy proven to be effective in the United States is also effective in the Latin American context, thus countering the argument that placebo controls are needed.

Equipoise

The ethically appropriate control group for a particular trial will also depend upon the requirement of equipoise. Equipoise refers to uncertainty about which of the treatments being compared in a research study is superior (Freedman, 1987). In other words, if there is reason to believe prior to the start of the trial that one of the treatment arms is superior, it is unethical to enroll subjects on the trial because some will receive an inferior treatment (Angell, 1999; Freedman, 1987; Weijer & Glass, 2002,). In cases where a proven effective treatment exists for the condition being studied, equipoise dictates that placebo controls should not be used because their use would mean giving one group of patients a treatment (or nontreatment) that is known to be inferior. In such a case, physicians would be faced with the ethical conflict of compromising the care of some subjects in the interests of conducting the research.

The equipoise condition is not met in the Surfaxin case because one of the three groups is a proven effective treatment, which is known to significantly decrease morbidity and mortality compared to no treatment. Even in less extreme cases where withholding the proven treatment does not result in serious harm, the investigator still has a responsibility to provide each research subject with a treatment that is considered at least as good as the proven treatment (Freedman, Glass, & Weijer, 1996; Rothman & Michels, 1994). Huston and Peterson (2001) also emphasize this "potential for a conflict of interest between the researcher and the subject each time treatment is withheld" (p. 913).

Local Versus Universal Standard of Care

Disagreement about the choice of control group for clinical trials in developing countries stems from debate about the meaning of "standard available therapy." Because of ambiguity about the meaning of "standard available therapy," a question arises in the international context: Are placebo-controlled studies ethically justified in situations where the proven treatment is not available to the population in which the research is conducted because of cost and other barriers to accessibility? There is controversy over whether a standard proven therapy was available in the Surfaxin case, and this controversy influences the ethical analysis of the trial.

Some argue for interpretation of "standard available therapy" to mean the most effective therapy that is available anywhere in the world (Lurie et al., 2001). On this basis, the Surfaxin trial design would not be acceptable because there is an effective treatment, although it isn't available to the proposed host population. Others call for a definition of "standard available therapy" such that the effective therapy must be available locally (Halsey, Sommer, Henderson, & Black, 1997; Levine, 1998). This definition leads to the conclusion that a placebo control may be used in contexts where no treatment is normally available, such as in the Latin American countries under discussion. Using the local standard of care rationale, placebo controlled trials, such as the Surfaxin study, would be ethical in these situations because subjects in the control group would be receiving the standard of care (nothing) and would not be left any worse off than if they hadn't participated in the research. Analysis of the Surfaxin case is complicated by the fact that surfactant *is* used in some hospitals in these countries, but isn't considered the standard of care because it is not available to the majority of people due to financial limitations.

Many who advocate for using the local available standard justify their position by an appeal to justice (discussed further below). New treatments should be compared to the best treatment available locally because that is the only means of obtaining results that are responsive to local health needs and have the potential to improve health care in that context (Ellenberg & Temple, 2000). These writers often cite the aforementioned HIV trials as examples of studies using this rationale. In these trials, most women in the countries where the studies were conducted did not have access to the proven effective zidovudine (AZT) regimen to reduce maternal–fetal transmission of HIV because it was too expensive and not feasible to implement given the realities of health care standards in these countries. Those conducting the trials argued that the appropriate research design would compare no treatment to a short-term, low-dose regimen that would be affordable and feasible to implement in developing countries. A trial comparing the short-course AZT regimen to the longer, proven regimen would not provide information that would be useful to the people in the developing countries (Macklin, 1999).

This rationale for using the local available standard does not apply to the Surfaxin case. As in the case of the HIV trials, the families in the Latin American countries being discussed do not have access to the proven effective therapy that is available in the United States. However, unlike the HIV trials that were testing a treatment specifically intended for women in Africa, the treatment being studied in the Surfaxin trial is not likely to be any more accessible to families in these Latin American countries than the four surfactant drugs already approved and available in the United States. It is therefore doubtful that the results of the trial will improve the health of people in these countries.

Respect for Persons

The principle of respect for persons incorporates the autonomy and individual rights of research subjects and is often applied through the doctrine of voluntary informed consent. International ethical codes, such as the Nuremberg Code, the *Declaration of Helsinki*, and the Council of International Organizations of Medical Sciences' guidelines, all require informed consent as the universal fulfillment of respect for persons. In pediatric research, informed parental permission for the child's participation is required and provides an important protection against the exploitation of research subjects. In the proposed Surfaxin study, the parents would be the sole decision makers because the subjects are premature infants unable to provide assent. In this situation, the protection of the subject becomes particularly critical because someone other than the child is making the decision about participation, and this decision is expected to be made in the child's best interests.

There are three components of informed parental permission that need to be fulfilled in every pediatric research study: disclosure and understanding of information, voluntariness, and the competence of the decision-maker. Achieving valid informed consent is always a very difficult, complex process, but informed consent for research in developing countries presents several additional challenges. Many discussions of informed consent procedures relating to placebo-controlled trials emphasize the need for information disclosure. For example, Emanuel and Miller (2001) point out that an adequate informed consent process would include the following explanations: (1) the reasons for including a placebo group in the trial design, (2) the fact that those who are randomly assigned to the placebo group will not receive standard effective treatment, and (3) the risks associated with not receiving effective treatment, which include death and severe morbidity in the case of RDS. Lurie et al. (2001) maintain that the consent process for the Surfaxin study would also need to include mention of the dozens of studies that have shown available surfactants to be effective in decreasing morbidity and mortality and an explanation of why some study subjects would not receive these surfactants.

The competence of the parent to make an informed decision must also be considered. In the context of the developing world, language and educational differences between the investigator and subjects/parents complicate the informed consent process. In addition, the ability of a parent to process complex trial information in order to make a decision may be seriously compromised due to situational factors. The circumstances surrounding the birth of a premature infant with RDS include a high physician and parental stress level, a need to make decisions and act quickly in response to the RDS, and a parent decision-maker that is in a weakened, perhaps semiconscious state. These circumstances are not conducive to obtaining informed parental permission, and the informed consent procedures may need to be altered to improve the decision-making context.

Obtaining informed consent from people in developing countries such as the proposed sites for the surfactant study may be problematic because of lack of understanding of the information provided. Some researchers contend that because of differences in explanatory models of disease causation and a general lack of education, many people in developing countries are incapable of understanding information that is disclosed to them about treatment alternatives, including trial participation (Christakis, 1988; Ekunwe, 1984; Kessel, 1984,). However, extra effort to address the differing explanatory models and translate information into culturally appropriate forms will increase the likelihood that parents of potential subjects are able to understand information necessary for them to make a decision (Christakis & Levine, 1995; IJsselmuiden & Faden, 1992; Kempf, 1996,). To this end, Barry (1988) calls for local community involvement to aid in making informed consent information understandable. McGrath and colleagues (McGrath, George, et al., 2001; McGrath, Mafigiri, et al., 2001) conducted interviews in Uganda prior to the initiation of an AIDS vaccine trial in order to assess the educational needs of the study population. This allowed them to tailor informed consent information to address concepts relating to vaccines that were not familiar to people. Cox and MacPherson (1996) suggest using a local mediator from the shared culture of the potential research subject to obtain verbal consent because verbal information may be tailored to the information needs of the patient. This helps ensure that the information provided is culturally relevant and understandable to the patient. These types of comprehension-building strategies would be necessary in the Latin American context of the proposed Surfaxin study in order to obtain informed parental permission.

The voluntariness of subjects to provide consent must also be taken into account. Lurie et al. (2001) highlight the potential for coercion in the setting of the proposed Surfaxin trial and suggest that the trial presents these economically disadvantaged parents with a choice that is not completely voluntary. These parents are likely to make a desperate choice to participate in the study in the hope of their child receiving one of the treatment arms because they would not otherwise have access to surfactant therapy. Lackey (2001, p. 9) presents the opposing argument that desperation does not invalidate consent because "the sick are desperate in every country" and this fact does not equal coercion. There *is* a real potential for coercion in situations where participating in a study is the only means of accessing care and getting otherwise unavailable treatment, and this potential needs to be factored into the ethical evaluation of the trial. While offering a study that provides potential subjects with treatments they could not otherwise get is not an actively or purposively coercive act, it does introduce the potential for undue influence on decision-making regarding trial participation. There is a level of desperation inherent in the illness state, but an honest evaluation of the discrepancies between the care available to people in developing versus developed countries suggests that the sick in some countries may be more desperate than the sick in others. Recognition of this is necessary to ensure that these desperate individuals are not exploited by subjecting them to unacceptable research risks.

In chapter 16 of this volume, Berg highlights the problem of the therapeutic misconception in pediatric research, which refers to the mistaken assumption that researchers act in the best interests of each subject rather than in the interests of the research (Appelbaum, Roth, & Lidz, 1982). She suggests that parents may be particularly prone to misunderstanding the difference between the goals of research and treatment because they are inclined to seize any opportunity to help their child and think of physicians as being solely interested in helping their child as well. The therapeutic misconception is likely to be even more prevalent in contexts where the only access to treatment of any kind is on a research study, such as in the Surfaxin case. A thorough disclosure process becomes even more critical to valid parental permission in cases like this where the therapeutic misconception is a common problem.

Another issue regarding informed consent in the international context is raised by the proposed Surfaxin trial. The ethical standard of informed consent that is adhered to in the United States and many other developed countries reflects the uniquely Western conception of a person and may not be meaningful to groups that adhere to more social or duty-based conceptions of personhood. For example, in some developing countries, individuals expect authority figures (physicians, community leaders) to make decisions for them. How can researchers from developed countries conduct ethical studies in developing countries whose norms regarding informed consent differ markedly from ours? Some have called for total tolerance of the ethical norms of others, and suggest that imposing our Western notions of informed consent on other cultures in which they are not meaningful is a form of ethical imperialism (Newton, 1990). Kleinman (1995) insists that our bioethical categories are derived from a Western philosophical tradition that lacks meaning in other settings, and therefore the ethical frameworks of other cultures must be interpreted on their own terms. Alternatively, others have argued that ethics developed in the West should be applied in all situations and settings (IJsselmuiden & Faden, 1992; Osuntokun, 1992).

Most, however, opt for the middle ground and require that the principle of respect for persons is a fundamental, universal standard that must be applied to all settings, but that the application of this principle does and should vary among contexts. For instance, Christakis (1988) asserts that rather than accepting culturally *relative* standards of research ethics, we make universal standards culturally *relevant*. He further states that beyond minimal standards, variability should be tolerated in such things as the particular content of the information disclosed, and the additional consent of community leaders or heads of household. Thus, the universal validity of the principles is not challenged, but a universal application of the principles is inappropriate because different contexts require different applications. At the core of this perspective is acknowledgement of distinct expressions of respect for persons that are shaped by particular social, cultural, and historical settings. Genuine respect for persons requires an understanding of the patient's or subject's cultural values and beliefs. Therefore, culturally relevant application of the principle of respect for persons "means broadening our view of autonomy so that respect for persons includes respect for the cultural values they bring with them to the decision-making process" (Blackhall, Murphy, Frank, Michel, & Azen, 1995, p. 825).

Other questions relating to respect for persons that arise in this case are: Did the countries agree to host the Surfaxin trial? Were the local communities involved in the development of the trial? There has been much discussion in the literature regarding the role of groups, such as communities, as gatekeepers to research (Juengst, 1998, 2000, 2003; Marshall & Rotimi, 2001; National Bioethics Advisory Commission, 2001; Sharp & Foster, 2000; Weijer, 1999). Sharp and Foster (2000) describe "community review" as having several forms, including community dialogue and consultation and formal community approval or disapproval. Regarding the latter, the NBAC suggests that in research conducted in developing countries "representatives of the host country, including scientists, public officials, and persons with the condition under study, should have a strong voice in determining whether a proposed trial is appropriate" (National Bioethics Advisory

Commission, 2001, p. 27). Getting permission from community leaders to conduct the research in developing countries shows respect for the local decision-making authorities and helps ensure the ethical acceptability of the research to the population. The fact that prior approval and support of local governments was sought before initiating the research on perinatal HIV transmission in Africa is often cited as evidence that the research was ethical (Resnik, 1998; Varmus & Satcher, 1999). While seeking support from local governments is a necessary preliminary step in international research, it should never be used as a substitute for the individual consent of research participants. In addition, the potential for community leaders who support the research to exert a coercive influence on individuals to participate must be addressed in every case (National Bioethics Advisory Commission, 2001).

In addition to community approval for research, community review includes dialogue and consultation. These refer to early discussions between investigators and communities about ways to minimize risks to subjects and maximize benefits by determining how the study can be designed to best respond to the needs of the community. This type of community review is referred to in CIOMS (2002) guideline 3: "The health authorities of the host country, as well as a national or local ethical review committee, should ensure that the proposed research is responsive to the health needs and priorities of the host country and meets the requisite ethical standards." The NBAC's recommendation 2.3 also discusses community participation: "Researchers and sponsors should involve representatives of the community of potential participants throughout the design and implementation of research project (National Bioethics Advisory Commission, 2001)."

The HIV trials are a good example of research that was developed with the participation of local communities. These trials involved communities in the identification of a crucial health problem and the development of a research question and trial design that responded to it in a manner appropriate to the local context (Varmus & Satcher, 1999). This type of community participation and approval of the local governments is necessary in the Surfaxin case in order to ensure the ethical acceptability of the trial for those being asked to participate.

Justice

Studies like the proposed Surfaxin trial highlight several issues of justice that concern research conducted in developing countries. The principle of justice refers to the fair distribution of the benefits and burdens of research in a given population. In the international context, justice requires that the people bearing the burdens of participation in the research and the larger community to which they belong are the primary recipients of the knowledge gained by the research. When investigators from the United States conduct research in a developing country, there is a concern that patients in the United States will be the beneficiaries of the research results rather than those who accepted the risks of participating in the research.

One aspect of justice in research relates to the need for research to respond to the health problems that are of major concern to the population being asked to serve as research subjects. Another facet of justice in research involves the researchers' responsibilities to make the treatment available to the study population after the research is completed. In international contexts, justice takes on great importance because of the concern that investigators from the United States will use vulnerable populations in developing countries as research subjects in order to get treatments approved quickly for commercial distribution primarily in the United States.

Many of the international ethical guidelines discuss these issues and provide recommendations for applying the principle of justice to the ethical evaluation of particular studies. Principle 19 of the *Declaration of Helsinki* states, "Medical research is only justified if there is a reasonable likelihood that the populations in which the research is carried out stand to benefit from the results of the research." Principle 30 further addresses this issue: "At the conclusion of the study, every patient entered into the study should be assured of access to the best proven prophylactic, diagnostic and therapeutic methods identified by the study (World Medical Association, 2000)."

The CIOMS (2002) guidelines regarding research in populations and communities with limited resources also articulate the ethical requirements of responsiveness and reasonable availability:

> Before undertaking research in a population or community with limited resources, the sponsor and the investigator must make every effort to ensure that:
>
> - the research is responsive to the health needs and the priorities of the population or community in which it is to be carried out; and any intervention or product developed, or knowledge generated, will be made reasonably available for the benefit of that population or community." (Guideline 10)

The NBAC's recommendation 1.3 states that: "Clinical trials conducted in developing countries should be limited to those studies that are responsive to the health needs of the host country." Recommendation 4.2 addresses the provision of post-trial benefits to the research population: "Research proposals submitted to ethics review committees should include an explanation of how new interventions that are proven to be effective from the research will become available to some or all of the host country population beyond the research participants themselves (National Bioethics Advisory Commission, 2001)."

Is the Surfaxin trial responsive to the needs of people in the Latin American countries in which it would be conducted? Four effective surfactants are now available in the United States, but they are not generally available in these developing countries (Flaherty & Stephens, 2001). There does not appear to be an urgent need for yet another surfactant treatment, and there is no reason to expect that a new treatment would be any more affordable or otherwise accessible to the people in the proposed host population. This begs the question of whether this is an important scientific question that is being asked to address a major health problem in these countries, or just a means for the pharmaceutical company to get approval for a new treatment that they will profit from by marketing the drug in the United States. Evaluation of the trial in light of the principle of justice does not demonstrate a fair distribution of the benefits and burdens of this research.

Another approach to the justice issue is to question whose interests are being served by the research and what the motivation for the study was. In the context of international pediatric research, a heightened level of suspicion for the motivation for research is necessary in order to ensure protection of vulnerable populations. The motivation for the proposed Surfaxin study appears to be the financial gain of the pharmaceutical company conducting the research, rather than answering a question intended to improve the health of the host population. With regards to this issue of responsiveness, the Surfaxin trial stands in contrast to the trials to reduce maternal-fetal transmission of HIV in Africa. The motivation behind these HIV trials was to test a treatment that was specifically for use in developing countries. The needs of the host population figured into the design of the trial, and the results provided information that was useful to the host population.

Economic considerations must be recognized in applying the principle of justice to this case. Justice requires paying attention to the economic circumstances of the research subjects and conducting research on treatments that will be affordable to them. Surfactant treatment for premature neonates with RDS in the United States costs between $1,100 and $2,400 and is therefore too expensive for the majority of people in these poor Latin American countries (Flaherty & Stephens, 2001). The cost of surfactant treatment, and the health care infrastructure needed to administer it, means that it would also not be feasible for the company to provide the population with Surfaxin in the long term. The sustainability of treatments being studied must always be assessed in light of local health care standards. The company proposing the Surfaxin trial partially addressed this issue of sustainability by promising such things as ventilators and neonatology training to the participating hospitals, but the fact that the treatment itself is unaffordable to most remains.

The second aspect of justice refers to making any treatments shown to be effective reasonably available to the population from which the research subjects came. The NBAC recommendations refer to this notion that investigators owe research participants something in return for their contribution to the research as "justice as reciprocity." When submitting the proposal for the Surfaxin trial, the pharmaceutical company agreed to provide neonatology training, equipment such as ventilators, and Surfaxin, if proven effective, at a discounted cost for 10 years throughout the countries in which the study would be conducted (Charatan, 2001). Unfortunately, it is not clear exactly what "discounted" means in this case. Given the extremely high cost of surfactant and the level of poverty in the host countries, in order to make it "reasonably available" the drug would need to be discounted to the point where the pharmaceutical company would not profit from its use in these countries. And while certainly laudable, the provision of treatment after the study is over can not be used as justification for the use of a placebo when withholding a proven treatment (available locally or not) leads to an increased risk of severe morbidity and mortality.

Many writers underscore the "perpetuation of inequities" that occurs in much research in developing countries (Piot, 1998; Schuklenk, 1998; Thomas, 1998). For example, Piot (1998) suggests that our primary concern should be the lack of access to treatment that exists in developing countries and that our efforts should be focused on making these treatments available to all. Thomas (1998) and Schuklenk (1998) describe how trade policies and the commercial interests of pharmaceutical companies perpetuate these global inequities and call for an ethical analysis that takes these into account. With regards to the Surfaxin case, our priority should be finding ways to make the surfactants that are already proven effective available to families in Latin America rather than testing yet another drug that will be unaffordable to them.

CONCLUSIONS

The above analysis demonstrates the complexity of the ethical issues involved in research conducted in developing countries. Many of the ethical principles discussed take on added significance in the international context because of the potential for exploitation of vulnerable populations. Proponents and critics of the Surfaxin trial both point to certain principles as justification for their ethical arguments. Pediatric research, however, must address all three principles in order to be ethically acceptable. For example, while obtaining informed parental permission is ethically and legally necessary, it can not take the place of a careful ethical analysis of the risk:benefit ratio for potential trial participants. Similarly, providing treatments to subjects after the conclusion of a trial does not compensate for conducting research that is not responsive to the needs of the host population.

As the above analysis shows, attention to the local socioeconomic, health care, and cultural context is of paramount importance when assessing the ethical acceptability of trials in developing countries. However, the local context cannot be used as justification for conducting trials that do not adhere to the ethical principles of beneficence, respect for persons, and justice. In the Surfaxin case, the company proposing the trial used the unavailability of surfactant treatment to the local population as a reason for conducting a placebo-controlled trial that presents an unfavorable risk:benefit ratio to subjects, does not address the health concerns of those being asked to participate in the research, and is motivated by the commercial interests of the pharmaceutical company. The bottom line is that the trial exposes children in developing countries to the risks of research that will primarily benefit the pharmaceutical company and children in the United States, and is therefore ethically unacceptable.

Questions for Discussion

1. Should research that is funded by American drug companies, but is not ethically permissible in the United States, be conducted in a developing country? If so, under what circumstances would this be acceptable?

2. The author concludes that the proposed Surfaxin trial is ethically unacceptable. Do you agree? Why or why not? How could the design of the trial be altered to make it more ethically justified? What would be the drawbacks of such a change?

3. Do you agree with the argument that placebo controls may be used in settings where subjects don't have access to proven effective treatments that are available elsewhere because those in the placebo group would not be left any worse off than if they had not participated in the research? Are there particular situations in which applying the locally available standard is in the subjects' best interests? How do the HIV perinatal transmission trials and the proposed Surfaxin trial differ from one another in this respect?

4. Who stands to benefit from the results of the proposed Surfaxin trial and in what ways? How do these potential benefits factor into the ethical analysis of this case?

5. What is the role of economic factors in the proposed trial? Discuss the ways in which economic factors influence your ethical analysis of this case.
6. Discuss the role of justice in international pediatric research. Is the Surfaxin trial responsive to the needs of the people being asked to participate in the research? Are the benefits and burdens of research fairly distributed? How does the pharmaceutical company's promise to provide Surfaxin at reduced cost after the conclusion of the trial impact your ethical analysis?
7. What are the difficulties with obtaining informed parental permission in developing countries? Discuss potential strategies for overcoming these difficulties. How can potentially coercive elements such as therapeutic misconception and the influence of community leaders be mitigated in the development and implementation of international research?
8. What contextual factors need to be considered in all international research? How do these factors shape the design and conduct of research in developing countries?
9. Why are children in developing countries considered to be an especially vulnerable population? How does this vulnerability change the ethical requirements for pediatric research in international settings?

References

Angell, M. (1998). Ethics of placebo-controlled trials of zidovudine to prevent the perinatal transmission of HIV in the third world: Reply. *New England Journal of Medicine, 338*(12), 843.

Angell, M. (1999). The ethics of clinical research in the Third World. In T. L. Beauchamp & L. Walters (Eds.), *Contemporary Issues in Bioethics* (pp. 770–772). Belmont, CA: Wadsworth Publishing Company.

Annas, G. J. D. (2003). The right to health and the Nevirapine case in South Africa. *New England Journal of Medicine, 348*(8), 750–754.

Appelbaum, P. S., Roth, L. H., & Lidz, C. (1982). The therapeutic misconception: informed consent in psychiatric research. *International Journal of Law and Psychiatry, 5*(3–4), 319–329.

Barry, M. (1988). Ethical considerations of human investigation in developing countries: the AIDS dilemma. *New England Journal of Medicine, 319*(16), 1083–1086.

Barry, M. (1991). Ethical dilemmas with economic studies in less-developed countries: AIDS research trials. *IRB: Ethics & Human Research, 13*, 8–9.

Blackhall, L. J., Murphy, S. T., Frank, G., Michel, V., & Azen, S. (1995). Ethnicity and attitudes toward patient autonomy. *Journal of the American Medical Association, 274*(10), 820–825.

Charatan, F. (2001). Surfactant trial in Latin America infants criticised. *British Medical Journal, 322,* 575.

Christakis, N. A. (1988). The ethical design of an AIDS vaccine trial in Africa. *Hastings Center Report, 18,* 31–37.

Christakis, N. A., & Levine, R. J. (1995). Multinational research. In W. T. Reich (Ed.), *Encyclopedia of Bioethics* (Rev. ed., pp. 1780–1787). New York: Simon & Schuster Macmillan.

CIOMS/WHO. (2002). *International ethical guidelines for biomedical research involving human subjects, revised.* Geneva: Council for International Organizations of Medical Sciences and the World Health Organization.

Cox, C., & Macpherson, C. N. L. (1996). Modified informed consent in a viral seroprevalence study in the Caribbean. *Bioethics, 10*(3), 222–232.

Curley, A. E., & Halliday, H. L. (2001). The present status of exogenous surfactant for the newborn. *Early Human Development, 61,* 67–83.

Ekunwe, E. O. (1984). Informed consent in the developing world: Case study commentary. *Hastings Center Report, 14,* 22–23.

Ellenberg, S. S., & Temple, R. (2000). Placebo-controlled trials and active-control trials in the evaluation of new treatments, Part 2: Practical issues and specific cases. *Annals of Internal Medicine, 133*(6), 464–470.

Emanuel, E. J., & Miller, F. G. (2001). The ethics of placebo-controlled trials- a middle ground. *New England Journal of Medicine, 345*(12), 915–919.

Flaherty, M. P., & Stephens, J. (2001, February 23). PA. firms asks FDA to back experiment forbidden in U.S. *Washington Post*, p. 3.

Freedman, B. (1987). Equipoise and the ethics of clinical research. *New England Journal of Medicine, 317,* 141–145.

Freedman, B., Glass, K. C., & Weijer, C. (1996). Placebo orthodoxy in clinical research II: ethical, legal, and regulatory myths. *Journal of Law, Medicine and Ethics, 24,* 252–259.

Freedman, B., Weijer, C., & Glass, K. C. (1996). Placebo orthodoxy in clinical research I: empirical and methodological myths. *Journal of Law, Medicine and Ethics, 24,* 243–251.

Guay, L., Musoke, P., Fleming, T., Bagenda, D., Allen, M., Nakabiito, C., et al. (1999). Intrapartum and neonatal single-dose nevirapine compared with zidovudine for prevention of mother-to-child transmission of HIV-1 in Kampala, Uganda: HIVNET 012 randomised trial. *Lancet, 354,* 795–802.

Halsey, N. A., Sommer, A., Henderson, D. A., & Black, R. E. (1997). Ethics and international research. *British Medical Journal, 315,* 965–966.

Huston, P., & Peterson, R. (2001). Withholding proven treatment in clinical research. *New England Journal of Medicine, 345*(12), 912–914.

IJsselmuiden, C. B., & Faden, R. R. (1992). Research and informed consent in Africa—another look. *New England Journal of Medicine, 326*(12), 830–834.

International Conference on Harmonisation of Technical Requirements for Registration of Pharmaceuticals for Human Use. (2000). *ICH Harmonised Tripartite Guideline. Choice of Control Group and Related Issues in Clinical Trials E10.* Geneva: International Conference on Harmonisation Secretariat, International Federation for Pharmaceutical Manufacturers Association.

Ishisaka, D. Y. (1996). Exogenous surfactant use in neonates. *Annals of Pharmacotherapy, 30,* 389–398.

Jobe, A. H. (1993). Pulmonary Surfactant Therapy. *New England Journal of Medicine, 328*(12), 861–868.

Juengst, E. T. (1998). Groups as gatekeepers to genomic research: conceptually confusing, morally hazardous, and practically useless. *Kennedy Institute of Ethics Journal, 8*(2), 183–200.

Juengst, E. T. (2000). Commentary: What 'community review' can and cannot do. *Journal of Law, Medicine and Ethics, 28*(1), 52–54.

Juengst, E. T. (2003). Community engagement in genetic research: the "slow code" of research ethics? In B. Knoppers (Ed.), *Populations and genetics: Legal and socio-ethical perspectives* (pp. 181–197). Leiden: Martinus Nijhoff Publishers.

Kempf, J. (1996). Collecting medical specimens in South America: A dilemma in medical ethics. *Anthropological Quarterly, 69*(3), 142–148.

Kessel, R. (1984). Informed consent in the developing world: case study commentary. *Hastings Center Report, 14,* 22–24.

Kleinman, A. (1995). *Writing at the margin: Discourse between anthropology and medicine.* Berkeley: University of California Press.

Kresch, M. J., Lin, W. H., & Thrall, R. S. (1996). Surfactant replacement therapy. *Thorax, 51*(11), 1137–1154.

Lackey, D. P. (2001). Clinical trials in developing countries: a review of the moral issues. *Mount Sinai Journal of Medicine, 68*(1), 4–12.

Lallemant, M., McIntosh, K., Jourdain, G., Le Coeur, S., Vithayasai, V., Lee, T.-H., et al. (1998). Ethics of placebo-controlled trials of zidovudine to prevent the perinatal transmission of HIV in the third world: correspondence. *New England Journal of Medicine, 338*(12), 839–840.

Levine, R. J. (1998). The "best proven therapeutic method" standard in clinical trials in technologically developing countries. *IRB: A Review of Human Subjects Research, 20*(1), 5–9.

Lurie, P., & Wolfe, S. M. (1999). Unethical trials of interventions to reduce perinatal transmission of the Human Immunodeficiency Virus in developing countries. In T. L. Beauchamp & L. Walters (Eds.), *Contemporary issues in bioethics* (pp. 766–770). Belmont, CA: Wadsworth Publishing Company.

Lurie, P., Wolfe, S. M., & Klaus, M. (2001). Letter to Tommy Thompson, Secretary of Health and Human Services, February 22, 2001. Retrieved July 20, 2004 from http://www.citizen.org/publications/release.cfm?ID=6761.

Macklin, R. (1999). *Against Relativism, Cultural Diversity and the Search for Ethical Universals in Medicine.* Oxford: Oxford University Press.

Marshall, P., & Rotimi, C. (2001). Ethical challenges in community-based research. *American Journal of the Medical Sciences, 322,* 501–513.

McGrath, J. W., George, K., Svilar, G., Ihler, E., Mafigiri, D., Kabugo, M., & Mugisha, E. (2001). Knowledge about vaccine trials and willingness to participate in an HIV/AIDS vaccine study in the Ugandan military. *Journal of Acquired Immune Deficiency Syndromes, 27*(4), 381–388.

McGrath, J. W., Mafigiri, D., Kamya, M., George, K., Senvewo, R., Svilar, G., Kabugo, M., & Mugisha, E. (2001). Developing AIDS vaccine trials educational programs in Uganda. *Journal of Acquired Immune Deficiency Syndromes, 26*(2), 176–181.

Miller, E. P., & Armstrong, C. L. (1990). Surfactant replacement therapy innovative care for the premature infant. *Journal of Obstetric, Gynecologic, and Neonatal Nursing 19(1):14–17.*

National Bioethics Advisory Commission. (2001). Ethical and Policy Issues in International Research: Clinical Trials in Developing Countries. Bethesda, MD Author.

National Commission for the Protection of Human Subjects. (1978). *The Belmont report.* Washington, DC: Author.

Newton, L. H. (1990). Ethical imperialism and informed consent. *IRB: Ethics & Human Research, 12,* 10–11.

Osuntokun, B. O. (1992). Biomedical ethics in the developing world: conflicts and resolutions. In E. Pellegrino, P. Mazzarella, & P. Corsi (Eds.), *Transcultural dimensions in medical ethics* (pp. 105–144). Frederick, MD: University Publishing Group, Inc.

Piot, P. (1998). Ethics of placebo-controlled trials of zidovudine to prevent the perinatal transmission of HIV in the third world: correspondence. *New England Journal of Medicine, 338*(12), 839.

Resnik, D. B. (1998). The ethics of HIV research in developing nations. *Bioethics, 12*(4), 286–306.

Rossello, J. D., Hayward, P. E., Martell, M., Del Barco, M., Margotto, P., Grandzoto, J., et al. (1997). Hyaline membrane disease (HMD) therapy in Latin America: impact of exogenous surfactant administration on newborn survival, morbidity and use of resources. *Journal of Perinatal Medicine, 25,* 280–287.

Rothman, K. J., & Michels, K. B. (1994). The continuing unethical use of placebo controls. *New England Journal of Medicine, 331*(6), 394–398.

Schuklenk, U. (1998). Unethical perinatal HIV transmission trials establish bad precedent. *Bioethics, 12*(4), 312–319.

Sharp, R. R., & Foster, M. W. (2000). Involving study populations in the review of genetic research. *Journal of Law, Medicine and Ethics, 28*(1), 41–51.

Temple, R., & Ellenberg. S. S. (2000). Placebo-controlled trials and active-control trials in the evaluation of new treatments, Part 1: Ethical and Scientific Issues. *Annals of Internal Medicine, 133*(6), 455–463.

Thomas, J. (1998). Ethical challenges of HIV clinical trials in developing countries. *Bioethics, 12*(4), 320–327.

Trials of war criminals before the Nuremberg Military Tribunals under Control Council Law No. 10, Vol. 2. (1949). Washington, DC: U.S. Government Printing Office.

U.S. Department of Health and Human Services. (1991, June 18). Subpart D: Additional DHHS protections for children involved as subjects in research. *Federal Register, 56,* 28032.

Varmus, H., & Satcher, D. (1999). Ethical complexities of conducting research in developing countries. In T. L. Beauchamp & L. Walters (Eds.), *Contemporary issues in bioethics* (pp. 773–776). Belmont, CA: Wadworth Publishing Company.

Verma, R. P. (1995). Respiratory distress syndrome of the newborn infant. *Obsterical and Gynecological Survey, 50*(7), 542–555.

Weijer, C. (1999). Protecting communities in research: philosophical and pragmatic challenge. *Cambridge Quarterly of Health Care Ethics, 8,* 41–52.

Weijer, C., & Anderson, J. A. (2001). The ethics wars, disputes over international research. *Hastings Center Report, 31*(3), 18–20.

Weijer, C., & Glass, K. C. (2002). The ethics of placebo-controlled trials. *New England Journal of Medicine, 346*(5), 382–383.

Wiswell, T. E., & Mendiola, J. Jr. (1993). Respiratory distress syndrome in the newborn: innovative therapies. *American Family Physician, 47*(2), 407–414.

World Medical Association. (2000). Declaration of Helsinki: Ethical principles for medical research involving human subjects. Adopted by the 18th World Medical Assembly, Helsinki, Finland, 1964, and as revised by the 52nd World Medical Assembly, Edinburg, Scotland, October 2000. Retrieved July 20, 2004 from http://www.wma.net/e/policy/b3.htm.

14

Research and Innovation in Pediatric Surgery: The Problem of Hypoplastic Left-Heart Syndrome

Erin Flanagan-Klygis and Joel E. Frader

CASE DESCRIPTION

Mary and John B. are expecting their first child. Mary's pregnancy is at 22 weeks of gestation. The couple has just learned that the fetus Mary carries has a congenital heart defect known as hypoplastic left-heart syndrome (HLHS). Mary's obstetrician suspected a problem on a routine ultrasound examination and then arranged for a more detailed, level 2 ultrasound and prenatal echo-cardiogram. The couple immediately consults with the cardiologist and cardio-thoracic (CT) surgeon at the nearby children's medical center. The cardiologist informs them about the options available when their infant is born. He recommends that, after the delivery, they provide comfort care and allow the baby to die, given the grave prognosis even with surgery. The CT surgeon strongly recommends staged surgical repair, which according to her would result in a good prognosis. According to this surgeon, allowing their infant to die without attempting surgical correction would be "unethical." Confused, the couple consults with other cardiologists and surgeons across the country, only to find no consensus on the management of HLHS. At some centers, team members believe a staged sequence of operations offers the best chance for survival. Doctors at other centers believe that heart transplantation works best and recommend placing the fetus on a transplant list while still in utero. In some centers, physicians favor a combination of initial surgical palliation followed by transplantation. Yet other groups counsel that they can make no clear recommendation, indicating that not doing surgery and providing comfort care constitutes an acceptable, perhaps preferable option.

When John asked one surgeon at an academic medical center how children do long-term after surgical palliation versus transplantation, the surgeon replied: "We don't really know if one is truly better than the other. We have no long-term survival and quality of life data. For that reason, we are participating in a multicenter randomized clinical trial [RCT] of heart transplantation versus staged surgical correction for infants with HLHS." After all their hours of consultation, the couple face a difficult series of choices. They have uncovered uncertainty and controversy surrounding the management of infants with HLHS. They feel confused and worried about how to proceed. Should they choose comfort care and protect their child from the pain, risk, and trauma of major surgery? If not, should they elect to pursue staged correction or heart transplant? Alternatively, should they consent to having their child enrolled on the RCT comparing the two operations?

ETHICAL ANALYSIS AND DISCUSSION

The Medical/Surgical Problem in HLHS

HLHS involves a spectrum of severe defects of the heart with a common problem: the main pumping chamber of the heart—the one that sends blood with a new supply of oxygen to the organs of the body—has not developed adequately. In addition, part of the body's main supply artery, the aorta, may be missing or underdeveloped. This problem does not matter during fetal life, as blood circulation in the fetus involves only the right side of the heart. Babies with HLHS can live for a time following birth, as long as a connection between the (normal) right ventricle (or pumping chamber) and the infant's aorta remains open. That opening normally closes hours to days following delivery, though medication can keep it open for weeks to months. Once the connection closes, the heart cannot deliver oxygenated blood to the tissues and the child will die.

In the last decades of the 20th century, surgeons began to use two quite different approaches to this previously "lethal" anomaly. One involves a series of two or three operations pioneered by Dr. William Norwood. This combination of surgeries is known, after its developer, as the Norwood sequence of procedures. The operations make it possible for the healthy right ventricle—which normally only pumps blood through the lungs and back to the heart—to do the work that usually two ventricles, working together, provide. The first Norwood operation can take place in the first days of life. If successful, it will sustain the baby's life for months and allow time for important growth and development. The alternative surgery is heart transplantation—removal of the defective heart with replacement by one with normal structure and function. Transplant surgery must wait for a donor heart to become available. Each pathway has its advantages and problems.

The Norwood palliative procedures do not afford complete correction or what most people would regard as "repair" of the heart. When successful, the surgeries provide sufficient cardiac function to support average or better daily activity for many years, probably into adulthood, possibly even middle age. At some point, the single pumping chamber may fail to provide everything an adult body needs. In addition, the series of operations themselves carry considerable risk of morbidity and mortality. One recent publication, based on a retrospective review of surgical results, showed a survival rate of 42% at 1 year and 38% at 5 years after Norwood procedures (Jenkins et al. 2000). The combination of repeated open-heart operations and the time the child's heart pumped poorly oxygenated blood to the brain and other organs also makes the child vulnerable to developmental and learning disabilities. At this point, doctors know relatively little about the quality of life experienced by survivors of palliative surgery for HLHS.

While transplantation will result in normal circulation and, in theory, more normal heart and blood vessel function, two difficulties stand out. First, organ transplantation agencies and transplant surgeons cannot provide as many hearts as waiting patients need. In practice, a large proportion of the infants awaiting a new heart die of complications of their disease and treatment while waiting for a new heart. Some babies succumb to infection related to the intravenous catheters needed to provide drugs that sustain circulation before surgery. Others die of heart or kidney failure. Second, medicine has yet to fully conquer the problem of organ rejection. While some babies who have had heart transplantation may, in the end, not need medication to suppress their immune systems' efforts to attack the "foreign" heart, many do require the medicines. Rejection and/or the medication to fight it can damage the new heart and may make the child more vulnerable to death from infection or cancer.

Both palliative surgery and transplantation involve long and complex courses of treatment. Neither option consistently results in a high percentage of children surviving for many years with good overall health and function. In this setting, many thoughtful persons feel parents and physicians may legitimately decide not to pursue surgery. Most importantly, the dilemma faced by parents of children with HLHS exemplifies what other parents considering pediatric surgery may encounter in their situations. The medical/surgical community has not conducted enough research to answer at least these pressing questions: (1) is putting the child through the surgery "worth it" and (2) what advantages and disadvantages do the alternative operations involve?

Research in Pediatric Surgery

Cooper, Garcia-Prats, and Brody (1999) addressed what Mary and John B. encountered. In a survey, they found major differences of opinion among cardiologists, neonatologists, and CT surgeons who manage infants with HLHS. The

authors noted differences among the groups in willingness to discuss and recommend specific therapies, perceptions regarding survival and quality of life after
transplant versus palliative surgery, and the local availability of treatment options.
Only research can resolve these differences, yet no one has done the needed
investigation. Why not?

In circumstances, as with HLHS, where death will occur without an intervention, surgeons and parents understandably try new ideas to affect a rescue.
Such desperation encourages creativity and innovation. Once one surgeon appears
to have promising success with an innovative technique, word gets out, creating
interest, excitement, and promise. Pressure builds for other surgeons to reproduce
the results. No one wants to take the time or make the effort to initiate clinical
trials (Frader & Flanagan-Klygis, 2001). Indeed, to the extent that an innovation
dramatically and plainly succeeds, formal research makes little sense—it might
even be inappropriate. This raises an interesting set of questions about what
counts as success. Is it survival alone? Does success mean survival for a certain
number of weeks, months, or years? Does survival with high rates of complications or residual disability spell success? Who should judge the degree of success?

Innovating surgeons will likely have considerable enthusiasm for their accomplishments, especially when it involves saving a child's life. The understandable bias of the surgeon can prevent recognition of unintended negative consequences arising from the new operation. The history of surgery contains many
such stories. New procedures arrive with considerable fanfare and then disappear
as experience or research reveal unappreciated harms or even show that the new
operation works less well than previously accepted surgeries. The only way to
assess whether a new treatment—including a new operation—works better than
the old is to compare two or more therapies in a systematic fashion.

Surgical Research Design

In order to generate reliable evidence that one treatment (a drug or an operation)
works better than another, physician/investigators need to compare the treatments
to one another or to a placebo (a similarly appearing but inactive intervention) in
a controlled manner. Ideally, this involves a controlled RCT. In such a design,
research subjects receive one of the alternative treatments by chance arrangement,
similar to the toss of a coin. This eliminates subtle influences in treatment assignment that might affect the results of the study. The best RCTs also involve
evaluation of treatment outcomes in a "blinded" fashion (i.e., where the treating
professionals and study evaluators do not know the particular treatment any individual study subject [patient] received). RCTs emerged in the 1940s and since
then have powerfully advanced the evaluation of new drugs. Surgeons have not

made equivalent use of RCTs to evaluate operations. In pediatric surgery, only 0.3% of more than 9,300 published surgical papers, reported on prospective RCTs (Hardin, Stylianos, & Lally, 1999).

Surgeons have typically let their colleagues and the world know the results of their innovative work through reports, in peer-reviewed journals, of a series of cases they have treated. Unfortunately, in most situations such case series cannot form the basis for a scientifically valid evaluation of the new operation. The selection of patients for the operation and the surgical team's enthusiasm for their innovative approach can lead to falsely positive or optimistic conclusions about the worth of the new surgery. Even when surgeons compare the results of the new operation on a new group of patients to the outcomes in a "control group" of patients previously treated with an older operation, the conclusions turn out to be wrong 40–60% of the time (Venning, 1982; Sacks, Chalmers, & Smith, 1982).

Comparative trials with adequate statistical power can permit systematic evaluation in surgery, much as they do with medical treatments. That is, the evaluation of outcomes in surgery does not differ *fundamentally* from outcome assessment of drugs treatments. People respond differently to medications, based on variable and sometimes genetically controlled differences in rates of distribution of the drug through the body, metabolism (use and breakdown) of the drug, and elimination from the body, just as individual bodies respond differently to similar operations. While individual surgeons differ with respect to skill and experience, statistical techniques, can, if a trial has an appropriate design, permit adequate interpretation of surgical results even when multiple surgeons are involved.

Experts in research design typically feel that a true test of a new intervention, including a new operation, requires testing the new treatment directly against "standard" care over the same limited period. As noted, the decision about which individual patient/research subject receives the experimental therapy or the older, more established one, should result from a random assignment to eliminate subtle, even unconscious biases regarding who gets which treatment. Furthermore, those responsible for *evaluating* the results of the treatments should not know the specific therapy any given subject received. Therefore, while one cannot keep the surgeon "blind" with respect to which operation she has done, someone other than the surgeon, using objective measures, can assess how well the surgery worked. Also, when comparing two or more different operations, it *is* sometimes possible that patients-subjects could agree ahead of time to remain unaware of specific surgical details. (Such an arrangement would not work in comparing Norwood procedures to transplantation for HLHS. The two treatment courses have too many differences to obscure.) Thus, many of the common objections to formal clinical trials in surgery do not hold up, though design and implementation of valid surgical research may offer somewhat greater challenges than studies involving medicines. Nonetheless, as one commentator, Haines, a surgeon, noted,

"To fail to use the best available (research) techniques merely because they are difficult and time consuming runs counter to the best traditions of medicine and surgery" (Haines, 1979).

However, barriers do exist to conducting research on surgery. One does not always know when, in the development of a new operation, to begin a comparative trial. If a study starts too soon, poor outcomes could reflect only insufficient experience with the new technique (i.e., not enough time for surgeons to master new skills for a novel operation). Many surgeons believe this "learning curve" phenomenon might have caused good operations, such as cholecystectomy (gall bladder removal) and coronary artery bypass grafting to be abandoned had they been subjected to RCTs in the early phases of their development (Bonchek, 1979; Sirrat et al. 1992; Troidl et al., 1991). Also, studies involving more than one surgeon do need to account for possible variability in skill between surgeons. For example, early results of the Norwood operation by surgeons other than the originator revealed far less success than Dr. Norwood reported.

Finally, controversy remains about when or even whether to enroll children as research subjects. While in many cases children cannot make independent decisions about whether to accept whatever risks might be associated with becoming a research subject, advancement of knowledge crucial to helping care for sick children requires their participation in research. Subjecting children to innovative techniques that have not withstood rigorous scientific testing may well prove the more hazardous course. Surgeons have abandoned many procedures that once seemed promising when experience or research showed them not to work or to offer no advantage over other approaches. Discarded procedures include tying off to internal mammary artery to increase blood supply to the heart muscle, freezing of the stomach lining to treat ulcers, and radical mastectomy for breast cancer. This history suggests that surgeons, like those who use medical therapies, have a duty of care to use formal assessments of new treatments in order to protect patients from dangerous and unproven therapies and to maintain the integrity of medical knowledge.

Ethics of the Trial Design and IRB Considerations

A randomized trial of HLHS surgical therapy comparing heart transplant with staged surgical correction presents a number of challenging ethical questions. These questions fall into three categories: trial design, appropriate category of institutional review board (IRB) approval, and questions around informed consent.

A large number of salient ethical concerns relate to the design of clinical trials, yet investigators, IRBs, and ethicists often overlook many of these issues. Excessive focus on consent documents obscures key questions in research ethics relating to study design. In this case, the randomized trial includes only two of the three potential approaches for children with HLHS; this is noteworthy and bears further analysis. Study design requires objective and comparable outcome measures in order to answer conclusively the critical research question(s). Heart transplantation and staged surgical correction may be compared with regard to outcome measures such as 1-year survival, 5-year survival, surgical complication rates, and cognitive outcomes for survivors. By contrast, a comfort care approach would not be amenable to these comparisons, since all infants would be expected to die without surgery. This does not suggest that comfort care has any less validity as a choice for parents or health care professionals caring for an infant with HLHS. However, comfort care cannot be included as a third arm of a "traditional" RCT. Without question, professionals and parents need the results of research on comfort care for infants with HLHS. Such studies would use different outcome measures, including assessments of any pain, dyspnea, or other symptoms the baby might have and parental/family psychological and social adjustment to the birth and subsequent death of their infant.

Another key requirement for the ethical design of clinical trials is the potential to answer the research question with valid and generalizable results. A robust research design balances the tension between strict eligibility criteria to provide valid results and more liberal eligibility criteria that allow for generalizability of findings to larger, more typical patient populations. In this case, the heart transplant arm of the RCT presents several complexities. The availability of donor organs, especially for small infants, presents a major challenge to the integrity of the study design. Could one ethically give enrolled infants a higher priority for available organs than babies waiting for a heart outside of a study? If so, would this unduly influence parents to participate? Could the knowledge gained from a successful study which would benefit future children with HLHS justify changes in the usual allocation of organs to waiting candidates? If donor organs are not readily available to those enrolled, the hazards of waiting for an organ could compromise the outcome for infants assigned to the transplant arm of the protocol, resulting in a falsely inferior result for this group. The supply of organs is also likely to vary over time, influencing the results of the study on an arbitrary basis. These considerations suggest the need to ensure donor organs for subjects randomized to the transplant arm, but at the same time raise other concerns about informed consent and undue inducements to participate.

IRBs will need to review the RCT and will face at least two important questions: whether to approve the study, and which category in the Federal Regulations best fits the protocol. HLHS is clearly an important problem and treatment options are very limited. The significance and need for the study is quite clear. The risks to the subjects in each arm of the study would appear to be reasonably in balance with potential benefits to the subjects. The experience of Mary and John in consulting multiple experts and receiving varied opinions supports the claim that there equipoise exists between the two arms of the study, providing a valid moral basis for the conduct of the RCT. Finally, the IRB could approve the trial under 45 CFR 405, research with the prospect of direct benefit to the subject.

Parents and the Need for Research in Surgery

Returning to HLHS, recall the radical variation in how infant heart specialists view alternative treatments for HLHS. This situation reflects, to a large degree, the lack of sufficient research on outcomes of surgical procedures. Without adequate data, the community cannot reach consensus about what to do. In HLHS, controversy continues about the mortality (death rates) and morbidity (complications and disability) associated with each of the surgical alternatives. A number of factors need to be better understood and weighed. These include the death rate for babies awaiting transplantation and how often deaths occur with each stage of the Norwood sequence, as well as how and why this may vary from one center to another, and the rate and severity of long-term deficits in intelligence, behavior, educational success, and social functioning in children surviving the surgical procedures. To date, no comparative studies, in the form of clinical trials, have attempted to address differences in outcomes between the two surgical approaches, even in the few centers that offer both transplantation and palliative surgery.

In the meantime, some researchers have examined the ethical tension parents feel with making decisions regarding surgery for HLHS. Vandvik and Førde (2000), in Norway, interviewed mothers of 10 children who survived the Norwood procedures as well as 10 mothers who chose "comfort care" (hospice) for their infants. The women had considered information about the available options and been told that the physicians expected the parents to decide how to proceed. The interviews for the study took place 2.5–6 years after the children were born. In the surgical group, 3 of the 10 children had normal mental function (intelligence and behavior). None of the mothers of infants who had had operations expressed regret over their decisions. In the comfort care group, the mothers noted they had primarily desired to prevent any suffering for their child. The authors concluded that the lack of long-term outcome data and the social expectation that one must "do something" for any sick child made parental decision making quite difficult. The authors called for greater professional guidance for parents facing such challenging decisions.

However, professional recommendations might also present problems. Recently, Kon, Ackerson, and Lo, (2000a) reported the results of a survey of physicians who care for infants with HLHS. They found substantial bias in the recommendations of cardiologists, surgeons, neonatologists, and pediatric intensive care doctors. The biases reflected the preferred interventions at each physician's center (the Norwood staged reconstruction surgery vs. transplantation vs. comfort measures) or the collective view of each subspecialty group at a given hospital (neonatologists more often recommended comfort care than did surgeons). In addition, the reported rate of surgery (greater than 85% of the babies underwent surgical intervention) exceeded the rate at which the physicians said they would choose surgery *for their own children* (39%). Doctors favoring operations for their own family member said they made clear recommendations to go ahead with surgery while those who would decline surgery for their own child indicated they would provide "nondirective" counseling for parents (Kon et al., 2000b)

Given our lack of direct comparative information regarding the outcomes of transplant surgery versus staged reconstructive surgery and given the diversity of opinions among physicians caring for infants with HLHS about what they might do for their own children, the failure to conduct comparative clinical trials itself raises serious ethical concerns. Doctors and parents alike can appreciate the value of organizing and conducting research designed to clarify the relative risks and benefits of the different approaches to HLHS. Clinicians might well approach parents, explain the nature of the uncertainty regarding which operation, if either, represents the "best" approach, and seek parental permission to enroll their infant into a study. While many parents would prefer the doctor to make a specific recommendation about which path the physician feels is best for their new baby, the most intellectually honest response would have to be that no one can know that without more research.

Again, the lack of scientifically sound data supporting the use of various operations prevents parents and physicians from having the information necessary to make the best choices for sick children. This fact reinforces the importance of professional and family support for high-quality research in pediatric surgery.

With the exception of the Norwegian study mentioned above, evaluating the psychological and ethical issues surrounding parental decision making regarding surgery or comfort care for children with HLHS, virtually no data exist comparing family functioning in situations where either surgical intervention or end-of-life comfort care remain morally acceptable options. Pediatricians and pediatric surgeons also have a moral obligation to undertake comparative studies of parental adaptation and feelings when the physicians and parents choose among substantially different alternatives. In other words, not only do we need prospective clinical trials of alternative therapies, we also need to study the effects of the alternative paths on the patients' families. A finding that many parents who elected to forgo potentially life-sustaining treatment had major regrets, suffered significantly higher rates of clinical depression, or had other negative outcomes would at least have to enter into the consent process prior to a decision for or against a particular surgical intervention.

The Research Imperative, Informed Consent, and Balance

Mary and John face a decision about how best to care for their child. Health care professionals struggle with how to provide the best surgical care for children with HLHS. While Mary and John may feel confused and desperate about what to do for their child, surgeons as a group are divided about the facts when it comes to the treatment of HLHS. The confluence of these situations provides the opportunity for, if not a duty to conduct, a clinical trial. The need for better information about this devastating anomaly is compelling.

The first surgeon Mary and John encounter stated that a choice of comfort care without surgical intervention would be "unethical." The use of this word in conversation with these parents is abhorrent, and represents thoughtless and arguably "unethical" behavior on the part of the surgeon. By contrast, the surgeon who offered enrollment in the RCT of heart transplant versus staged surgical correction engaged in morally praiseworthy behavior. The informed consent process for such a trial would ideally include thoughtful, supportive counseling for the parents, allowing ample time for them to ask questions and seek advice from other sources. Specifically, parents of other children with HLHS could be a valuable resource for Mary and John, and those offering the clinical trial may wish to consider building such a possibility into the consent process. There are several advantages to this approach to informed consent. These include the fact that experienced parents can empathize with Mary and John in a way that health care professionals may not be able to, may be able to provide information on both practical and quality-of-life issues, and are likely to be less intimidating and potentially less directive than physicians. Many parent advocates strongly support clinical research, and physicians should take care to assure that the parents in an advisory role refrain from inappropriate attempts to influence new parents and present a balanced view. It might be desirable to introduce Mary and John to parents who elected comfort care rather than surgical intervention to be certain this perspective is included. Experienced parents can provide a powerful adjunct to the informed consent process in difficult circumstances such as this.

CONCLUSION

Modern pediatric surgery would not have achieved considerable success without the creative energies of innovative surgeons. Without question, innovation in the art and practice of surgery makes further progress possible. However, good hunches and the best of therapeutic intentions give insufficient justification for surgical innovations without following up with well-designed clinical trials. Children, parents, and the community of pediatric surgeons deserve high-quality data supporting the efficacy of proposed operations. Surgeons, like other physicians, have a scientific and ethical responsibility to assess their therapeutic interventions with valid, formal outcome measures. Conducting good research not only protects patients from dangerous and unproven therapies, it also fosters and maintains the integrity of medical and surgical knowledge.

Questions for Discussion

1. Morbidity and mortality rather than quality of life has been defined as the primary outcome for most clinical trials. Why should studies of pediatric patients that survived HLHS after palliative surgery and/or transplantation assess quality of life?

2. The authors of this chapter raise an interesting set of questions about what counts as success in HLHS. Had you been an investigator conducting empirical research to measure the success of new treatments, what criteria would you utilize to determine what counts as a successful treatment?

3. Do you think the common objections to formal clinical trials in surgery justify the alternative of publishing case series rather than conducting a RCT?

4. How would you handle the obstacles of conducting research on surgery, discussed by the authors?

5. Can you propose a creative solution to the ethical dilemma raised by the randomized trial of HLHS surgical therapy comparing heart transplant with staged surgical correction?

6. The authors argue here that "[a] large number of salient ethical concerns relate to the design of clinical trials, yet investigators, IRBs and ethicists often overlook many of these issues. Excessive focus on consent documents obscures key questions in research ethics relating to study design." What could be the reason that IRBs and ethicists, either in the medical setting in general or in the specific case of HLHS, emphasize consent issues and neglect concerns regarding the trial design? Do you find this phenomenon justifiable?

7. What is the ethical dilemma related to the availability of donor organs in the case of HLHS according to the chapter? Does the utilization of a scarce resource like infant sized donor hearts change your level of support for a randomized clinical trial (RCT)? If so, does this use contribute to or diminish justification for the trial? Are clinical trials a good use of a scarce resource?

8. In the outset case, considering the radical variation in how infant heart specialists view alternative treatments for HLHS, how should Mary and John weigh the different options? Why is it so difficult to compare transplantation, palliative surgery, and comfort care?

9. Do you find the authors' view that parents of other children with HLHS could be a valuable resource for Mary and John persuasive? Explain your answer, and discuss potential problems with this approach.

—

References

Bonchek, L. I. (1979). Are randomized trials appropriate for evaluating new operations? *New England Journal of Medicine, 301*(1), 44–45.

Cooper, T. R., Garcia-Prats, J. A., & Brody, B. A. (1999). Managing disagreements in the management of short bowel and hypoplastic left heart syndrome. *Pediatrics, 104*(4), 1–7.

Frader, J. E., & Flanagan-Klygis, E. (2001). Innovation and research in pediatric surgery. *Seminars in Pediatric Surgery, 10*(4), 198–203.

Haines, S. J. (1979). Randomized clinical trials in the evaluation of surgical innovation. *Journal of Neurosurgery, 51,* 5–11.

Hardin, W. D., Stylianos, S., & Lally, K. P. (1999). Evidence-based practice in pediatric surgery. *Journal of Pediatric Surgery, 34,* 908–913.

Jenkins, P. C., Flanagan, M. F., Jenkins, K. J., Sargent, J. D., Canter, C. E., Chinnock, R. E., et al. (2000). Survival analysis and risk factors for mortality in transplantation and staged surgery for hypoplastic left heart syndrome. *Journal of the American College of Cardiology, 36: 1178–1185.*

Kon, A. A., Ackerson, L., & Lo, B. (2000a). Counseling parents on treatment options for children with hypoplastic left heart syndrome: Factors which influence physician advise [Abstract]. *Critical Care Medicine, 28*(Suppl.), A59 (Abstract 106/M12).

Kon, A. A., Ackerson, L., & Lo, B. (2000b). Treatment options for hypoplastic left heart syndrome: An ethical perspective. *Critical Care Medicine, 28*(Suppl.), A60 (Abstract 108/M14).

Sacks, H., Chalmers, T. C., & Smith, H. (1982). Randomized versus historical controls for clinical trials. *American Journal of Medicine, 22,* 233–240.

Sirrat, G. M., Farndon, J., Farrow, S. C., Fardon, J., & Dwyer, N. (1992). The challenge of evaluating surgical procedures. *Annals of the Royal College of Surgeons of England, 74,* 80–84.

Troidl, H., Spitzer, W. O., McPeek, B., Mulder, D. S., McKneally, M. F., Wechsler, A. S., Balch, C. M., et al. (1991). *Principles and practice of research: Strategies for surgical investigation.* New York: Springer-Verlag.

Vandvik, I. H., & Førde, R. (2000). Ethical issues in parental decision-making. An interview study of mothers of children with hypoplastic left heart syndrome. *Acta Paediatrica, 89,* 1129–1133.

Venning, G. R. (1982). The validity of anecdotal reports of suspected adverse reactions—the problem of false alarms. *British Medical Journal, 284,* 249–252.

15

Near the Boundary of Research: Roles, Responsibilities, and Resource Allocation

Christopher Church, Victor M. Santana, Pamela S. Hinds, and Edwin M. Horwitz

---

CASE DESCRIPTION

A 7-year-old female with infantile malignant osteopetrosis was referred to a pediatric research center for enrollment on a research protocol to study hematopoietic stem cell transplantation (HSCT) as a potentially curative effort. Osteopetrosis is a rare, heritable skeletal disease in which the lack of normal osteoclast function results in a gradual and cumulative formation of bone, resulting in excessive bone deposition. Medical complications include numerous bone fractures, growth failure, delayed tooth eruption, blindness, and other sensory and neurological impairments. Because osteopetrosis obliterates the marrow space and is itself associated with defective leukocyte function, chronic infections that are refractory to treatment are common. If left untreated, children with osteopetrosis are severely impaired, and only 30% survive to 6 years of age. Recent but limited research findings suggest that HSCT may ameliorate the gradually progressive disease. However, no therapy has been identified as unequivocally curative. Because osteopetrosis is an uncommon disease, most patients are referred to academic or research centers.

Originally diagnosed and treated in a developing country, this child came to a university hospital in the United States at 6 years of age. There, the child received megadoses of vitamins and gamma interferon to ameliorate the sequelae of osteopetrosis, and she was placed on chronic antibiotics for recurring infections. Because the parents were uninsured aliens, the university hospital did not offer the more expensive, but potentially curative, treatment option of HSCT. One year later, the physician at the university hospital referred the child to a pediatric research center, after learning that that center's active research program included rare metabolic diseases and that its policy was to provide care without respect to ability to pay.

Information provided at the time of the referral indicated the child might be eligible for an open protocol, so the child was accepted as a patient at the research center "sight unseen." Subsequent evaluation at the pediatric research center found the child to have a chronic bacterial infection of the jaw bone (osteomyelitis) and to have difficulty maintaining her weight because of an inability to swallow solid foods. These impairments rendered the child ineligible for enrollment on the research protocol. The research center remained committed to the child as a patient, and the chief investigator continued as the child's attending physician.

Following discussion with other physician-researchers in the transplant clinical service, the attending physician told the parents that the only potentially curative intervention was HSCT. Active infection is usually a contraindication to HSCT; however, it was thought that her advanced disease and associated immune deficiency made it impossible to provide successful definitive treatment for the infection. Given this difficult conundrum, the transplant clinical service suggested that it would be reasonable to proceed with HSCT. Because the attending physician understood the offer of HSCT outside the research protocol to be a "single patient treatment plan" and not research, he did not request approval from the hospital's institutional review board (IRB).

The child was still quite active and playful and apparently took joy in her life. Though her face was dysmorphic, a few minutes of watching her at play would convince most observers that she was a child much like any other. She was able to dance and climb from lap to lap for hugs from family and staff, despite the fact that she was blind. Her parents knew her as a "miracle child" who had beaten the odds more than once when physicians had given a dismal prognosis for survival to discharge.

The child's only sibling, a 3-year-old brother, was found to be a perfect match for HSCT. The parents understood the risk to both the donor and recipient and provided informed consent to proceed with transplant. HSCT was offered "as per" the research protocol, with modifications to accommodate the patient's impairments and to reduce potential adverse effects during the course of treatment. No data existed on the efficacy of HSCT for an osteopetrosis patient with chronic infection or disease so advanced that she had little marrow space available for engraftment. The parents understood the gravity of the patient's situation; she had outlived most children with osteopetrosis and had neurologic impairment associated with advanced disease. They understood that her blindness was not reversible. Her parents also understood that if she did survive transplant, she would need surgery to reconstruct her jaw—care that likely would be unavailable in her own country.

In multiple interviews, the parents indicated full understanding of the increased risk the transplant option presented to their daughter, in light of her impairments and the team's lack of experience with similar patients. Repeatedly, the patient's parents asked not to be informed of less-aggressive options for their daughter's care, such as comfort-only measures. However, the attending physician insisted that the parents be informed of the full range of reasonable options, including no further attempts at cure. The parents were resolved to pursue transplant as their daughter's only hope, and they adamantly opposed a palliative approach to care.

Based on these considerations, a decision was made to proceed with HSCT. Prior to the transplant, the patient received intravenous antibiotics and hyperbaric oxygen to contain the chronic localized infection and treatment to improve her nutritional status. The transplant team modified the preparative regimen to reduce the anticipated toxicity of chemotherapy and to avoid risks related to the active infection. The patient had few complications and tolerated the rigors of transplant better than the treatment team expected.

Two months posttransplant, the patient suffered graft rejection, developing low peripheral blood counts and a hypocellular bone marrow. No data existed on the efficacy of a second transplant for a child with osteopetrosis; however, the physician concluded that the patient likely would not live beyond 3 months to 1 year unless she received a second transplant. The transplant team physicians concurred that a second HSCT should be offered. Other members of the bedside care team questioned the prudence of this plan. Again, the parents rejected the proposal for a palliative care plan and expressed a desire for a second transplant. The brother could not serve as a donor again because of his young age and the short time since the previous donation. One parent was tested and found to be a potential donor (partial match).

The chief medical officer was asked to "sign off" on the parent's role as donor, since hospital policy did not permit a parent to consent to be a donor *and* to grant permission for a child to receive HSCT, without independent review of risks to the donor. At this point, medical administrators and others at the research center questioned the medical and ethical appropriateness of the second transplant, including whether a second transplant was in the child's interest and whether this effort was a responsible use of institutional resources. Medical administration referred the matter to the ethics committee. Because the second transplant would not be possible without use of an investigational device required to manipulate the stem cells of mismatched donors, the attending physician sought both IRB and Food and Drug Administration (FDA) permission to proceed.

ETHICAL ANALYSIS AND DISCUSSION

When is the use of a nonvalidated treatment justified? Does categorizing a treatment as "research" change its ethical acceptability? How are responsibilities altered when a nonvalidated means is used solely for the potential benefit of a single pediatric patient? When does the balance of anticipated burdens and benefits to a pediatric patient no longer justify use of a nonvalidated means aimed at cure?

The National Commission (1977) recommended that "radically new procedures" (i.e., those that represent "significant" departures from standard medical practice) should be incorporated into a formal research project. The commission's intent was to foster timely, evidenced-based medicine. Generalizable knowledge gained from timely clinical trials is critical for two reasons. Patients can be harmed by continuing exposure to nonvalidated interventions that later prove to be ineffective or even harmful and by delayed access to as yet nonvalidated interventions that clinical trials ultimately demonstrate to be effective.

From the regulatory perspective, a patient who is not eligible to participate in a clinical investigation (trial) may be able to have access to the experimental agent through one of two mechanisms (21 CFR 312–313, §§ 312.34, 312.35, 312.36 and 312.83). First, under special circumstances a patient may be treated with an investigational drug under a "compassionate use" protocol.[1] A different situation arises in the case of a patient with a serious immediately life-threatening disease (defined as expectation of death in a matter of months) for which the treating physician believes that a promising new drug or treatment offers some potential of benefit. Under this alternative to obtain and use an investigational drug, the physician must file a single patient or emergency investigational new drug (IND) application directly with the FDA. This must be done with the cooperation and permission of the drug supplier.[2]

For both of these mechanisms, there is an evidence burden prior to initiating the treatment protocol. If the available scientific evidence taken as a whole fails to provide a reasonable basis that the investigational drug may be effective for the patient or if the investigational drug would expose the patient to unreasonable or significant additional risk of illness or injury, the FDA may deny its use.[3]

Regarding this case, the patient was ineligible for the investigational HSCT protocol since she had undergone a matched sibling donor HSCT previously (i.e., this would be a second HSCT, which is excluded in the eligibility criteria). However, HSCT as definitive treatment for osteopetrosis per se is not completely investigational, and this patient had the potential of benefit from such therapy. Moreover, the first HSCT used a very mild chemotherapy-conditioning regimen; therefore, the risk of regimen-related morbidity was not anticipated to be significantly greater than if it were the first HSCT. The medical care team, then, decided that a second HSCT was a reasonable therapeutic option for this patient.

Despite the fact that HSCT is not investigational, this particular protocol employed a medical device that had not been approved by the FDA. Therefore, the entire protocol was arguably investigational and required oversight by the local IRB and by the FDA. Since the patient was ineligible for the (investigational) protocol but had a reasonable expectation of benefit from the intervention, the attending physician applied to the IRB and FDA for a compassionate use protocol as outlined above.

Questions of Beneficence

With the shift from the anticipated research context to the context of nonvalidated, innovative therapy using an investigational device off-protocol, some key roles shifted. The anticipated investigator became the physician-innovator. Gone was the investigator's responsibility to advance science, although the innovator was required to report adverse events to the IRB and FDA. What remained in the innovative therapeutic context was the duty to promote the child's interests, whether by access to the innovation, by protection from its risks, or by careful balancing of both. Since HSCT is a well-recognized therapy for leukemia, more was known about the risks associated with HSCT than about possible efficacy in treatment of osteopetrosis. European HSCT studies reported success in treating infants with osteopetrosis; however, it was uncertain whether similar results could be obtained with a much older child. In this case, many individuals made a risk: benefit analysis regarding a second HSCT for this child. These perspectives included (1) the attending physician, (2) HSCT clinical care staff, (3) the IRB and FDA, which needed to approve or reject the use of the investigational device, (4) the child's parents, (5) medical administration, and (6) the institutional ethics committee.

The Attending Physician. The patient's attending physician communicated that the chance of the child benefiting from HSCT was very slight, but represented the child's only hope for long-term survival. Nonvalidated interventions that pose "more than minimal risk" may be justified by the prospect of direct benefit to the child, particularly if the anticipated benefit exceeds that of available alternatives. For advanced-stage infantile malignant osteopetrosis, no "standard of care" exists. HSCT remained the only potentially curative option; limited experience with younger patients offered promise, but the *advanced* stage of the patient's disease, including neurological sequelae, tempered hope for survival. The first attempt at engraftment using cells from the matched sibling was not successful. A second HSCT using partially matched cells from a parent would necessitate use of an investigational device not yet approved by the FDA. The attending physician conjectured that if the child engrafted, her bones might remodel and, thus, some deficits associated with osteopetrosis, such as brittle bones and an impaired immune system, might be remedied. Her neurological deficits, including blindness, were thought irreversible; here, the best outcome would be survival at the current level of neurologic functioning. Other deficits (i.e., the dysmorphic jaw and difficulty swallowing solid foods) could be corrected only by subsequent surgeries. Therefore, the attending physician felt justified in offering a second HSCT, using the investigational device, as a reasonable medical option. The *Declaration of Helsinki* (World Medical Association, 1964) supports recourse to medical innovation in such cases.[4]

The HSCT Clinical Care Staff. There had been some lack of consensus among the HSCT service physicians regarding the reasonableness of the first offer of transplant, given the patient's advanced disease and comorbidities. Some felt that the balance of risks to probable benefits for this child disfavored recourse to HSCT; others felt that even a slight possibility of cure could effectively outweigh grave risks. After some expected problems did not arise and/or in response to a challenge by medical administration, the attending physician reported consensus or near-consensus among the HSCT physicians. However, the entire team of diverse disciplines did not support the second transplant option. For example, some nurses felt trapped, obligated by the physician and parents to provide care that they believed to be, on balance, harmful to the child.

Discord over treatment decisions can be disruptive to an interdisciplinary team's efforts to provide excellent care to patients. In clinical care situations, physicians are empowered to present reasonable medical options to patients or, most often in the pediatric setting, to parents. Parents are empowered to choose for their children so long as their choices are neither abusive nor neglectful. Other members of health care teams (i.e., nurses, social workers, and chaplains) have less voice in decision making, but not less responsibility to advocate for the patient. These team members' contributions to patient care are not expendable; teamwork is particularly important in transplantation. The potentially harmful effects of discord over a treatment decision forced upon a team is a form of social cost of bilateral decision making (by only physicians and parents), although clearly far less of a cost than that faced by the patient (and family).

When making recommendations to the family about innovative treatment, members of the direct care team should have an opportunity, in the family's absence, to voice their opinions and feelings. This goal is best accomplished by a multidisciplinary case conference, including physicians, nurses, social workers, chaplains, and others involved in the care of the child. Use of innovations associated with high risk and questionable benefit call for the same degree of ethical justification and exceptional teamwork as decisions involving withholding or withdrawing life-sustaining interventions.

The IRB. Cowan and Bertsch (1984) found that no federal regulation classifies innovative therapies as research per se; no regulation requires that innovative practices "be conducted according to the norms of research absent inclusion in a formal research project." However, Singer et al. (1990) noted, "the ethical assessment of innovative therapies falls in a gray zone between research (which requires IRB approval) and practice (which does not)." Further, "whether federal regulations for the protection of human subjects in medical research apply to innovative therapies is not completely clear" (Singer et al., 1990). However, if (as in this case) the medical innovation entails the use of an investigational drug or device, then FDA regulations apply.

Although IRB oversight is limited to clinical research rather than clinical practice, many pediatric subjects participating in sound clinical research simultaneously receive the high quality of clinical care and treatment, as has been demonstrated over the last three decades in the field of pediatric oncology. When the treatment activity does not clearly entail research (or the use of an investigational drug or device), the practicing physician has great leeway in exercise of clinical judgment. However, when a clinical innovation represents a degree of departure from accepted practice similar to that found in research protocols, role of IRB oversight becomes a legitimate question.

Given our patient's impairments and poor prognosis, she might be viewed as even more vulnerable than those patients eligible for enrollment in the protocol on which her care was modeled. Therefore, her participation in an innovative intervention was also deserving of institutional oversight. We would argue that maintaining a clear distinction between research and clinical care is an important goal. For this reason, we suggest that ethics committee review is generally a more appropriate form of oversight than the IRB for cases like this. The FDA and IRB review is required for this particular case only because of the investigational device needed to manipulate the donor stem cells.

Parents. Parents who are offered a nonvalidated innovation with potential of direct benefit for their child face a difficult choice. It may be unreasonable to expect parents to understand the technical, scientific questions raised by this option. Even clinicians are sometimes hard pressed to evaluate complex options. The question of a second HSCT for this child is no less daunting. Ethics committees may be able to assist parents in navigating the *terra incognita* of a nonvalidated innovation with potential of direct benefit and possible harm to the child.

An ombudsperson or other advocate can also assist vulnerable parents in negotiating complex decisions.

These parents' past experience with fallible physicians who offered inaccurate and dismal prognoses for survival likely led them to downplay the frank disclosure of grim prognosis by their current doctor. The parents were asked to weigh the unlikelihood of real benefit from the innovative intervention (preservation of their child's life at its current quality) against the greater likelihood of grave harms, such as death from infection, graft failure, and graft-versus-host disease. The risks associated with a second HSCT using an investigational device were thought more likely than were benefits, though some anticipated risks of HSCT did not materialize with the initial transplant. The parents were asked to compare the risks and benefits of comfort care only, which was a reasonable end-of-life care option. However, the parents consistently preferred a more intensive and potentially curative approach, and refused to consider comfort-only measures.

According to Ross (1998), "when treatment has a low probability of success, is likely to result in poor quality of life, or is experimental, the parents are free to decide whether the benefits outweigh the risks and costs. It is a value-laden, quality-of-life decision that should be theirs to make" (p. 142). The "received view" is that in cases of certain death, almost any risk, even those associated with nonvalidated innovations, is acceptable. This received view is less problematic in adult medicine than in pediatrics.[5] The pediatric context is more complex; benefits and burdens are born not only by the child patient but also by the parents, whose own interests are tied to the child's in multifarious ways. If the child dies, parents grieve perhaps the greatest personal loss known and must live with their decisions regarding treatment. Their grief may be compounded by regret for the suffering the child experienced in the course of ineffective treatment. If the child survives with significant impairment, parents and siblings may continue to live as hostages to the child's disorder. Therefore, parental decisions to forgo treatment, even if motivated by a desire that the child experience a good death, are subject to criticism of neglect of the child's interest for the sake of other family interests. If the child not only survives but also shows marked improvement following innovative treatment, parents may feel vindicated in their choice, but that is a small matter; those parents still have their child and their hopes for their child.

Parents vary not only in their values but also in their comfort with risk (degree of risk aversion).[6] If someone wins big when the odds are clearly a long shot and the risk of loss is small, we may say, "You were fortunate." We may be tempted to judge the risk post hoc as a savvy move. If someone loses who had little to lose on the gamble, we don't regard this as a great misfortune. However, applying this lottery model to a high-stakes pediatric case is problematic. First, in this pediatric case, what the gamblers (i.e., parents) risked was not merely their own, even if it was "their child"; what they risked was their child's present quality of life for the sake of a remotely possible future. Second, the child *did* have something significant to lose if the parents gambled on a cure: the child would loose the opportunity to live a different life while dying, a life outside the hospital, possibly with a few more active weeks, a life off the ventilator, or a life surrounded by extended family in their country of origin.

Medical Administration. The administrative leadership of the research hospital questioned whether the proportionality of anticipated benefits to expected harms favored the second HSCT. They expressed strong doubts about exposing a child to what were perceived as grave risks for very uncertain gain. The chief medical officers believed the intervention was very unlikely to provide any real benefit to the child, given her advanced disease and the contraindications, such as chronic infection. They feared that transplant was almost certain to contribute to a more immediate and difficult death than if the child did not receive the intervention. They also raised issues about the child's quality of life in light of her various impairments and whether prolongation of life might paradoxically harm the child. These concerns would be even more profound with a mismatched HSCT and its increased risk of graft-versus-host disease. Dissatisfied with the parents' preference for curative high risk approaches, medical administration suggested that a guardian *ad litem* be appointed to make an independent judgment regarding the child's best interests. Recognizing the potential for conflicts of interests in their role as stewards of institutional resources, medical administration agreed to abide by recommendations of the ethics committee. The ethics committee did not find the parents' actions either neglectful or abusive (although many members felt the choice of high-risk curative means rather than a palliative tack was unwise in this case). Thus, the ethics committee did not recommend recourse to the courts.

Questions of Respect for Persons

In a pediatric context, respect for persons entails both protection of the vulnerable child and respectful listening to the voices of the key stakeholders: the child and parents. Protections of vulnerable children include required risk-benefit analyses (i.e., by an IRB, the FDA, or an ethics committee), some limitations on risk to which a child may be exposed without expectation of direct benefit to the child (thus limiting the options available for parents' consideration), as well as the requirements for parental permission and of the child's assent. We use respectful listening rather than respect for autonomy because of the nuances of the pediatric settings.[7] Which factor is most weighty, either protection from risk or respect for a stakeholder's choice, is context dependent: Sometimes the degree of risk is determinative, other times the likelihood of benefit, sometimes parental wishes, and still other times the child's.

With the shift to an innovative therapeutic context, the parents' duty remained to further their child's interest and to balance those interests with the family's needs. The consent process was modified to highlight increased risks and uncertainties of the innovation for this patient. This showed respect for the parents' role as decision makers for their child. Both parents and the attending physician had a duty to involve the child in decision making in an age-appropriate way and to the degree the child desired such. Physicians and parents involve a child at this developmental stage in decision making primarily by communicating what they have judged best serves the child's interests, by listening to the child's concerns, and seeking the child's assent.

Institution. For the decision addressing the second HSCT using an investigational device, hospital administrators, IRB, and ethics committee members were involved in weighing of the burdens to the patient against potential benefits as a way of providing additional protection to the child. Institutional concerns included the promotion of the patient's interests, including protection from unjustified harms in the course of medical interventions, respect for family autonomy tempered with concerns for the burdens of aggressive interventions on the child, and protection of the adult donor.

Parents. Some members of the HSCT clinical care staff sensed that the parents felt pressure from their community of origin to be a strong advocate for the child, interpreted as demanding curative measures and rejecting comfort-only care. Formal hospice care is not well established in the country of origin, where more deaths are experienced in the home. Religious factors were involved, because the parents interpreted the child's survival of repeated life-threatening episodes as evidence of divine deliverance. The parents hoped that if they persevered, God would intervene. If their child's recovery were not the will of Providence, the parents would be guiltless if they had been aggressive advocates and would accept that outcome. The parents' interpretation of their faith tradition made them suspicious of quality-of-life judgments. They viewed preservation of life as a sacred duty.

Paternalism is justified on that the grounds that the parents are generally in a better position than is a not-yet-mature minor to identify a full range of options, to balance both short-term and long-range benefits and harms, and thus to promote the child's welfare. School-aged children tend to focus on the immediate, lived experience as the hospitalized child, weighing current burdens more heavily than parents do. In comparison, parents generally have known the child before he/she

became a patient and have hopes and responsibilities for their child after anticipated discharge. Therefore, parents tend to weigh the desired or feared future
more heavily than the child's recent experience of burdensome interventions and/
or diminished quality of life. In cases of research offering potential for direct
therapeutic benefit, parental permission is necessary to authorize children's research participation (45 CFR 46.405), just as it may authorize a standard therapeutic practice.

In this case, the parents never wanted to hear a discussion of shifting care
goals from curative means to comfort-care only. The physician-innovator was,
however, right to insist that the parents hear of less-intensive options at each point
it was appropriate for them to consider such choices for their child. In cases
involving competent adults, respect for autonomy favors a personal preference
rule for informed consent (or refusal; i.e., adults should receive as much information as they want, and no unwanted information should be forced on them).
However, if guardians refuse to hear all information a prudent patient (or surrogate) would desire, the refusal seems a failure of fiduciary responsibility to be
well-informed in making choices for vulnerable others. In a pediatric context, a
physician-innovator has a fiduciary responsibility to the child-patient to ensure
that parents have all material information needed to deliberate over what interventions will promote the child's interests. Here the physician-innovator's duty to
the pediatric patient overrides respect for the parents' refusal of information regarding end-of-life care options. Indeed, the refusal to be fully informed may be
an attempt to evade the parental fiduciary responsibility to make difficult decisions
on behalf of the child.

Parents are generally empowered to choose for their children, as long as their
choices are neither abusive nor neglectful. These choices are especially difficult
when efforts at treatment have failed to arrest the progress of their child's catastrophic disease. Ross (1998), who generally advocates for parental autonomy,
cautions as follows:

> The question remains whether there comes a point when physicians should
> override patient or surrogate decisions because the likelihood of benefit is so
> low or the potential benefit can yield only a very poor quality of life; that
> is, when treatment is both "virtually futile and inhumane." Even if treatment
> can achieve some physiological goals, the pains, harms and costs to the pa-
> tient prohibit parents from authorizing treatment because the treatment is not
> consistent with the modified principle of respect [for children as developing
> persons]. (pp. 142–143)

As undocumented aliens from a developing country, the parents and child
being treated "off-protocol," might be viewed as vulnerable on multiple counts:

(1) language barriers, (2) educational level, (3) economic status, (4) immigration status, (5) separation from support networks of extended family, religious community, and village, and (6) lack or scarcity of health care resources in the country of origin. All these factors may impinge on carefully considered, voluntary decision making. Here, the family spoke a regional Spanish dialect but had learned some English during the year they had spent at the referring university hospital. A staff physician who is a native speaker of Spanish provided translation services for informed consent discussions. The family was of modest means and did not have health insurance. The pediatric research center provides families with a wealth of ancillary services—housing near the center, meal cards for the cafeteria, and transportation to appointments, among others benefits.

These ancillary services raise the possibility of at least some parents' being partially influenced to enroll their children in research (or continue to permit their children to participate) for the sake of secondary gains for the family. In the context of a research protocol, the question whether such assistance might rise to the level of undue inducement to research participation is germane. (Since the patient in question was not enrolled in a research protocol, the research center did not benefit at her expense.)

The question of undue influence can remain in the context of single-patient, nonvalidated innovations. Decisions whether to permit a child's participation "off-protocol" on-site, where a full range of ancillary services are provided, are constrained when the alternative is transfer to a facility in a developing country, where parents may face the difficult task of caring for a dying child without comparable institutional support. The balance of benefits and risks changes if medically appropriate aftercare will be unavailable due to financial reasons (i.e., the parents are uninsured, uninsurable, and destitute) or lack of resources (i.e., in the patient's country of origin). Attending physicians and other staff members have an obligation to work for continuity of care by providing appropriate referral and discharge planning for all. If a return to the country and community of origin is anticipated, additional issues (i.e., how to care for an immunosuppressed child in a community without safe drinking water and sanitary waste disposal) arise.

The Child. Most 7-year-old children would be considered to have developing decisional capacity, from whom assent is sought.[8] The American Academy of Pediatrics (1995) urged that pediatric "patients should participate in decision making commensurate with their development; they should provide consent to care whenever reasonable."[9]

In this case, the child was not a "formal research" participant because she did not meet eligibility requirements for the protocol. These requirements excluded the child, at least in part, because she was at high risk given her comorbidities and she had not engrafted with the first HSCT. The planned intervention (second HSCT, using an investigational device) was less likely to benefit the patient than those enrolled in the protocol cohort on which her care was modeled. Arguably, here the chance of direct therapeutic benefit from the medical intervention was not very different from the slight chance of unexpected benefit from participation in a phase I trial. Had she dissented, serious questions regarding the ethical weight of her dissent would have ensued.[10] However, the patient was apparently willing to defer decision making to her parents (as is common with younger school-aged children and with members of the patient's ethnic group) and proved to be cooperative with the care team. In cases in which the chance of direct therapeutic benefit is very slight, an ombudsperson or other child advocate not involved in the research program might safeguard the child's voice (and interests) in deliberations dominated by, perhaps overly optimistic, staff and family.

Both pediatricians and parents have a fiduciary duty toward the child-patient to further his or her interests. The poignancy of such a responsibility for the child's welfare is seldom (if ever) greater than when "treatments" have failed to generate the hoped for benefits for a child with a catastrophic illness. The rules regarding the weight of a child's dissent (binding for nontherapeutic research, nonbinding for research offering potential for direct therapeutic benefit, non-binding for standard therapies) are efforts to further the child's own interests: society rather than the child benefits from nontherapeutic research, so such participation must be voluntary; however, the child *may* benefit directly from "therapeutic" research or standard therapies, so the child may be treated against her or his will (although certainly efforts should be made elicit the child's assent). However, faced with (repeated) therapeutic failure and/or very low expectations for therapeutic success of interventions under consideration, a child's dissent should be strongly considered, if not binding. The temptation to continue unwanted, burdensome interventions out of concern for the parents should be resisted.

Ethics Committee. The ethics committee determined that the parents had made a morally reasonable choice as they had chosen an option (a second HSCT, using an investigational device) offered to them by an expert in the specialty of transplantation. No noninvestigational curative alternatives existed; the decision to forgo the innovative therapy would be acceptance of their child's death. Absent of evidence of neglect or abuse, the ethics committee found no grounds for seeking a guardian *ad litem*. Although many committee members expressed the opinion that a comfort-only treatment plan would be more consistent with the child's best interests, they were willing to defer to the parents.[11] The parents' insistence on a second HSCT could be seen as their risking the child's present quality of life for the sake of a remotely possible future.

Questions of Justice

With the shift from the anticipated research context to the context of innovative therapy using an investigational device off-protocol, some responsibilities also shifted. For the decision addressing the second HSCT, hospital administrators and ethics committee members were involved in weighing of the costs of various options for the institution. Here, institutional responsibilities and concerns included allocation of resources on what would likely be ineffective or "virtually futile" care. This concern relates to the administration's responsibility to support the institutional mission of research and care by setting research priorities and securing funds for open protocols. The organizational ethics of the research center's commitment of extraordinary resources to this child with advanced disease and serious complications included a strong sense of the mission to cure, institutional responsibility for desperate clinical situations, and a desire to be good stewards of institutional resources that exceed what other health care settings have available for their uses.

As administrators of a pediatric hospital, the chief medical officers questioned expenditure of further resources in a case of "virtual medical futility." As administrators of a research center, they questioned expenditure on a case unlikely to further institutional research goals. The chief medical officer requested that the ethics committee review the case with an eye to these concerns (i.e., balance of benefit and harms and just allocation of resources). Both chief medical officers opposed the allocation of resources for this second transplant. Administrators at private pediatric research centers are involved in institutional ethics in multiple ways. These personnel provide administrative frameworks for (1) recruiting and appointing qualified researchers who are respected for their contributions to science, their commitment to research ethics, and their excellence as clinicians; (2) developing in-house research staff through continuing education that promotes scientific growth and ethical sensitivity; (3) financing the research and treatment programs in responsible ways; (4) setting institutional priorities for research allocation that support the institution's mission; (5) avoiding waste and inefficiency, thereby proving to be good stewards of charitable gifts and public funds; (6) instituting research oversight (i.e., by ensuring funds for adequate staffing of the IRB and acknowledging its statutory charge); and (7) by ensuring adequate staffing of an ethics committee and by giving it the leeway to offer independent review of cases. Finally, administrators contribute to setting the ethical tone of the institution.

Some members of the ethics committee indicated that the research center had been very generous in providing the first transplant and could not be faulted for not providing a second transplant; other members stated the center could be criticized in denying the transplant in light of the perceived availability of resources at the center. The attending physician played the role of "ideal advocate" by arguing that "the life of a blind child is worth saving."[12] However, some observers might conclude the physician perhaps gave insufficient weight to the extreme unlikelihood of treatment success—something a "restricted ideal advocate" would accept.

The pediatric research center in the present case could be viewed as a closed system. The center is a hospital of last appeal—its research participants-patients would not find the center's cutting-edge clinical options available from other providers. The chief medical officer of the research center estimates that the center would have to quadruple available beds to meet the needs of all U.S. children who might benefit from participation in the center's protocols. Even with the wealth of resources at the center's disposal, such expansion is impossible; a situation of moderate scarcity arguably exists.[13] Had the second bone marrow transplant been denied as an inefficient use of resources, those resources might have been redirected to other, higher priority institutional needs (i.e., care of other patients or requirements of basic research). However, there was no certainty that such a justified reassignment would occur. According to Daniels (1987), denials of care under a rationing plan can be just under two conditions:

> First, weighing the opportunity cost of one class of treatments or technologies against another must take place in a *closed* system. When beneficial care is denied it must be because the resources will be used better elsewhere in the system. Second, principles of justice must govern the decisions about priorities within this closed system—and thus define what counts as "better" uses of services. (p. 76)

Daniels (1987) suggests "some expanded role for hospital ethics committees" may be in order. Committees "might consider ethical issues involved in decision making under cost restraints. This would provide a broader, more public forum in which disputes between physicians and hospital administrators might be aired. (p. 79)" In our case, the ethics committee provided such a venue for the attending physician to appeal care that hospital administrators judged inappropriate. The ethics committee was unwilling to recommend rationing of care on an ad hoc basis. The committee concurred that any denial of care based on virtual futility should be grounded in a policy applicable to like situations.

Reasonable Care: Who Decides?

Who determines what care is reasonable or beneficial (a question of *locus* of authority), and what criteria distinguish unreasonable care from reasonable yet innovative (or nonvalidated) care? Those defining reasonable care might include (1) physicians and other members of the health care team, (2) the parents of the minor patient, (3) hospital administrators, and (4) third-party payers. Conflicts among these groups stem from differing commitments and values. Parents may demand burdensome care that physicians or other health care professionals judge is medically inappropriate, or physicians may recommend medically necessary care beyond what administrators or third-party payers desire to fund. Such conflicts are not merely over who decides but over the basis for decision making. These various parties do not always share the same set of care goals.

In the pediatric research hospital context, perhaps the more interesting question is what criteria distinguish care as unreasonable to various parties. First, research physicians likely will not understand reasonable to mean customary or even cost effective. Perhaps reasonable means in part supported by science whereas unreasonable may designate approaches that lack a scientific basis. Certainly, reasonable includes what is medically appropriate (i.e., what contributes to realization of various, widely recognized goals of medicine).[14] However, that goal-oriented understanding of "reasonable" raises the related issue of what are the goals or ends of medicine that can possibly (or likely) be realized in the present case.

Second, when a child suffers from a catastrophic illness, parents may take reasonable to mean anything that might help my child, no matter how burdensome the treatment or unlikely the benefit. Parents may feel that they have failed their children if they are not aggressive advocates who push caregivers to do everything possible. In this case, the parents' cultural group reinforced this imperative to fight until the end. Parents may need permission, even encouragement, to let go of hope for a cure. Here, children and parents may be best served by a strong recommendation from doctors to change the goals of care, giving priority to the quality of the child's remaining life over efforts to provide cure. Often, there will be a negotiation to come to agreed upon, shared goals. Even when curative options no longer exist and death is anticipated in the near future, much remains to be done to relieve symptoms, pain, and suffering; to improve or maintain compromised functional status; and to avoid harms to the patient in the course of what is in fact end-of-life care. Education and counseling of parents regarding their child's present condition and what to expect are no less important at the end-of-life than they were when parents were first asked to permit their child's participation in a research protocol or nonvalidated innovation.

Third, hospital administrators and third-party payers have goals in addition to patient care; they are concerned with allocation of resources, ideally in the service of patient populations. Here, "reasonable" may well mean "customary" or even "cost-effective." In regard to research hospitals, the goal is the benefit of future generations by developing cures, treatments for management of disease, and means of prevention. In this situation, it may be justified to deny a second HSCT to this child.

CONCLUSIONS

Medical innovation is neither an unqualified boon nor an unquestionable bane. Exigencies sometimes favor action beyond what has been customary under like circumstances. Such is likely the case when a condition is life-threatening or severely debilitating, when no validated intervention has outcomes acceptable to the parents, child patient and treatment team, *and* when it is reasonable to theorize that the innovation might offer significant prolongation of life and/or improvement in quality of life. Sometimes exigencies favor conformity to established practice, including hospice philosophy care. However, when innovative practices are used, careful reflection should be given to how recognized ethical duties can be fulfilled in an unfamiliar landscape.

—

Questions for Discussion

1. The authors discuss two regulatory mechanisms that are available for a patient who is not eligible to participate in a clinical investigation and yet seeks to access the experimental agent.
   a. What is the evidence burden necessary for both of these mechanisms prior to initiating the treatment protocol?
   b. According to the authors of this chapter, which of the two mechanisms was more appropriate in this case? Do you support their position?
2. What change in key roles occurred with the shift from the anticipated research context to that of nonvalidated, innovative therapy using an investigational device off-protocol? What, if any, are the ethical implications of this shift?
3. Do you agree with the authors' concerns about the negative implications of conflict over treatment decisions in an interdisciplinary team's efforts to provide excellent care to patients?
4. In terms of beneficence, do you agree with the authors' position as to the desired approach of each party (the attending physician, the HSCT clinical care staff, the IRB, the parents, the medical administration)? Had you been any of those parties, would you have decided differently?
5. What is the role of the health care team when making recommendations

to the family about innovative treatment? How is this role different than the team's role in decisions involving withholding or withdrawing life-sustaining interventions?

6. According to the authors, "when a clinical innovation represents a degree of departure from accepted practice similar to that found in research protocols, the role of IRB oversight becomes a legitimate question." Where would you draw the line between innovative therapies and research per se? Should IRBs have jurisdiction over clinical innovation?

7. In terms of respect for persons, do you agree with the authors' position as to the desired approach of each party (the attending physician, the HSCT clinical care staff, the IRB, the parents, the medical administration)? Had you been any of those parties, would you have decided differently?

8. Do you agree with the idea of respectful listening as a replacement for the concept of respect for autonomy in the pediatric context? What are the implications of this substitution?

9. What criteria distinguish care as "unreasonable" to various parties (research physicians, parents, hospital administrators and third-party payers)? Had you been the ethics committee in this case, which criteria would you adopt?

10. What would you consider to be the most defensible and just decision in this case? Should the second transplant go forward?

———

Notes

1. This would necessitate that the patient be *ineligible* for the investigational new drug (IND) protocol currently available but have an expectation of benefit from the intervention. These determinations are made on a case-by-case basis and involve the sponsor and the FDA.

2. Filing a single patient or emergency IND carries the same responsibilities as any IND in that the local IRB must be notified and approve, and adverse events, clinical updates, and an annual report must be filed with the FDA. Other conditions that must be met for an emergency IND are that there is no comparable satisfactory or alternative drug available for treating that stage of the disease in the intended patient. However, the drug must also be under investigation in a controlled clinical trial or all other clinical trials have been completed and the sponsor of the controlled clinical trial is actively pursuing marketing approval of the investigational drug with due diligence.

3. The same safeguards and reporting requirements that apply to any other IND study apply to these situations. The protocol (i.e., treatment plan) is required to contain an explanation of the rationale for the use of the investigational drug as well as a list of what available regimens should be tried prior to its use or an explanation of why the use of the investigational drug is preferable to the use of available marketed treatments.

4. According to the *Declaration of Helsinki* (World Medical Association, 1964), (1) "[i]n the

treatment of the sick person, the doctor must be free to use a new diagnostic and therapeutic measure, if in his or her judgment it offers hope of saving life, reestablishing health or alleviating suffering," and (2) "[t]he potential benefits, hazards and discomfort of a new method should be weighed against the advantages of the best current diagnostic and therapeutic methods."

5. There, competent adults are free to assess relative risks and benefits, given their own level of comfort with risk (degree of risk aversion) and their own conceptions of a good life, including quality-of-life judgments.

6. Some discussions of distributive justice distinguish persons who are risk-averse (i.e., who like to "play it safe") from those who accept great risk (i.e., who are "willing to gamble"). Daniels (1985) noted "we have no conception of the good life that embodies just one degree of risk aversion" (p. 157).

7. With the exception of emancipated minors and, in some instances, mature minors, pediatric patients are not autonomous individuals (i.e., they are not empowered to choose based on their own values); parental permission is generally required. Neither are parents acting as surrogates for their children autonomous in the same sense as when they make decisions regarding their own medical care or research participation; rather, in choosing for their children, parents exercise paternalism (rather than autonomy). Furthermore, parents are somewhat constrained in the options they may consider for their children; for example, in the Unites States, parents may not authorize a child's participation in nontherapeutic research that entails more than minimal risk, though parents would be free to volunteer for such research themselves. Similarly, competent adults are free to refuse likely life-saving interventions for themselves, but parents are generally not free to refuse such for their child, even on religious grounds.

8. The American Academy of Pediatrics categorizes children as (1) those who lack decision-making capacity, (2) those with a developing decisional capacity, and (3) those who have decision-making capacity for health care decisions.

9. That statement further advised that "pediatricians should not necessarily treat children as rational, autonomous decision makers, but they should give serious consideration to each patient's developing capacities for participating in decision making, including rationality and autonomy. If physicians recognize the importance of assent, they empower children to the extent of their capacity."

10. In a nontherapeutic research context, the child's dissent would be legally binding. As the chance of benefit to the individual child approaches zero, the distinction between innovative practice and formal research (at least with respect to anticipated outcome for the individual patient or research participant) fades.

11. Again, Ross (1998) is instructive: "Given a liberal community's toleration of a wide range of conceptions of the good, state intervention is only justified if the parents' decision is abusive, neglectful, or exploitative, not if an alternative is better" (p. 93).

12. Daniels (1987) contrasts an unrestricted ideal advocate with a restricted one. Traditionally, physicians are enjoined to make clinical decisions uninfluenced by judgments about the patient's social worth. This proscription of judgments based on social worth "is interpreted by some to mean that the physician should not put a price on a patient's life—should not decide how much it is worth to save or extend a particular patient's life. More narrowly interpreted, [this prohibition] bars a physician from considering factors other than medical need or likelihood of treatment success in making clinical decisions for a particular patient" (p. 71).

13. Daniels (1987) acknowledges that given conditions of moderate scarcity, individuals have no "basic right to have all their health care needs met. Rather, there is a social obligation to provide individuals only with those services which are part of the design of a system that on

the whole protects equal opportunity" (p. 76). Daniels predicts that "providers will not be able to be the unrestricted advocates of their patients, but will have to do the best they can for them under the restrictions that exist in the system" so that "a more equitable distribution of resources overall results" (p. 76). In this new world, as it was also in the ancient Hippocratic world, "there will be some things that providers cannot do for their patients." Physicians can act as 'gatekeepers' only if they are "abiding by a just social decision" and not their "own determination that it is not worth the resources to treat a particular class of patients in a particular way" (p. 77).

14. Jonsen, Seigler, and Winslade (1998) offer the following enumeration: (1) promotion of health and prevention of disease, (2) relief of symptoms, pain and suffering, (3) cure of disease, (4) prevention of an untimely death, (5) improvement of functional status or maintenance of compromised status, (6) education and counseling of patients [and their parents] regarding their condition and prognosis, and (7) avoiding harms to the patient in the course of care.

References

American Academy of Pediatrics, Committee on Bioethics. (1995). Informed consent, parental permission, and assent in pediatric practice (RE9510). *Pediatrics, 95*(2), 314–317.

Cowan, D. H., & Bertsch, E. (1984). Innovative therapy: The responsibility of hospitals. *Journal of Legal Medicine, 5*(2), 219–251.

Daniels, N. (1987). The ideal advocate and limited resources. *Theoretical Medicine, 8,* 69–80.

Daniels, N. (1985). *Just Health Care.* Cambridge: Cambridge University Press.

Jonsen, A. R., Seigler, M., & Winslade, W. J. (1998). *Clinical ethics.* New York: McGraw Hill.

Ross, R. F. (1998). *Children, families, and health care decision-making.* New York: Oxford University Press.

Singer, P., Siegler, M., Lantos, D., Emond, J., Whitington, P., Thistlethwaite, R., & Broelsch, C. (1990). The ethical assessment of innovative therapies: Liver transplantation using living donors. *Theoretical Medicine, 11*(2), 87–94.

World Medical Association. (1964). *The Helsinki declaration.* Revised Edinburgh, Scotland, (2000).

16

Children and Placebos

Jessica Wilen Berg

___

CASE DESCRIPTION

Many children suffer from psychiatric illnesses, and yet few studies have been done on the available medications. In one case a research trial is proposed involving children suffering from attention deficit–hyperactivity disorder (ADHD). ADHD is not life-threatening but may result in significant learning and social disabilities. Standard therapies, such as Ritalin, are available. The trial is designed as a double-blind placebo-controlled study. Subjects in the placebo arm would be without medication for a 2-month period.

Pediatric research is a subject of controversy, as evidenced by the chapters in this book. Placebo-controlled trials are a hotly debated issue (Hoffman, 2001). The combination of the two—use of placebos in pediatric research—is certain to raise ethical concern in both the scientific and lay communities. This chapter explores the ethical aspects of using placebo controls in pediatric research trials, drawing on the study described above to demonstrate the range of issues raised. It begins with a brief discussion of placebos and outlines the arguments supporting their use in pediatric populations, starting from the assumption that placebos are ethical in some studies with competent adult subjects and in fact may be necessary in order to obtain good scientific data regarding new treatments (Leber, 2000). Analysis of the debate about placebo use in general is left to others (Miller & Brody, 2002; Rothman & Michels, 2002). After providing this brief background on placebo use in pediatric research, the chapter then identifies the current legal and ethical guidelines that apply to such use. Finally, it considers the ethical issues raised by the placebos use and explores how those issues play out when the subjects in question are children. It does not seek to provide definitive answers on the use of placebos in pediatric research trials, but rather to identify the range of ethical concerns that may help evaluation of different protocols.

Placebos

The word placebo is derived from the Latin phrase "to please." Technically, a placebo is an inactive substance that is usually designed to resemble an active substance. The use of placebos in the context of clinical treatment is very different from the role of placebos in research. In the clinical treatment context placebos are generally given to patients in order to facilitate psychological aspects of healing. In the research context placebos can function to eliminate bias and help distinguish true from false pharmacological effects of an experimental intervention. A placebo-controlled double-blind study is one in which at least some of the subjects receive an inactive substance or intervention, but the allocation of active and inactive substances is not known to either the subjects or the investigators. Contrary to popular belief, subjects in the placebo-arm of a study may, in fact, receive some benefit (Gilbert & Packer, 1995). This can include such things as increased attendant care and monitoring, or standard treatments that do not interfere with the study design. However, subjects do not receive the experimental treatment that the study is designed to investigate.

The scientific rationale for the use of placebos in research trials is based on the concept of "placebo effect." The placebo effect is the measurable positive response that patients or subjects demonstrate to an inactive intervention. It may entail pain relief and/or resolution of symptoms. It is often discussed in terms of percentages, in the same way that the positive effect of an experimental intervention is framed. For example, in one meta-analysis of studies of new treatments for major depression, an average of 30% of subjects responded to a placebo (Walsh, Seidman, Sysko & Gould, 2002). Interestingly the same analysis found that the placebo response rate varied considerably from year to year and has increased significantly in recent years. In fact, in some studies subjects receiving an inactive substance have as good if not better outcomes than subjects who received an experimental substance (Enserink, 1999). Estimates of the prevalence of the placebo effect vary, ranging from 35% to 75% of subjects deriving a positive benefit from an inactive substance. Although the effect appears to be especially evident in drug studies, it can also be seen in clinical trials of new surgical methods that employ a "sham surgical" arm (Freeman, Leaverton, Godbold, Hausner & Goetz, et al., 1999). Sham surgeries are surgeries that entail everything but the actual surgical intervention—including preoperative care, anesthesia, incisions, and postoperative care. Given the high rates of placebo response, it is extremely difficult to know if the positive effect of a new treatment is due to pharmacological or physical properties of the experimental substance, or due to the symbolic or comforting effect of receiving some intervention, or even due to the natural history of remission. Thus, studies that fail to compare an active treatment arm to a placebo control risk providing false data regarding efficacy.

This concern about the placebo effect of pharmacologically or physically "ineffective" interventions combined with the very real risks and potential side effects of many treatments have led some commentators to argue that clinical trials that fail to include a placebo arm are unethical (Cohen, 2002). Moreover, the use of a placebo control arm may provide better incentives for investigators to engage in careful research since even a small showing of effectiveness for an experimental intervention when compared with a placebo may be sufficient to achieve Food and Drug Administration (FDA) approval (Hoffman, 2001). Furthermore, the use of a placebo arm is less costly, enabling larger trials and thus potentially faster results (Hoffman, 2001).

Because of all of these factors, the FDA considers placebo-controlled studies to represent the "gold standard" of research. Although there may be some controversy over their use in any circumstance, the primary objections to placebo-controlled studies focus on cases in which a standard treatment of proven efficacy is available. As Miller (2002) states: "A consensus exists that placebo-controlled trials are unethical if patients risk death or irreversible serious morbidity as a result of having standard treatment withheld" (p. 708). Moreover, he notes that, "[w]hen no effective treatment exists for a given disorder, it is not ethically problematic to conduct a trial comparing placebo with an experimental agent" (p. 708). In the absence of an effective standard treatment, comparison with placebo may be ethically required since it would not be known whether the experimental intervention (with all of its attendant risks) has any potential benefit (Fost, 2001). In a situation where the investigator has some evidence (but perhaps not conclusive evidence) that the experimental intervention will be beneficial, one ethicist suggests use of a cross-over design where all subjects have an opportunity to receive the active treatment (Hyman, 2000).

However, it is important to stress that even when a standard treatment is available, it may not be completely effective. For example, it may not alleviate all symptoms, or fail to do so for all patients. In addition, many standard treatments may entail significant and unpleasant side effects that prompt the search for new and better treatments. In some cases the risks involved in providing a standard treatment combined with concerns that the subject pool in question will not benefit from the standard treatment weigh strongly against using an active control (Temple & Ellenberg, 2000). For example, in a number of studies of new psychiatric medications, the subject pool may be comprised of individuals for whom the current standard therapy is ineffective, or for whom the side effects pose too great a risk. It might be considered unethical to require these individuals to receive the current standard therapy as part of a clinical trial testing a new experimental therapy, since they would be exposed to the potential risks of the standard therapy without any (or enough) potential for benefit.

The rationales for conducting research trials and including placebo-control arms are applicable to studies involving pediatric populations. Recent controversy over pediatric drug testing highlights the significant lack of information regarding pediatric medications and the absence of drug studies involving children (Albert, 2002). Many drugs that are commonly used in treating children have never been subjected to formal research investigation, except with adult populations (107th Congress 2001). One article recounts the numerous innovative treatments that have been used in children without being tested in clinical trials and the widespread harms that followed (Fost, 2001). A recent study suggests that between 1997 and 2000, almost 4,000 deaths of children younger than 2 years may be attributable to medication. The author stresses that additional studies of medication effects on young children are crucial and that these must include placebo-controlled trials. More specifically, a 1999 editorial in the journal *Pediatrics* reviews the evidence regarding narcotic use in ventilated neonates and concludes that the lack of proven benefit requires that placebo-controlled trials be conducted for this population (Kennedy & Tyson, 1999). Other authors have stressed the need for placebo-controlled trials for psychiatric treatments (Malone & Simpson, 1998), particularly for children with mood disorders (Fisher & Fisher, 1996; Pellegrino, 1996) or schizophrenia (Armenteros & Mikhail, 2002). Especially problematic is the continued use of antidepressants despite consistent studies showing no benefit over placebo (Fisher & Fisher, 1996). Moreover, "subjects in child and adolescent trials often have a high rate of response to placebo" (Malone & Simpson, 1998, p. 1413) and thus placebo controls may be essential in certain circumstances (Emanuel & Miller, 2001). However, it may be that placebo response rates vary with cognitive development, at least to the extent that placebo responses are linked to the belief that one is obtaining treatment (and thus depend on awareness of treatment). If so, placebo-controlled studies may be more important to conduct in some pediatric populations than in others.

Legal and Ethical Guidelines for Placebo Use in Pediatric Research

Most research protocols involving children in the United States are required to comply with regulations promulgated by the Department of Health and Human Services (45 CFR 46.401). These regulations do not mention placebos. They state in broad terms the circumstances under which research is permissible, separating research into three primary categories: (1) minimal risk, (2) greater than minimal risk with potential for direct therapeutic benefit, and (3) greater than minimal risk with no potential for direct benefit but likely to yield generalizable knowledge.[1] The first category of clinical trials may be conducted as long as parental (or guardian) consent is obtained, along with the child's assent where appropriate (Code of Federal Regulations, 45 CFR 46.404, 2001). Research involving greater than minimal risk (into which category presumably most drug studies involving placebos would fall) is permissible if there is a possibility of direct therapeutic benefit from the intervention, or a likely increase in well-being due to the monitoring procedures, if certain conditions are met (45 CFR 46.405, 2001). Institutional review boards (IRBs) considering the protocol must find that:

- The risk is justified by the anticipated benefit to the subjects;
- The relation of the anticipated benefit to the risk is at least as favorable to the subjects as that presented by available alternative approaches; and
- Adequate provisions are made for soliciting the assent of the children and permission of their parents or guardians (45 CFR 46.406).

For research without direct benefits for subjects, additional restrictions are imposed (45 CFR 46.406). Many of the pediatric research trials that include a placebo arm will fit into the second category of greater than minimal risk but potential for direct benefit. This is true of the ADHD study described at the outset of this chapter. Some subjects in the study will receive an active treatment that may provide a therapeutic benefit.

It is not clear, however, whether the guidelines are to be interpreted to require that all subjects individually have the potential for direct benefit from the intervention, or whether the study is to be considered as a whole. For example, all subjects who participate in a study that randomizes participants between an active treatment arm and a placebo arm have a potential for a direct benefit because all have the potential (when considering the study from the outset) to be assigned to the active arm. Thus, in one study that tested a placebo against an active treatment (i.e., growth hormone injections), the National Institutes of Health review panel interpreted the language of the regulations to require pre-randomization analysis of potential benefit (Williams, 1996). But a recent article argues that the "entire protocol" approach is inappropriate and that risk:benefit determinations should be made individually, for each arm in question (Miller, Wendler, & Wilfrond, 2003). As a result, placebo trials would only be allowed when the placebo (and other) arms fit within one of the three categories identified above. Although the authors list a number of factors that need to be taken into account, the individual arm evaluation requirement would result in more limitations on placebo use. For example, considered in its entirety, the ADHD study described at the outset would entail a potential therapeutic benefit since some of the subjects will be randomized to the group receiving the experimental drug. But considering each arm individually, subjects in the placebo arm would not get the potential for benefit from taking the experimental medication and thus to fit within the guidelines either another source of benefit would need to be identified, or additional restrictions would be imposed.

For those studies using a cross-over design, in which subjects are switched from one arm of the study to another at some midway point, all subjects will eventually receive the active treatment and thus the potential for benefit. In such a case the risk:benefit ratio would be determined by evaluating the entire protocol, since each arm would be exposed to all interventions. In other situations, a high rate of placebo response might be considered a potential benefit that can offset risks, although this may not be what was intended by the federal regulations. Even if the potential for direct benefit via access to an active treatment is in question, the monitoring procedure used for the study may be likely to contribute to subjects' well-being, thus fitting into the second aspect of permissible nonminimal risk research (45 CFR 46.405). However, IRBs may be uncomfortable relying on indirect benefit from increased monitoring to balance out risks, and thus as a practical matter it may be difficult to gain study approval. Finally, when there is no potential benefit, placebo controls may still be permissible under the regulations depending on the type of risk in question and the availability of standard treatment, issues discussed in more detail in the last part of this chapter. All of this is not to say that every pediatric study should be approved, but merely demonstrates that the inclusion of a placebo arm is theoretically permissible under the federal regulations.

Although the framework of the U.S. Federal Regulations would not bar the use of placebos, there are a number of ethical codes and guidelines that may be less permissive. The oft-cited Nuremberg Code can be interpreted as suggesting a complete prohibition of research involving children (or any other incompetent population). It makes no specific mention of placebos. Neither is there language in the *Belmont Report* (www.fda.gov/oc/ohrt/irbs/belmont .html, accessed 7/20/04) (from which the federal regulations are derived) specifically covering the use of placebos. However, the *Declaration of Helsinki*, promulgated by the World Medical Association (WMA), does specifically consider placebo use and restricts them to situations where "no proven prophylactic, diagnostic or therapeutic method exists" (World Medical Association, 2000). This would raise concerns regarding the ADHD study since there are medical treatments available. In 2001, the WMA issued a "note of clarification" on its placebo position, stating that placebo-controlled trials may be ethical "(1) where for compelling and scientifically sound methodological reasons its use is necessary to determine the efficacy or safety of a prophylactic, diagnostic, or therapeutic method, or (2) where a prophylactic, diagnostic or therapeutic method is being investigated for a minor condition and the patients who receive placebo will not be subject to additional risk of serious or irreversible harm" (World Medical Association, 2001). Arguably, in all cases where a placebo effect is present, and particularly those situations where the effect is significant (i.e., psychiatric treatments), placebos are permissible under the first category. But the first condition merely restates the debate—are placebos necessary from a scientific standpoint to prove efficacy? The second category is more helpful since it appears to allow for placebo use, even when standard therapy is available, as long as the risks are low. But interpreting such a provision is not simple, as discussed further below. For example, it is not clear whether ADHD may be considered a "minor" condition, or whether the subjects would be exposed to a risk of "serious or irreversible" harm. The *Helsinki Declaration*'s position on placebos remains extremely controversial, and the document itself has no particular legal force.

The American Academy of Pediatrics (AAP) continually emphasizes the need to include children in clinical studies of drugs (American Academy of Pediatrics, 1995). According to the AAP, placebos are considered permissible "if their use does not place children at increased risk." Although the notion of increased risk is not developed in the AAP's position statement, the academy does provide a list of five conditions that may justify the use of a placebo in pediatric drug research:

- When there is no commonly accepted therapy for the condition and the agent under study is the first one that may modify the course of the disease progress;
- When the commonly used therapy for the condition is of questionable efficacy;
- When the commonly used therapy for the condition carries with it a high frequency of undesirable side effects and the risks may be significantly greater than the benefits;
- When the placebo is used to identify incidence and severity of undesirable side effects produced by adding a new treatment to an established regimen; or
- When the disease process is characterized by frequent, spontaneous exacerbations and remissions and the efficacy of the therapy has not been demonstrated.

The list includes most situations in which placebos would be permissible for adult populations. For example, although standard treatment exists for ADHD, there may be concerns with the efficacy and side effects. Furthermore, many mental illnesses are cyclical in nature, becoming better and worse over time. This make it difficult to know whether remission is due to disease cycle or the positive effect of a new treatment, making comparison of a new therapy to placebo particularly important.

Although placebos can be analyzed under the federal regulations and the AAP provides more specific guidelines, no document provides a full ethical analysis of the issues raised by the use of placebos in pediatric research. Because of this absence, it is worthwhile to consider placebo use in light of the ethical precepts that are thought to guide research in general—in particular, those outlined in the *Belmont Report*.

___

ETHICAL ANALYSIS AND DISCUSSION

Exploring the Ethics of Placebo-Controlled Pediatric Research Trials

The National Commission for the Protection of Human Subjects of Biomedical and Behavioral Research issued the *Belmont Report* in 1979. It eventually formed the basis of the federal regulations discussed previously. The report identifies three primary ethical principles that should guide research: respect for persons, beneficence, and justice. Respect for persons is framed in terms of consent and may involve protections for vulnerable populations who lack capacity to consent. Beneficence includes both preventing harm (nonmaleficence) and maximizing benefit. Justice in research entails fair distribution of both the burdens and benefits. Although the concept of justice has significant implications for pediatric research as a whole, the two primary ethical issues raised by the use of placebos (in any population) are consent and beneficence/nonmaleficence. When the concepts are applied to pediatric research additional concerns are raised. The following sections discuss each of these—consent and beneficence—in turn.

Respect for Persons: Consent. Application of the doctrine of informed consent generally satisfies the requirement for respecting persons involved in research. Thus subjects who consent to participate, and consent to placebo use, are respected as ends in themselves, and not merely as means to gain research knowledge. But numerous empirical studies over the years since the doctrine developed have shown the limitations of informed consent. One particular concern in the research context is the prevalence of the so-termed "therapeutic misconception" (Appelbaum, Roth, Lidz, Benson, & Winslade, 1987). The therapeutic misconception refers to subjects' consistent failure to understand the differences between research and treatment, even when full disclosure is made regarding these differences. It affects ill subjects whose disease is under investigation. (Healthy subjects do not expect any treatment since they are not suffering from a disease and thus should not be affected by the therapeutic misconception.) These research participants often erroneously believe that a study is designed specifically to help them, and that the physician-investigators are engaged in treating their illness.

In one of the most widely reported demonstrations of the therapeutic misconception, subjects from two studies were interviewed (Appelbaum, Roth, & Lidz, 1982). In both studies the subjects were given an explanation of the process of randomization, the presence of a placebo-arm, and the notion of a double-blind study, and yet in the subsequent interview process, few (if any) could accurately describe how subjects were assigned, whether a placebo would be given, or whether the investigators were aware of which treatments the subjects would receive. Most telling was an interview with one of the subjects who understood the ideas of "randomization," "double-blind," and "placebo" in the abstract but either could not or refused to accept that these methods would be applied to her participation in the research protocol. The authors note, "In this subject's case, despite an understanding of randomization, and a momentary recognition that random assignment would be used, the subject's conviction that the investigators would be acting in her best interests won out" (Appelbaum et al., 1982, p. 327). The consistent failure, regardless of information disclosures, to understand the framework of research, and particularly the notions of placebo and randomization, significantly undermines the use of informed consent as a justification for allowing research to occur. The therapeutic misconception may be so strong that it is impossible to gain informed consent regarding placebo use, and thus alternative justifications for allowing such research to continue should be explored.

For young children, the presence of the therapeutic misconception is confounded by at least two factors—their lack of capacity and parental decision making. In most research studies children are asked to "assent" to participation, and full "consent" is obtained from parents or guardians (Koren & Carmeli, 1993). Children are even less likely than competent adults to understand complex terms such as randomization and placebo, although this varies considerably by age and maturity (Leikin, 1993) and illness experience. Moreover, children may be more likely to suffer from the misconception that physician-investigators are focused primarily on promoting their best interests and thus fail to understand their role in a research study (Leikin, 1993). In one case, for example, 13-year-old twins, one of whom suffered from ADHD, were recruited to participate in a nontherapeutic study to determine whether the twin with ADHD had other psychiatric illnesses (Gordon & Bonkovsky, 1996). Despite repeated explanations, both children failed to understand that the study was not going to entail treatment.

Even more troublesome in this context is the effect of the therapeutic misconception on the parental decision makers. In the study described above, there is some indication that the parents also failed to understand the purpose of the protocol. There is no reason to think that the misconception does not function for proxy decision makers, and thus even if parents are better able to understand the concepts in the abstract, they may still believe that the research endeavor is designed to help their child. In fact, parents may be more susceptible to the misconception since they are likely to grasp any chance to help their child and be less inclined to accept that the physicians involved in the research are not focused on that task.

In one study of parental attitudes toward research involving their children, the authors found that the parents demonstrated an "inordinate faith in the medical system to protect their children" and a "natural tendency to deny and downgrade risks in such ventures" (Harth & Thong, 1995, p. 90). Interestingly, another study by the same authors found that parents who agreed to enroll their children in research were "significantly less well-educated and less well-represented in professional and managerial occupations . . . had significantly less social support and displayed greater health-seeking behavior and used more habit forming substances" (Harth, Johnston, & Young, 1992, p. 90). They concluded that the volunteering parents "may be more predisposed to enrolling their children as a way of coping with having young children with a distressing illness" (Harth et al., 1992, p. 90). These findings raise significant concerns about why parents consent to their child's participation in research and whether their consent is sufficient. Although these concerns about consent are prevalent in any study involving children, they may be less troublesome when there is no available treatment for a disease and participation in a research trial testing an experimental therapy is the only option. Parental consent to research participation when there is a standard effective treatment available, such as the ADHD study, are more problematic.

Beneficence. In addition to concerns about consent, placebo use in pediatric research trials also raise significant concerns relating to beneficence. First, there may be a special responsibility to avoid doing harm since children are a vulnerable population. Glantz (1996) points out the difficultly in determining a child's best interests when considering enrollment in a research protocol, particularly in the context of placebo-controlled trials. Although there are arguments against the use of placebo controls for any population when a standard proven therapy exists, their use may be especially problematic in the pediatric context (Miller & Shorr, 2002). There are at least three issues here. First, is there a standard proven therapy available? Second, what are the risks of harm of a non-treatment placebo arm? Third, can a child be wronged without being harmed while participating in a placebo-controlled trial?

The question of whether a standard, proven effective therapy is available is not as straightforward as it may seem. How should we determine whether a therapy is "proven," "effective," and "available"? In many cases, the standard therapy has never been subjected to clinical trials, and this is especially true for children where most medication use is "off-label" (i.e., the medication has been approved by the FDA for one use, usually for adults, but not the specific pediatric use). Although some treatments may be clearly effective, despite not having been tested in a research protocol, many others are not so obvious. There is some debate as to whether any treatment should be considered "proven" if it has not been subjected to randomized double-blind studies. The placebo effect is fairly significant and may be more evident in some areas than in others. This is exactly the problem that placebo-controlled trials are designed to combat—providing evidence that the treatment in question is, in fact, effective based on its pharmacology rather than its psychological impact. But it may be extremely difficult to get parents, patients, and physicians to reconsider the effectiveness of a standard therapy that has been used for a long period of time.

In addition to concerns about how to evaluate whether a treatment is "proven," there are also concerns about what counts as "effective." Should a treatment that merely delays the onset of symptoms or treats some symptoms, but does not cure the underlying disorder be considered effective? This issue is particularly pertinent in the treatment of some diseases (i.e., HIV infection) where the administration of current medications may render later developed medications ineffective. Thus, some people may want to forgo current therapy in favor of trying an experimental one, in the hope that it will be more effective. In other situations the standard therapy entails serious side effects that patients may want to avoid. Thus, many individuals participating in trials of new psychotropic medications may wish to avoid the risks attendant with standard therapies. In fact, the people who choose to participate in the trials are likely to be ones for whom the standard therapy does not work and thus a placebo control entails a better risk:benefit ratio than a standard therapy control. Of course, this assumes that the "nocebo" effect—the potential that subjects in the placebo arm will manifest the risks of the experimental treatment—is lower than the potential that the risks will manifest in the active treatment arm. This is very likely to be true in young pediatric populations who are not even informed about potential risks (although there may be some problems with parental reporting of risk manifestation). Moreover, for subjects who are informed, the nocebo effect (if there is any) may not survive eventual unblinding of placebo assignment after completion of the study. Unfortunately, there is little data on the nocebo effect, and there are no reported evaluations of its impact on pediatric populations. Assuming the nocebo effect is minimal in the pediatric context, and since the side effects of active treatments may be largely unknown, the mandate to "do no harm" may support comparison of an experimental treatment to placebo, in order to meet legal and ethical requirements to minimize risks.

Finally, issues relating to the notion of "availability" of treatments raise both beneficence concerns and justice concerns. Some proven treatments may be generally unavailable (outside a research trial) to the population in question because of cost or geographic location or even supply. If a proven treatment is "unavailable" in these senses are placebo controls warranted? This issue has been raised most recently in the context of international research protocols. One example entailed a trial of a new surfactant drug in Latin-American newborns in which the new drug is compared to both a placebo arm and an active treatment arm (Charatan, 2001). The trial would likely not be considered ethical in this country because of the availability of standard treatment. This issue is discussed in detail in another chapter of this book. Another study involved an evaluation of a new acellular vaccine against pertussis involving infants in Sweden and Italy (Cagliano, & Traversa, 1995). One justification that was put forth for allowing comparison to placebo was the low national average of vaccination (40%) compared to the number vaccinated in the study (90%). Other authors have pointed out the problems with using placebo-controlled trials of zidovudine (AZT) to prevent HIV transmission from mother to infant in Africa when there is a treatment available in this country (Cark, 1998; Kaiser, 1997; Lie, 1998). It is not clear how to evaluate placebo controls in a world where there are vastly different standards of care depending on geographic location (Studdert & Brennan, 1998).

The issue of risk of harm is more straightforward. There is a general consensus that a placebo is not warranted when there is a serious risk of harm from nontreatment (Hoffman, 2001; National Depressive and Manic-Depressive Association, 2002). Risks of death and serious permanent disability appear to fall into this category, but the concept of risk is 2-fold. It entails both evaluation of the magnitude of the risk (i.e., bruising vs. death) and the probability that the risk will manifest (i.e., 1% likelihood vs. 75% likelihood). Do so-called "serious" risks include all those of significant magnitude, regardless of probability? For example, some people argue that it is unethical to use placebo controls for pediatric trials of new asthma medications, since the untreated disease can be fatal (Ferdman, 1999). Not only may there be difficulty in determining how to categorize serious risks, but the acceptability of other risks, such as pain and suffering, may be problematic. These may be of particular concern when dealing with children who may be unable to understand either the temporary nature of the discomfort or the reasons for it. Thus placebos may be inappropriate in the ADHD trial described at the outset since the children in the control group will "suffer" during the 2-month washout period (i.e., a period of time during which all medications are stopped to ensure that any drugs are "washed out" of the patient/subject's system to avoid undesirable drug interactions).

Finally, children may be wronged without being harmed. Placebo use in young children inevitably requires deception that may be justified in the clinical context by direct benefit to the child, but raises serious ethical concerns in the research context. Without the ability to obtain informed consent or solicit meaningful assent, young children receiving placebo may be misled into thinking they are receiving active medication. This violates the obligation to be truthful with children, and may put children at risk for losing trust in the health care system if they feel deceived. Although no actual physical harm may occur, the child may have been wronged in a morally significant way.

CONCLUSION

Placebo use in research continues to be controversial and its inclusion in studies involving pediatric populations is certain to be a source of debate. This chapter takes the position that placebo use is ethically acceptable and may even be ethically required in some research trials, including those that involve children. However, it recognizes that there may be additional ethical concerns raised when dealing with pediatric populations. In particular, children's lack of capacity and the addition of parental decision makers may exacerbate undesirable effects such as the therapeutic misconception, thus undermining a primary justification for allowing placebos. In addition, risks of harm may be more difficult to quantify for children and there may be less comfort with exposing children to risks of even temporary pain and suffering. The age and relative capacity of the children in question will surely make a difference in any ethical analysis. This chapter does not attempt to provide definitive answers to the questions raised by the use of placebo controls, rather it is designed to serve as an impetus for further discussion.

Questions for Discussion

1. Many studies point out the high benefit of using placebo, either due to the positive effect that placebo has on patients or due to the development of improved alternative treatments following the use of placebo. Should this fact play a role in policy making regarding the use of placebo? For this matter, should there be a difference between children and adults subjects?

2. Is there a stronger justification to use placebo in minimal risk studies as opposed to more than minimal risk studies with the prospect of direct benefit?

3. Is there a stronger justification to use placebo in studies where all subjects are exposed to all the interventions?

4. Should high rate of placebo response be considered a potential benefit that can offset risks?

5. When there is no potential benefit to the subject, should placebo controls still be permissible?

6. Which one of the four discussed guideline documents (Nuremberg Code, *Belmont Report*, *Helsinki Declaration*/World Medical Association, or American Academy of Pediatrics) would you consider the best ethical code guiding the use of placebos in pediatric research?

7. What would be the difference in applying the principles of respect for persons and beneficence to children, as opposed to adults, when dealing with the ethical dilemma of using placebo in research? What about the use of placebo in the nonresearch, purely clinical context?

8. As a policy maker, where would you draw the line between research and treatment? Why and to what extent is it important that the subject understands the framework of research, and particularly the notions of placebo and randomization?

9. Does the fact that the subject is a child mitigate or amplify concerns about therapeutic misconception?

10. Is the case of parental permission to participate in research where a standard effective treatment is already available more problematic than parental permission for a research trial testing an experimental therapy that is the only tenable option?

11. How do you define "serious risk of harm from nontreatment" when considering children in research? Would you argue for a restrictive or permissive definition? Explain and defend your answer.

12. How would you analyze the case of the placebo-controlled randomized trial for ADHD presented in this chapter?

13. Do the ethical concerns raised by the author in her conclusion necessarily undermine the primary justification for allowing placebos? Can you think of other arguments that strengthen the justification?

———

Note

1. There is also a category of research "not otherwise approvable" that is not discussed here (45 CFR 46.407).

References

Albert, Tanya (2002, November 18). Federal court overturns FDA pediatric drug testing rule. *AM News*. Retrieved 7/20/04 from www.ama-assn.org/amednews/2002/11/18/gvsc1118.htm

American Academy of Pediatrics. (1995). Guidelines for the ethical conduct of studies to evaluate drugs in pediatric population. *Pediatrics, 95,* 286–294.

107th Congress. (2001) *Hearings Before the Sen. Comm. on Health, Education, Labor and Pensions. (2001). Better pharmaceuticals for children: Assessment and opportunities* 19 (statement of Sen. DeWine).

Appelbaum, Paul S., Roth, Loren H., & Lidz, Charles W. (1982). The therapeutic misconception: Informed consent in psychiatric research. *International Journal of Law and Psychiatry, 5,* 319–329.

Appelbaum, Paul S., Roth, Loren H. Lidz, Charles W., Benson, Paul, & Winslade, William (1987). False hopes and best data: Consent to research and the therapeutic misconception. *Hastings Center Report, 17,* 20–24.

Armenteros, Jorge L., & Mikhail, Ashraf G. (2002). Do we need placebos to evaluate new drugs in children with schizophrenia? *Psychopharmacology, 159,* 117–124.

Cagliano, Stephano, & Traversa, Guiseppe (1995). Letter to the Editor. *New England Journal of Medicine, 332,* 60.

Charatan, Fred (2001). Surfactant trial in Latin American infants criticized. *British Medical Journal, 322,* 575.

Clark, Peter (1998). The ethics of placebo-controlled trials for perinatal transmission of HIV in developing countries. *Journal of Clinical Ethics, 9,* 156–166.

Cohen, Peter (2002). Failure to conduct a placebo-controlled trial may be unethical. *American Journal of Bioethics, 2,* 24.

Emanuel, Ezekiel J., & Miller, Frank G. (2001). The ethics of placebo-controlled trials: A middle ground. *New England Journal of Medicine, 345,* 915–919.

Enserink, Mary (1999). Can the placebo be the cure? *Science, 284,* 238.

Ferdman, Ronald M. (1999). Letter to the Editor. *Journal of Pediatrics, 134,* 251.

Fisher, R., & Fisher, S. (1996). Antidepressants for children: Is scientific support necessary? *Journal Nervous Mental Disorders, 184,* 99–102.

Fost, Norman (2001). Ethical issues in research and innovative therapy in children with mood disorders. *Biological Psychiatry* 49: 1015–1022.

Freeman, Leaverton, P. E., Godbold, J. H., Hauswer, R. A., Goetz, C. G., & Aoanow, C. W. (1999). Use of placebo surgery in controlled trials of a celluar-based therapy for Parkinson's disease. *New England Journal of Medicine, 341,* 988–992.

Gilbert, Edward, Packer, Milton (1995). Letter to the Editor. *New England Journal of Medicine, 332,* 41.

Glantz, Leonard (1996). Conducting research with children: Legal and ethical issues. *Journal American Academy of Child Adolescent Psychiatry, 34,* 1283–1291.

Gordon, V. M., & Bonkovsky, F. O. (1996). Family dynamics and children in medical research. *Journal of Clinical Ethics, 7,* 349–354.

Harth, S. C., Johnston, R. R., & Young, Y. H. (1992). The psychological profile of parents who volunteer their children for clinical research: A controlled study. *Journal of Medical Ethics., 18,* 86–93.

Harth, S. C., & Thong, Y. H. (1995). Parental perceptions and attitudes about informed consent in clinical research involving children. *Social Science Medicine, 40,* 1573–1577.

Hoffman, Sharona (2001). The use of placebos in clinical trials: Responsible research or unethical practice? *Connecticut Law Rev, 33,* 449–501.

Hyman, S. E. (2000). An NIMH perspective on the use of placebos. *Biological Psychiatry, 47,* 689–691.

Kaiser, J. (1997). Bangkok study add fuel to AIDS ethics debate. *Journal of the American Medical Association, 278,* 1553.

Kennedy, K. A., & Tyson, J. (1999). Narcotic analgesia for ventilated newborns: Are placebo-controlled trials ethical and necessary? *Journal of Pediatrics, 134,* 127–129.

Koren, G., & Carmeli, D. B.(1993). Maturity of children to consent to medical research: The baby-sitter test. *Journal of Medical Ethics, 19,* 142–148.

Leber P. (2000). The use of placebo control groups in the assessment of psychiatric drugs: An historical context. *Biological Psychiatry, 46,* 699–706.

Leikin, S. (1993). Minors' assent, consent, or dissent to medical research. *IRB, 15,* 1–7.

Lie, Reidar (1998). Ethics of Placebo-Controlled Trials in Developing Countries, Bioethics 12(4), 307–311.

Malone, R. P., & Simpson, G. M. (1998). Use of placebos in clinical trials involving children and adolescents. *Psychiatric Services, 49,* 1413–1417.

Miller, F. G. (2002). Placebo controlled trials in psychiatric research: An ethical perspective. *Biological Psychiatry, 47,* 707–716.

Miller, F. G., & Brody, H. (2002). What makes placebo-controlled trials unethical? *American Journal of Bioethics, 2,* 3–9.

Miller, F. G., & Shorr, A. F. (2002). Ethical assessment of industry-sponsored trials: A case analysis. *Chest, 121,* 1337–1342.

Miller, F. G., Wendler, D., & Wilfond, B. (2003). When do the federal regulations allow placebo-controlled trials in children? *Journal of Pediatrics, 142,* 102–107.

National Depressive and Manic-Depressive Association. (2002). Consensus Statement on the Use of Placebo in Clinical Trials of Mood Disorders. *Archives General Psychiatry, 59,* 262–270.

Pellegrino, E. (1996). Clinical judgment, scientific data, and ethics: Antidepresssant therapy in adolescents and children. *Journal Nervous Mental Disorders, 184,* 106–108.

Reidar. K. L. (1998). Ethics of placebo-controlled trials in developing countries. *Bioethics, 12,* 307–311.

Rothman, K. J., & Michels, K. B. (1994). The continuing unethical use of placebo controls. *New Eng. J. Med, 331,* 394–398.

Studdert, D. M., & Brennan, T. A. (1998). Clinical trials in developing countries, scientific and ethical issues. *Medical Journal of Australia, 169,* 545–548.

Temple, R., & Ellenberg, S. E. (2000). Placebo-controlled trials and active-control trials in the evaluation of new treatments: ethical and scientific issues. *Annals of Internal Medicine, 133,* 455–463.

Walsh, B. Timothy, Seidman, Stuart, Sysko, Robyn, Gould, Madelyn (2002). Placebo response in studies of major depression. *Journal of American Medicine, 287*(14), 1840–1847.

Williams, P. (1996). Ethical principles in federal regulations: The case of children and research risks. *Journal of Medicine and Philosophy, 21*(2), 169–186.

World Medical Association. (2000). Declaration of Helsinki: Ethical principles for medical research involving human subjects. Retrieved 7/20/04 from www.wma.net/e/policy/b3.htm

World Medical Association. (2001) Note of Clarification. Retrieved 7/20/04 from www.wma.net/e/policy/b3.htm

17

When Eligibility Criteria Clash With Personal Treatment Choice: A Dilemma of Clinical Research

Benjamin Wilfond and Fabio Candotti

CASE DESCRIPTION

Joshua is a 15 year old with a congenital immune disorder that has resulted in moderate chronic lung disease (Lung function [FEV_1] is 50% predicted) and poor growth (height < third percentile). His lung function and growth have been stable for the last 4 years, and he has not had significant life-threatening infections. His current treatments include daily oral antibiotics and monthly injections of intravenous immune globulin (IVIG). Recently the cause of his immune disorder has been identified as adenosine deaminase deficiency (ADA), a form of severe combined immune deficiency (SCID; Hershfield & Mitchell, 2001). SCID is usually diagnosed shortly after birth and generally results in high susceptibility to recurrent and life-threatening infections. Transplantation of allogeneic hematopoietic stem cells (HSCT) can be curative for ADA-SCID and is highly successful when HLA-identical sibling donors are available. Unfortunately, most patients do not have a matched sibling donor, and the results of HSCT from haplo-identical parental donors is much less satisfactory (Antoine et al., 2003). An alternative form treatment for patients lacking an HLA-identical donor is represented by enzyme replacement with polyethylene-glycolated adenosine deaminase (PEG-ADA), given as a weekly intramuscular (IM) injection.

Joshua does not have siblings and his family declined a mismatched HSCT that was offered to them before the diagnosis of ADA deficiency was made. His primary immunologist now recommends that Joshua begin PEG-ADA. Joshua refuses because he is concerned about the pain of weekly IM injections. He is satisfied that his current treatment plan has kept him stable. His parents are supportive of his decision. They have learned that PEG-ADA will not work in 20% of the cases and that in the remaining cases it will provide protective, although not normal, immunity. They feel Joshua's current clinical management is also providing protective treatment and that there are no guarantees that PEG-ADA will improve his conditions. The only sure thing, they state, is that PEG-ADA treatment will cause additional pain. The parents are generally skeptical of physicians and perceive that others in the community are not sensitive to the needs of living with a chronic disease. They have not acted upon clinical recommendations for a feeding gastrostomy tube to improve his growth or to use daily airway clearance exercises to manage his lung disease. They have also had frustrating experiences with insurance companies, social service agencies, and law enforcement.

The family finds out about a phase I gene transfer research (GTR) study at the National Institutes of Health (NIH) that involves ex vivo gene transfer in hematopoietic stem cells for patients who are currently receiving PEG-ADA. The reason for this "additive" study design is that PEG-ADA is considered conventional therapy for all patients who do not undergo HSCT. The family wants to enroll Joshua but does not want him to receive PEG-ADA because they believe that GTR offers the best clinical alternative to their current supportive approach. The investigators are sympathetic to the family's request on scientific grounds, because of indirect evidence from previous human studies that GTR is more likely to work in patients who are not taking PEG-ADA (Aiuti et al., 2002; Kohn et al., 1998). Thus, this patient offers them a rare opportunity to explore a scientific hypothesis that was outside the boundaries of the initial research design. The investigators obtain an ethics consult and consider their options. The ethics consultant identifies three potential courses of action. First, the investigators could tell the family that the current research protocol requires that the subject also be taking PEG-ADA, and that Joshua could be enrolled *only* if he began PEG-ADA therapy. Second, the investigators could request that the institutional review board (IRB) grant a special one-time exception to the protocol to allow Joshua to enroll. Finally, they could amend the current research protocol to include subjects who are not taking PEG-ADA.

ETHICAL ANALYSIS AND DISCUSSION

How should investigators respond to a family's request to forgo conventional interventions of likely but potentially limited efficacy in favor of research that holds out an unlikely but possible prospect of direct benefit? As a clinical issue, there would be little controversy that Joshua's wish to forgo PEG-ADA should be respected, even if like the decision to forgo the feeding tube or airway clearance, this decision is not in his medical interest. However, it is much less clear whether it is appropriate for the investigator or the IRB to agree to allow Joshua to participate in the research. The goals of research and the obligations of researcher, while sometimes overlapping with clinical care, are distinct (Miller & Rosenstein, 2003). Analysis of the ethical questions in this case turns on that distinction.

This chapter focuses on the particular dimensions of the research nature of the intervention. However, it is important to point out that even though this phase I study offered an unlikely prospect of direct benefit to the subject, the family viewed the GTR as a clinical intervention that offered the best prospect of benefit for their child. Therefore, we will begin by asking two standard clinical ethics questions: (1) What is in Joshua's best interest? (2) Should Joshua's preferences be respected? We will then consider how the benefits of this study should be considered within the regulatory framework of 45 CRF 46 Subpart D.

Interests

First we should consider whether taking PEG-ADA is in Joshua's interest. In classic ADA deficiency, PEG-ADA results in protective although not normal cellular immune function in 80% of patients. However, the drug is derived from cows and some patients develop an immune response to PEG-ADA. This immune response diminishes the drug's efficacy in such patients and may also cause adverse effects requiring that the drug be discontinued (Hershfield & Mitchell, 2001).

It is difficult to predict how beneficial PEG-ADA will be for Joshua. He has had a less severe clinical course than usual, so it is possible that PEG-ADA will provide little additional benefit to his immune function. Further, because of the milder immunodeficiency, there is a higher likelihood of developing an immune response to PEG-ADA. His most significant clinical manifestations, moderate lung disease and poor growth, are not reversible with PEG-ADA. While forgoing PEG-ADA could expose Joshua to some risk of life threatening infection, he has a 15-year history without serious infection, suggesting that this risk is not high. In summary, while taking PEG-ADA may be in Joshua's interest, it is far from clear that forgoing this treatment will be associated with significant harm.

Second, we should consider if GTR is in his interest. The first clinical trial of GTR was conducted at the NIH in 1990 on a subject with ADA deficiency. There have been more than 500 clinical trials of GTR for a broad range of conditions. Among these trials, there has been very limited evidence of efficacy and some notable adverse events, some of which were lethal. However, some of the most promising results have been in ADA deficiency and other forms of SCID. There have been 17 subjects with SCID (including four with ADA deficiency) who have had significant long-term clinical improvements as a result of GTR

(Aiuti et al., 2002; Cavazzana-Calvo et al., 2000; Hacein-Bey-Abina et al., 2002). However, with greater efficacy, more adverse effects have also occurred, including a leukemia-like complication in two subjects (Hacein-Bey-Abina et al., 2003). It is difficult to predict the likelihood of success of GTR in Joshua, and the historical odds are not favorable, although most recent results seem to indicate that GTR may have progressed to a level where there is a reasonable possibility of clinical benefit for ADA-SCID. On one hand, he may be more likely to benefit from GTR than other subjects in this trial because he is not on PEG-ADA. However, it may be less likely to be successful because of his relatively old age, which may translate as ineffective thymopoiesis. While successful GTR would improve his immune function and may reduce his need for IVIG, it is not likely to have a significant impact on his lung disease and it is not clear that it will improve his nutritional status.

PEG-ADA and GTR each have potential for benefit and potential to harm Joshua in comparison to his current clinical care. For this reason, consideration of his interests alone does not point in a particular direction in a compelling fashion. Because Joshua and his family clearly prefer GTR, we next turn to the question of whether these preferences should be respected.

Preferences

Although Joshua is not an adult, the wishes of adolescents with decision-making capacity should be respected unless these preferences are profoundly dangerous. In addition to acknowledging their developing decision-making capacity, this respect is also based on the practicality that it is often difficult to "compel" adolescents. Second, even if Joshua's decision is not the most prudent choice, it may not be completely unreasonable. Finally, by fostering a relationship between the researchers and the family, Joshua may be more willing to consider PEG-ADA at a future date.

However, there are other considerations suggesting that his wishes should not prevail. The primary reason is that he does not meet the eligibility criteria of the research protocol. The investigators' primary obligation is to conduct sound research; the provision of clinical care is a secondary obligation, albeit one that cannot be compromised in a way that harms subjects. In fact, modifying the protocol to include Joshua may reinforce Joshua and his family's view that that primary goal of the research is to help Joshua (Appelbaum, Roth, Lidz, Benson, & Winslade, 1987). Additionally, his current refusal of PEG-ADA therapy suggests that he may not be an ideally compliant research subject. He may require extraordinary amounts of staff time and may not be willing to follow-through on other recommendations. As a result, this may place Joshua at an increased clinical risk (i.e., he may refuse hospitalization for worsening infection) or may diminish the value of the research (i.e., he may refuse research related blood draws). Third, his reasons may not sound compelling (not wanting the pain of IM injections) and be perceived as adolescent manipulations. Finally, if Joshua has an adverse outcome from study participation, it might be very easy to retrospectively criticize the decision to enroll him. Given Joshua and his family's unsatisfactory experiences with health care providers, an adverse event could also result in litigation. In this sense, Joshua's enrollment in the study has the potential to place the entire research program at risk.

While the investigators may be concerned about enrolling Joshua for the reasons cited above, they may also desire his participation because it may offer a unique scientific opportunity to understand how the GTR would work in the absence of PEG-ADA. In order for Joshua to be included in the study, the IRB would have to approve his participation. This would require the investigators to propose either a one-time exception or an amendment to allow subsequent subjects to be enrolled without ADA therapy. In either case, the investigators and IRB must determine which category of research would pertain under the Additional Protections for Children in the Code of Federal Regulations (Subpart D).

Prospect of Direct Benefit

Section 46.405 of Subpart D pertains to research that offers a prospect of direct benefit to the subject. This protocol has been classified as a phase I study, where the scientific objective is generally to establish the safety and maximum tolerated dose of a new drug. However, in reality, phase I trials are a more heterogeneous group of studies (Agrawal & Emanuel 2003). At one end of the phase I spectrum are studies in otherwise healthy subjects given a single dose of an experimental agent that has never been used in humans. At the other end are studies involving subjects who have serious illness and limited effective treatment options, who are given approved drugs in new combinations, with goal of improving the outcome. While the lack of prospect of direct benefit is clear in the first case, the second case is analogous to innovative clinical practice. Thus, prospect of direct benefit cannot easily be evaluated on the basis of a study being categorized as phase I but is contingent on the particular details and context.

To determine if a study intervention offers a prospect of direct benefit, it is useful to distinguish between four dimensions of benefit: nature, likelihood, magnitude and duration (King 2000). The *nature* of benefit refers to the way the benefit is experienced by the subject. *Clinical benefits* are those that the subject subjectively experiences, such as less frequent infections or exacerbations, or a decreased need for other medicines such as IVIG. Other benefits are laboratory markers, and these may or may not be a result of subjective clinical benefits. An example of such *surrogate benefits* would be laboratory evidence of improved immune function. A surrogate marker should not be considered a direct benefit when deciding which section of the regulations apply, unless there is close correlation between the surrogate marker and a relevant clinical outcome.

The *likelihood* of clinical benefit from GTR is possible but remote. However, to determine if the likelihood is sufficient to be considered a reasonable "prospect," it should be compared to the likelihood of benefit from other clinical options. In this case, benefits from GTR and PEG-ADA are both highly speculative because there is very limited empirical data that would apply to this specific clinical situation.

The *magnitude* of benefit of GTR could range from partial to complete immune reconstitution, which is greater than the magnitude of benefit of PEG-ADA even in classic ADA deficiency. The duration of the GTR benefit has the potential to be greater than PEG-ADA in that it could be permanent. Not only might there be clinical improvement in response to infections, but Joshua may be able to discontinue other potentially toxic medications. In addition, GTR can provide a cure after one single treatment, while for PEG-ADA to be effective it will have to be administered life-long.

One challenge in assessing the various dimensions of benefit relates to the quality of evidence that is available. Similar to other fields of clinical experimentation, emerging data from GTR clinical trials are often discussed at scientific meetings before the data are published in peer-reviewed journals with consequent widespread public diffusion. Thus, it may be difficult for investigators and IRBs to make such judgments with confidence.

In fact, one of the unresolved issues in evaluating the ethics of pediatric research is deciding when there is a sufficient likelihood and magnitude of benefit that an early phase study should to be considered under section 45 CFR 46.405. Because there is spectrum of research that is labeled "phase I," from some research that has no possibility of benefit to some research that offers the best chance of benefit, there are some studies in the middle of this spectrum where the prospect of direct benefit is quite ambiguous, and there may be disagreement about which regulatory section applies.

If such studies are not considered under 45 CFR 46.405, but instead under 45 CFR 46.406 (no prospect of benefit), then the primary requirement is that the study not pose a risk that is greater than a "minor" increase over minimal risk. While this criteria may be no less ambiguous (Shah, Whittle, Wilfond, Gensler, & Wendler, 2004) than "prospect of direct benefit," using this category may allow IRBs for IRBs and investigators to be clearer about the limited expectations of direct benefit in both the justification for the research and in communication with the subjects. This, in turn, may minimize any therapeutic misestimation of the benefits of research (Horng & Grady 2003). However, if the risks of such research include the potential for serious adverse effects, as may be foreseeable in GTR, or experienced occasionally, as in oncology research, it may not be reasonable to consider such risks as only a "minor increase over minimal risk." The issue of what counts as sufficient benefit to be considered a "prospect of direct benefit" and how much risk is more than a minor increase have not been resolved in a compelling fashion.

In this case, the authors believe that potential benefits are sufficient (based on the experience of the four previous ADA patients) to consider the intervention as offering a prospect of direct benefit. However, it is necessary to consider the two additional requirements that must be satisfied before an intervention can be approved within the category of "prospect of direct benefit" in subpart D. First, the potential benefits must be justified by the risks. Second, the risk:benefit ratio must be as favorable as the alternatives.

Are the Potential Benefits of GTR Justified by the Risks?

The main benefit of GTR is the potentially permanent improvement in immune function. The main risk of GTR *alone* is to forgo a conventional treatment of likely but potentially small magnitude of benefit. In this case, the prospective subject has already decided to forgo this conventional treatment, so this risk may be less relevant. Regardless, risk:benefit judgments are subjective and it is difficult to articulate *absolute* standards for such judgments. However, the second requirement of the regulations, that the risk:benefit ratio be as favorable as the alternatives, is a *relative* standard, and it is more feasible to make such relative comparisons.

Favorable Alternatives

In order to make such relative comparisons, it is necessary to determine what interventions should be considered as the baseline for the comparison. To address this question, Table 17.1 shows that the four possible interventions for comparison include the current clinical management (supportive care, S), a *conventional* approach, PEG-ADA (P), and two *experimental* interventions, GTR alone (G) and GTR in the presence of PEG-ADA (GP). To determine if one of the experimental interventions has a favorable risk:benefit ratio, it is necessary to select the appropriate comparison.

TABLE 17.1 Potential Comparisons for Determining If There Is Favorable Risk-Benefit Ratio for a Study Intervention

	Current study	Proposed study
Experimental intervention	GP (GTR/PEG-ADA)	G (GTR)
Nonexperimental care	P (PEG-ADA)	S (Supportive care)

The Original Trial Design

In the original trial design, all subjects would receive GP. The comparison that was used to demonstrate that this trial had a favorable risk:benefit ratio was between the experimental intervention, GP and a conventional approach, P. This initial trial design was chosen precisely because GP offered what was considered a favorable risk:benefit ratio for patients compared to P. The potential benefits to both groups are similar and potentially greater for the GP. There were risks from the GTR itself. As an "add-on" trial, there are no risks related to forgoing "conventional treatment." An alternative experimental intervention arm of GTR alone was not considered because at the time of protocol development the available scientific information suggested this option not to be appropriate because it would involve the risks of forgoing PEG-ADA in a setting where this was the conventional treatment for life threatening immune deficiency.

The Family's Request

The family's request to change the experimental intervention from GP to G alone suggests that the assessment of favorability be based on the comparison between the two experimental interventions, G and GP. The risks of GTR itself are not relevant since both arms include GTR. Thus, the balance is between any additional benefits of GTR alone with any risks of no PEG-ADA.

In this particular situation, both the benefits and risks are uncertain in terms of likelihood and magnitude. The potential for benefits of G compared to GP may be greater. Further, while the risks of G (from forgoing PEG-ADA), compared to GP, are greater in general, the relative increase of the risks with GTR alone may be less in Joshua than it is in infants. The duration of risk from forgoing PEG-ADA is limited, since the trial will only last for 2 years and Joshua could decide to begin PEG-ADA at a later time. Thus, the risk:benefit ratio of G may be as favorable as GP.

However, perhaps this is not the appropriate comparison because Joshua is not willing to take PEG-ADA. From the perspective of Joshua and his family who claim that they would never even consider PEG-ADA, the comparison should be between the supportive care approach, S, and an experimental approach, G. The benefit of G is the potential to be able to forgo S at a later time. There are the additional risks of S from infection by forgoing PEG-ADA, but these risks present regardless if Joshua were to enroll in the modified study. Thus, there does appear to be a favorable risk:benefit of G compared to S. However, Joshua's decision to not take PEG-ADA could possibly be influenced by the possible availability of GTR. Suppose the investigators were firm that GTR alone was not an option? Might Joshua and his family then decide to consider PEG-ADA?

Resolution

Should the family be told that Joshua is not eligible for the study unless he agrees to take PEG-ADA? Should the study be modified to allow Joshua to enroll without taking PEG-ADA, either as a special exception or as general amendment for this class of individuals? Based on the prior analysis, both scientific issues and ethical issues do not clearly point in one direction or the other. In fact, we are sympathetic to enrolling Joshua in the study without being on PEG-ADA, because of respect of the family's wishes and the possible scientific value. Conversely, were Joshua and his family to agree to begin PEG-ADA, this would be welcome news as it might minimize risk for Joshua and for the study.

A central concern is whether the family's decision to forgo PEG-ADA is somehow related to the availability of the GTR study. In other words, if there was no question that Joshua will not take PEG-ADA, regardless, then the GTR study would not pose additional risks compared to those currently in the study. One way to establish this would be to consider a two-phase process. First would be to clearly communicate (verbally and in writing) that PEG-ADA is the clinically recommended therapy and Joshua is not currently eligible for the study unless he is on PEG-ADA. If the family responds to such definitive statements and they were to change their mind at this point to begin PEG-ADA, the problem of whether it is acceptable to enroll Joshua would be resolved. Even if they did not change their mind, it would more clearly address the question that their decision was not related to the study and thus offering the study to Joshua without PEG-ADA would not incur the "risk" of forgoing PEG-ADA, since that decision had been made independently.

However, the problem with this approach is that it is disingenuous. It requires misleading the family about the possibilities in order to see how they respond. This is not the way to build a trusting relationship. Alternatively, the investigators could affirm the importance of PEG-ADA and explain that in order for Joshua to enroll without PEG-ADA, it would require the approval of the IRB and FDA, which might take months and is not necessarily guaranteed.

The investigators and IRB would still be faced with the decision about whether to approve Joshua's enrolling without being on PEG-ADA. One way to approach this issue is to consider the general case of people who are not taking PEG-ADA. As this case demonstrates, some ADA deficient patients do not take PEG-ADA because of personal preferences, financial considerations or intolerable side effects. There is also scientific value in conducting GTR research on this population. The risks of GTR in this population do not appear to be greater than other populations. Thus, an amendment to include such individuals could be approved under 46.405 because the risk:benefit ratio was as favorable. Developing and justifying an amendment that defines the scientific objectives, risks, and benefits of enrolling children not on PEG-ADA is preferable than just making a special exception for Joshua for several reasons. First, it allows for a more general dispassionate evaluation of the scientific and ethical issues. Second, it emphasizes that the ethical issues are the concerns about enrollment of children in research, rather than the clinical concerns of interests and preferences.

CONCLUSION

This case illustrates several important issues related to risk:benefit assessments in pediatric research ethics. First is the issue of whether phase I studies can be evaluated under 45 CFR 46.405 which requires that an intervention offer a "prospect" of direct benefit. This is a contingent issue that will depend on the details of the study. This may be appropriate when there is sufficient clinical data to suggest that there is a reasonable chance of efficacy. Further, what is a "reasonable" chance may depend of the likelihood of standard interventions being efficacious. Finally, this may be more appropriate when the intervention is offered as an "add on" to conventional treatments. However, this may not be appropriate when there is very limited applicable clinical data, or when the intervention is not provided in a dose, duration, or manner that makes clinical efficacy a plausible possibility.

Second is the issue of accounting for subject and family preferences. Benefit to subjects is not the primary objective of research and while respecting preferences is central in the clinical setting, this is not the case in the research context. It is important to keep clear that the main purpose of the study is to determine if the GTR approach is safe and effective. While a desire to respect the preferences of the subjects adds to the investigators motivations, the enrollment of subjects like Joshua offers clear scientific opportunities.

To emphasize that any change in the protocol is primarily motivated (and justified) by scientific concerns, it is important to make a general modification of the protocol to allow some subjects who are not on PEG-ADA to be enrolled. This allows the decision to be made based on scientific considerations, as well as based on determining that the modification does not expose subjects to an unfavorable risk:benefit ratio. This also suggests that although the approach to such dilemmas can be informed by the particulars of a case, including the families preferences, the justification should be robust enough to be generalizable for all similar subjects. In fact, if such a modification could not be justified, it would not be appropriate to allow the family to enroll as a "compassionate-use exception."

Finally, this case illustrates how a particular request can result in the investigators reexamining the ethical basis for the original study design. But what is important is that resolution of the request is not based solely on clinical ethics considerations such as interests and preferences, but with research ethics considerations such as favorable risk:benefit assessment (Emanuel, Wendler, & Grady 2000). This may seem like a subtle difference, but it emphasizes that there may be times when these perspectives may diverge, and that the IRB needs to be engaged in the deliberations. Keeping these justifications distinct may help the investigators and the IRB be clear about their primary scientific objective, while at the same time trying to protect subjects from harm or exploitation.

Questions for Discussion

1. Does a decision to participate in the research fit within the range of decisions that are consistent with Joshua's best interests? Who should get to determine the boundaries of that range in this case? What do you think the boundaries should be?

2. The authors argue as follows: Joshua's current refusal of PEG-ADA therapy suggests that he may not be an ideally compliant research subject. Consequently, he may require extraordinary amounts of staff time and may not be willing to follow through on other recommendations. This may place Joshua at an increased clinical risk and/or may diminish the value of the research. Do you think these arguments justify excluding Joshua from the study? What is the significant ethical difference between the two arguments?

3. Do you find the argument for allowing Joshua's participation because it may offer a unique scientific opportunity to understand how the GTR would work in the absence of PEG-ADA persuasive?

4. According to this chapter, in order for Joshua to participate in the study, special IRB approval is required. The investigators will have to propose either a special exception or an amendment to allow subsequent subjects to be enrolled without ADA therapy. Which of the two options would be do you find more appropriate?

5. Are you comfortable with the ambiguity surrounding the prospect of direct benefit for some phase I studies, or would you favor a more rigorous definition that might exclude any potentially therapeutic study from the phase I category?

6. Do you agree with the comparative analysis of the four treatment alternatives (G, P, GP, S) presented in this chapter and with the conclusion regarding the most favorable alternative in this case? What are the strengths and weaknesses of this analytic approach?

7. Do you favor the "two-phase process" suggested by the authors to address the concern that the family's decision to forgo PEG-ADA is somehow related to the availability of the GTR study?

8. The authors discuss the question whether phase I studies can be evaluated under 45 CFR 46.405, which requires that an intervention offers a "prospect" of direct benefit. Do you agree with their analysis of risk:benefit ratio? What about their final conclusion with regard to Joshua's case?

9. According to the authors, why is the distinction between clinical ethics considerations and research ethics considerations so significant? What are the ethical, legal, and practical implications of the distinction in Joshua's case?

___

References

Agrawal, M., & Emanuel, E. J. (2003). Ethics of phase 1 oncology studies: Reexamining the arguments and data. *Journal of the American Medical Association, 290*(8), 1075–1082.

Aiuti, A., Slavin, S., Aker, M., et al. (2002). Correction of ADA-SCID by stem cell gene therapy combined with nonmyeloablative conditioning. *Science, 296(5577)*, 2410–2413.

Aiuti, A., Vai, S., Mortellaro, A., et al. (2002). Immune reconstitution in ADA-SCID after PBL gene therapy and discontinuation of enzyme replacement. *Nat Med., 8*(5), 423–425.

Antoine, C., Muller, S., Cant, A., et al. (2003). Long-term survival and transplantation of haemopoietic stem cells for immunodeficiencies: Report of the European experience 1968–99. *Lancet, 361*(9357), 553–560.

Appelbaum, P., Roth, L., Lidz, C., Benson, P., & Winslade, W. (1987). False hopes and best data: Consent to research and the therapeutic misconception. *Hastings Center Report, 17*(2), 20–24.

Cavazzana-Calvo, M., Hacein-Bey, S., de Saint Basile, G., et al. (2000). Gene therapy of human severe combined immunodeficiency (SCID)-X1 disease. *Science, 288*(5466), 669–672.

Emanuel, E. J., Wendler, D., & Grady, C. (2000). What makes clinical research ethical? *Journal of the American Medical Association, 283*(20), 2701–2711.

Hacein-Bey-Abina, S., Le Deist, F., Carlier, F., et al. (2002). Sustained correction of X-linked severe combined immunodeficiency by ex vivo gene therapy. *New England Journal of Medicine, 346*(16), 1185–1193.

Hacein-Bey-Abina, S., Von Kalle, C., Schmid, M., et al. (2003). LMO2-associated clonal T cell proliferation in two patients after gene therapy for SCID-X1. *Science, 302*(5644), 415–419.

Hershfield, M. S., & Mitchell, B. S. (2001). Immunodeficiency diseases caused by adenosine de- aminase deficiency and purine nucleoside phosphorylase deficiency. In C. R. Scriver, A. L. Beaudet, W. S. Sly, & D. Valle (Eds.), *The metabolic and molecular bases of inherited disease* (pp.). New York: McGraw-Hill.

Horng, S., & Grady, C. (2003). Misunderstanding in clinical research: Distinguishing therapeutic misconception, therapeutic misestimation, and therapeutic optimism. *IRB, 25*(1), 11–16.

King, N. M. (2000). Defining and describing benefit appropriately in clinical trials. *J Law Med Ethics, 28*(4), 332–343.

Kohn, D. B., Hershfield, M. S., Carbonaro, D., et al. (1998). T lymphocytes with a normal ADA gene accumulate after transplantation of transduced autologous umbilical cord blood CD34+ cells in ADA-deficient SCID neonates. *Nat Med., 4*(7), 775–780.

Miller, F. G., & Rosenstein D. L. (2003). The therapeutic orientation to clinical trials. *New England Journal of Medicine, 348*(14), 1383–1386.

Shah, S., Whittle, A., Wilfond, B., Gensler, G., & Wendler, D. (2004). How do institutional review boards apply the federal risk and benefit standards for pediatric research? *Journal of the American Medical Association, 291,* 476–482.

18

Involving Children With Life-Shortening Illnesses in Decisions About Participation in Clinical Research: A Proposal for Shuttle Diplomacy and Negotiation

Myra Bluebond-Langner, Amy DeCicco, and Jean Belasco

CASE DESCRIPTION

Just a few a months shy of his 13th birthday, Jeremy Foster, a mentally gifted, social, and artistically talented boy, was diagnosed with an anaplastic astrocytoma, a malignant brain tumor (high-grade glioma).[1] Due to its location the surgeons were able to remove only a portion of the tumor. Even when fully resected, the prognosis for this tumor type is poor. With only a partial resection of his tumor, Jeremy had only a 20% chance of surviving five years.

After surgery, his treatment options were radiation alone or radiation with chemotherapy. There were no open clinical trials at the time. Jeremy received radiation for approximately 40 days, followed by PCV therapy—a combination of three chemotherapy agents—procarbazine, vincristine (Oncovin), and lomustine (CCNU) used for high-grade gliomas.[2] Eleven months later, chemotherapy was stopped due to persistent thrombocytopenia.[3] The plan was to continue with regular blood tests, monthly examinations in the clinic, and MRI scans every 3 months.

Three months later, 14 months after diagnosis, Jeremy, now almost 14 years old, had clearly moved into puberty. There was fuzz on his lips and his voice cracked. Despite improvements made with intensive physical, occupational, and speech therapy, permanent brain damage persisted. Doctors noted during his regularly scheduled monthly visits that Jeremy still had "significant expressive and receptive aphasias"[4] such as word finding and reading impairment, as well as a myriad of neurologically derived physical problems such as a "right-sided hemiparesis,[5] right-sided muscle atrophy, a right steppage gait[6] and a facial droop." He wore a brace on his leg and took Risperdal, which controlled tumor-induced behavior problems such as poor impulse control. In addition to attending school regularly he also continued regular sessions of physical, speech, and occupational therapy.

As planned, Jeremy went from the oncology clinic to the radiology department for an MRI scan. The MRI revealed that the tumor had recurred in the tumor bed and had progressed into the temporal lobes. At recurrence, the prognosis for this type of tumor is very poor. The Fosters were contacted and asked to come to the hospital for a family meeting.[7] The nurse practitioner who called them suggested that the Fosters not bring Jeremy with them for the meeting.

The next day, Jeremy's parents crammed into the small windowless conference room in the out patient clinic along with Jeremy's neuro-oncologist, Dr. Sumner, and the social worker, Alex Rankin.[8] Dr. Sumner began the meeting by telling the Fosters that Jeremy's tumor had "come back." She gave a detailed medical description of the tumor progression. Mr. Foster immediately asked, "So what do we do?" Mrs. Foster asked, "Is it terminal?" Variations of these two questions and Dr. Sumner's response, along with questions of what to tell Jeremy, of what his life would be like, and of the possibility of miracles, would be woven through the hour-long discussion of the options that were available for care and treatment.

After explaining to the parents that further surgery or radiation were not possible, Dr. Sumner then presented and described three cancer-directed options: a currently available phase I clinical trial of a new treatment SU5416,[9] a soon to be available phase I/II clinical trial of a newer drug STI571,[10] and a slightly older medication, temozolomide.[11] In terms of non-cancer-directed therapy options, Dr. Sumner said, "Some families don't want any medicine and that's not giving up."[12] By medications Dr. Sumner meant, and Mr. and Mrs. Foster understood, that she was referring to clinical trials or other cancer-directed therapies. She did not mean that there would not be medications for pain and symptom control. On the contrary, she was quite emphatic and direct in response to Mr. Foster's questions about pain management. "There are many, many, many things we can do to prevent pain. There are many things we can use to keep someone incredibly comfortable. So I don't expect him to suffer pain at all. Because we will have plenty of things we can use to prevent that. And we will stay committed to that. The thing that we have the least ability to prevent is [phrase not completed], save his life."

The issue of the possibility of cure and long-term survival were handled somewhat differently than the issue of pain management. For example, after discussion of the various cancer and non-cancer-directed therapies and Dr. Sumner's suggestion that they go home and think about them, Mrs. Foster said, "I just feel like, okay, we have this information. It's our decision. It's confusing to me."

Dr. Sumner replied, "Maybe because . . . I think that you've been living in, we all have, in the hope that he is going to survive this. And as soon as, in talking this through, that it's clear that his tumor is bad and you are faced with it; anybody, I couldn't even imagine, you ask questions that are at the heart of the matter: 'Is he going to die?,' 'Is this a terminal cancer?' you want to ask. You really have cut to the chase. And now that you have those answers, options begin to swirl around and not make any sense. And I think that, I think uh, you could just need more time, to just sort of let it settle a little bit. Because I think you, you do get a mixed answer. On the one hand, you get an answer that the cancer is incurable, medically incurable, that he will die short of a miracle, but in the same breath, there's well, here are other treatments you can do. And that's somewhat contradictory. And I think that, as your husband said, the treatments are about life. Well, they are. And that would be the only reason we would offer them, not in terms of trying to hurt him, but to gain life, good life and a longer life. Then again, but the issue of quality of life is the most important thing. Then I think that once you look through the options, focusing on the quality as well as a possible link, it may become more clear as to what you are to think. Maybe needing more time and more talking."

"Well," Mrs. Foster began, "have you seen the situation such as this where there has, just say in a situation very similar to Jeremy's, this kind of anaplastic astrocytoma. Have you seen another case where kids at least got more years and quality years?"

"You mean quality of time?" Dr. Sumner asked.

"Time—like months?" Mrs. Foster clarified.

"Or a couple of years, even?" Dr. Sumner asked, probing. "I think that I, I think that for most parents, what we all want is longer, long years."

"Well I never wanted long, long. I wanted . . ." said Mrs. Foster starting to cry.

"Even getting into adulthood," said Dr. Sumner finishing her sentence.

"I wanted that. I wanted him to experience (*crying*) a girlfriend, experience sex, experience driving a car. I didn't necessarily want him to live to be 30, 40. I want him to experience that. I'm so, you know, it's something we have to go home and talk about. But if you're talking about maybe just buying more months?" Mrs. Foster voice rose.

"Or maybe longer?" Dr. Sumner said, a bit of a question still in her voice. "But you know, I think it would be wrong to say that these medicines will now have a track record that could give him 10 plus years. Medically speaking that's not going to happen. That doesn't mean you couldn't gain months, a couple years. And then again, I think the chances of even a couple of years are really slim. Can that happen? Yes. Does it rarely happen? Rarely."

"Then can you say where a tumor, where you did another MRI, the tumor was just gone?" Mrs. Foster asked.

Dr. Sumner answered, "I've seen some kids that I have no idea why . . . not with this particular tumor . . . because I think that I've seen two different kinds of miracles. The miracles we always want, which are for a cancer that is there to go away. And I've seen that. What it means is I don't know. But when you ask if I've seen miracles? Yes. Do I see that often? No. The more common miracle is that we can survive."

"So this is really, his particular tumor location, that's a pretty, pretty rotten deal."

Dr. Sumner nodded and said nothing.

Mrs. Foster wondered out loud what they should tell Jeremy. Mr. Foster felt that there was no need to tell him anything "We don't have to say anything."

"But we have to tell him something," Mrs. Foster replied. "When he knows what he'll have to be getting, what else he'll be getting."

"We are not telling him anything. I don't want him told." Mr. Foster rejoined.

"What do you mean? Ever?" Mrs. Foster asked.

"Not right now."

"That's what I'm talking about. Not right now. But we don't have a lot of time. We have got to make some decisions."

"So let him take it." Mr. Foster stated.

The decision of what to tell Jeremy was part of the discussion of how to make the decision of which course(s) of care and treatment to pursue and of the other input that they would seek. Mrs. Foster wanted to know if then "should they discuss all of this with Jeremy?"

Mr. Foster said flatly, "No."

Mrs. Foster turned to Mr. Foster, "But he's a smart kid."

"Well, I don't think you have to have a discussion about it," Mr. Foster replied.

Eleven days later, Jeremy's parents came to clinic with Jeremy for "clearance to get his line placed."[13] As soon as Dr. Sumner came into the examining room, before she took her usual seat at the desk, Mrs. Foster told Dr. Sumner that, "We talked to Jeremy and told him that he has a little spot of something on his MRI, and that he would need to go back on medicine, that he needs a little more treatment."

Dr. Sumner swiveled her chair around so that she was facing Jeremy. He was in his usual place—perched on the examining table facing her desk, his legs dangling below him.

"Jeremy, do you have any questions about that?" Dr. Sumner asked.

Jeremy had lots of questions and managed to get them all out despite his difficulties with speech and word finding. He started by asking, "What will the line be like?" Dr. Sumner explained the type of line they would use, where it could placed—arm or chest—the choice was his, the procedure for inserting the line, and that with a port he wouldn't "need to be stuck."

"I hate IVs," he said as she closed her remarks with the advantage of the port being "not needing to be stuck each time."

Dr. Sumner waited as Jeremy formed the next question, "What does a spot mean?"

Putting her hands on Jeremy's knees, she looked right at him and began, "It means your tumor's back. The tumor that you had when I first met you has grown back, is growing back."

"How did you know I had cancer?" Jeremy asked.

Mrs. Foster moved forward in her seat about to speak as Dr. Sumner went on, "Do you mean the cancer that's growing back now?"

"When it started," Jeremy clarified.

Mrs. Foster started to answer, "Well your right side was weak."

"Your Mom is right, Jeremy," Dr. Sumner said before Mrs. Foster could say much more. "And remember when I first met you?"

Jeremy nodded.

Dr. Sumner continued, not taking her eyes off Jeremy. "You are a very, very, very bright young man. We found out you had cancer because of the weakness on your right side, but also you were having some trouble at school."

Jeremy's eyes lit up. He laughed and turned to his parents seated by the door, "And you said I was bad."

Everyone laughed and Dr. Sumner went on, "Jeremy, I'm glad you raised this question. It's a really good question. I really need you to know that it was your cancer. It was not your fault. It's because of where your tumor is. You still are very, very, very smart and you are who you are, but you know you've had to work real hard, really hard in terms of getting some of the things back.

"You're a 14-year-old boy now," Dr. Sumner affirmed. "A lot of 14-year-old boys lose their tempers sometimes and are a little moody, and that can be normal. But if you're having trouble, you've worked really hard to get back what you've gotten back, but if you find that you are having trouble, or that your moods are really bothering you because they're not within normal, that's not your fault. It's your cancer.

"Jeremy you know yourself better than anybody, and you know if it's in the range of what you feel all right with, it's OK. But if you feel like you're losing your temper and this is not you, it's because of your cancer; then you need to let us know because then we can adjust your medicines so we can make it better."

Jeremy nodded.

Dr. Sumner then started to examine Jeremy. During the examination, Mrs.

Foster asked, "If this treatment doesn't work, does this prevent us from getting other treatments?"

Before Dr. Sumner could answer, Jeremy asked, "Other medicines?"

Later that day when Bluebond-Langner questioned Dr. Sumner about what had occurred during the clinic visit, Dr. Sumner commented that when Jeremy asked the question, "Other medicines?" she had wondered if his parents had told him about temozolomide, or only about SU5416 that was available through clinical trials.[14] She said that she had assumed the latter.

In fact, Mrs. Foster had told Jeremy only about the SU5416. In addition, she had explained it as a "chemotherapy treatment," not as a trial. Mrs. Foster also said to Bluebond-Langner after the examination, "When you interview Jeremy just say chemotherapy treatment because that's what it is—chemotherapy. He's a kid, you know. You know they're young. You know they're like [they would ask], 'A trial, what do you mean a trial?' So, we tell him it's just your treatment like before. I just wanted to give you a heads up."

Mrs. Foster continued unprompted, "He basically knows everything except that this is a clinical trial. But like I shared with you, we have a very strong faith and I believe, I've seen miracles with medicine with family members. So I know they do exist, so you know we keep a positive spin on it, that's what you have to do. And we felt like telling him it's a clinical trial, it's just so harsh."

When Bluebond-Langner asked Mrs. Foster about whether she had involved Jeremy in the decision about participating in the clinical trial, Mrs. Foster replied, "To be truthful, I didn't really involve him, um, cause I just feel at that age, I don't, I don't think totally he's not informed enough to make his own decision. Maybe if it is a teenager, 17, 18, I think you can involve them, but for a child, I think the parents do have to kind of make the decision what they feel is going to be best for their child.

"We did tell him that it's just a different type of chemo. We never did use the word clinical trial because we didn't want him to think of this as some experimental drug that may or may not prove helpful. He is only 13, almost 14 in 3 weeks. We just didn't feel that that's something he needed to know.

"I think they don't need to know everything. If they're a child of 16, 17, 18, well, maybe you can get a little more involved, but I, I think anyway these children, as I said before, have an insight about what is going on. And I think it's just, um, a spiritual ability that God gives children who are sick—to know if things are going to maybe not work out for them."

Mrs. Foster returned to her former theme, "Yes, I don't think you need to go into uh, a long involved process at that age, because they are still children and at that age they're still children. And, why give them something that's so heavy on them—a heavy burden to deal with. I just think let them enjoy their childhood, however long we don't know its going to be. So, we opted not to tell him that it was a clinical trial. We opted not to ask him if he wanted to even to participate. Because, again, at that point we did not know what other options we had. I mean Dr. Sumner did tell us an option, "You can just do nothing."

"You can just do nothing," she repeated. "And I guess, you know, we, we prayed about it and we felt, why do nothing when this might be a miracle in the making, this drug might show promise. I mean the drug now that is allowing AIDS patients to live longer, somebody had to experiment with that, you know."

Her views on what to tell Jeremy were not limited to what a researcher should say or what she and her husband should or shouldn't say, but also extended to what the medical staff should say in front of Jeremy. "I don't want him to hear anything that's really, um, how can I put it? Something that is a real negative, I would rather it be discussed with my husband and I first and we in turn explain it to him. That's, that's what I would prefer.

"Now if the child asks, I don't think you should ever lie, but there are ways you can tell the child that are, are, I guess, are effective for that age. You know, I mean, I think personally kids grow up too fast nowadays anyway and they, they don't need to know such heavy things, you don't lie but there's ways, you know."

Thinking about one of those heavy things and how to talk about them, Bluebond-Langner asked Mrs. Foster, "If Jeremy asked you, do you think I'm going to die? What would you tell him?"

"Well, I would say, 'Honey we're all going die, all of us, that's a sure fact, but the illness you have probably, um, this illness has shown that children, you know, do have a shorter life span, but only God knows when that would take place.' And I think to get caught up in saying 'Yes' we would be trying to play God, because we don't know. Only God knows. That's one sure thing. Only God knows when we're going to leave this planet. And uh, to get caught up in, you know, when; we don't know. I mean I could go before he goes. You know you can get into a car accident. You can have a heart attack. You know, you don't know so. . . .

"And we've already told him. He has asked that question. And we told him, that only God knows. And we said, 'We're about the positive. We're about living. We're not about discussing dying.' And we told him, 'You just enjoy each day, cause tomorrow is not promised to anyone.'

"He even said to Dr. Sumner one time [a few months after diagnosis, while receiving radiation therapy], he says, 'Well, if this tumor doesn't shrink, I'm going to die, right?' And Dr. Sumner said, 'No, that is not necessarily so, Jeremy. Why are you saying that?' And he's like 'Well, its okay.' So, he knows the severity of this, but he also knows that we as a family rely on our faith, that you know only God knows."[15]

Quiet, but for a moment Mrs. Foster continued, "Jeremy knows he has cancer. He knows some people die with cancer. But, we try to have him rely on faith, that you have people praying for you, you pray for yourself, um, and it doesn't necessarily have to mean that. But he knows.

"Sometimes we're watching the news and something comes on about cancer and he's like 'No Mom! Mom' [when Mrs. Foster would turn the T.V. off]. He wants to listen. Sometimes, I don't want him to hear, you know, cause he is still a kid. But, um, I think most of these kids here [at the hospital], they, they have, I really think when kids get sick that there's like an intuition that they develop, that I think sometime that they know more than the parents think they know, but they are trying to protect the parent."

In a voice that sounded as much as thinking out loud as a statement, Mrs. Foster continued, "Yea, I think they know. For Jeremy even to say to Dr. Sumner, 'Well if my tumor doesn't shrink that means I'm going to die, right?' I mean he said it so, like I was shocked. I never heard him say that before. And I ran over to hug him, I'm like, 'Oh Jeremy', I want to say, 'Don't think that.' And he's like 'Mom,' pushing me away, 'It's okay.' [It was] almost like he was saying, 'If that's what it comes down to, so be it.' "

"Sometimes," Mrs. Foster went on, "When I really want to probe Jeremy and talk to him, he doesn't really want to go really deep into things. I think, because he feels he wants to maybe protect. They want to protect the parents. I think they know."

After the physical examination, Dr. Sumner asked the Fosters if they had the consent form. They hadn't brought it with them. They had kept it "for their files, for the information." Dr. Sumner went and got another. She gave it to Mr. Foster. He signed and passed it to Mrs. Foster, who signed on the line "2nd parent or guardian" and passed it back to Dr. Sumner.

Dr. Sumner looked at Jeremy. "You can do whatever you want. This is up to you. You can sign that you consent to this. And if you don't want to it's fine because you know you're saying it's OK to be treated because you are 14 and you're fine with it."[16]

Jeremy looked surprised. He looked at his parents. He took the paper and signed below his parents, on the line "Signature of Person Obtaining Assent." There was no line for the child giving the assent to sign.

——

ETHICAL ANALYSIS AND DISCUSSION

Children are not allowed to consent, as an adult would, to participation in clinical research. In order to secure the participation of a child in a study a researcher must, among other things, follow his/her institution's institutional review board (IRB) directives about soliciting assent from children. Assent is defined as the child's "affirmative agreement" and is explicitly distinguished as more than "mere failure to object" to participate.

The IRB determines whether it is appropriate to seek assent from the children who could be involved in a particular protocol. The regulation (45 CFR 46.408, subpart D) states that in doing so the IRB "shall take into account the ages, maturity, and psychological state of the child involved." One applauds the federal regulators for erring on the side of flexibility rather than establishing their own implied view of child development. But, their statements still suggest that there *is* an appropriate age for participating in decisions about participation in a given study, even if that is to be determined locally.

In this chapter, we argue that criteria such as age and maturity are problematic in determining whether a child with a life-limiting illness can be a participant in decision making about enrollment in clinical research related to his or her disease. Further, we take the position that a quest focused on the acquisition of assent shows a lack of understanding of the social roles and relations of parents and children. A child may be perfectly capable of understanding the possible outcomes and side effects of participation in a trial and be capable cognitively of making a decision yet simply acquiesce to the course that the parents select (Bluebond-Langner, 1978, 1996; Bluebond-Langner, Belasco, & Goldman, 2003). The reasons for this are more complicated than an aversion, which many children have, for conflict with their parents. The reasons for a child's silence are related to the fact that children often will not show, in front of their parents, that they understand the gravity of their illness or know their prognosis to be death (Bluebond-Langner, 1978, 1996; Bluebond-Langner et al., 2003). Parents' interpretations of their own roles also affect the extent to which they will allow discussion of the options for care, treatment, and the prognosis with their child. Any regulations governing the decision-making process must recognize and deal with these facts (Bluebond-Langner, 1978, 1996; Bluebond-Langner et al., 2003). Not insignificantly, there is also an essential ethical dimension to the relation between parents and children that can not be overlooked. Regulations aimed at securing the ethical treatment of human subjects must respect and protect these relations in the process.

Children respect and act to preserve the social order of their families. Regulations that do not take these realities into account are not useful in facilitating children's involvement in decision making or in fostering whatever autonomy they possess. They may, in fact, if enthusiastically applied, do harm.

In the second part of this chapter, we propose a model for decision making that is based upon recent empirical studies of children and their families. The model provides a meaningful role for children by focusing on what we take to be the primary factor affecting their participation. That factor is not their abilities, but the social realities of family life, which constrain their participation. The model also allows a role for the physician, who seems to have been excluded from the process. The reality of an ethical relation of trust and reliance by the parents and the child upon the physician (whether investigator or not) needs to be brought back into the process of decision making. The proposed model also facilitates parents and children being as informed as possible about the issues that they must face.

Current Policy and Practice: Practical Realities We Need to Address

Children's Knowledge and Understanding

Federal regulations require that the IRB take into account "age, maturity and psychological state of the children involved." According to Leiken (1993), using developmental stages as the sole or major criteria is problematic because "there is considerable difference in the rate of development of each [developmental] trend in each individual. These variations make it difficult to speak of a certain age, or stage, at which minors have or do not have the cognitive capacity for decision making" (p. 2). And yes, while studies have shown that children do not understand all of the elements of the research study in which they are enrolled, studies also have shown that adults' understanding of the research study in which they are enrolled is poor.

Using age as criteria for involving children in decision making becomes even more problematic when the child has a life limiting illness that she/he has lived with for some time. In some situations living with an illness can lead to increased knowledge about the illness. For example, the nine year old in the first rounds of induction chemotherapy may know far less than a six year old who has relapsed and is being considered for a bone marrow transplant (Bluebond-Langner 1978). In other situations, as in the case of Jeremy Foster, the illness can lead to cognitive deficits, but not necessarily decreased understanding of his condition or the options available.

Even for those who are confident about the cognitive abilities of children in this context, there are a number of obstacles to assessing what a child really understands about his condition and situation. One such factor, which is also an issue with adults, is that children can hold different and even inconsistent views of their condition and prognosis. Children, irrespective of age, exhibit different views on different occasions, or in response to different events or questions. For example, Bluebond-Langner et al. (2003) found that while the children might acknowledge that other children with the same disease, treated in the same way have died, that didn't mean that they thought that they themselves would die. They believed or hoped that there were things that could be done and that they would get better. For example, while Lakshmi, age 5, and I were coloring in the playroom of the hospital where she was sometimes admitted, Lakshmi casually remarked, "Leah died. You don't know her. She had JMML just like me. I am going to get more cells."

"Oh," I said, and let it go at that as we continued to color. Lakshmi was not one to talk about her disease and would usually ignore you if you asked too many pointed or direct questions.

Lakshmi broke the silence, ". . . from my mom and be all better," and continues to color.

The children were not the only ones who separated what happened to them from what happened to others. Their parents did as well. For example, 2 days after Lakshmi died her mother said, "It wasn't until we were in the hospital this last time that it hit me that all the children we knew died. And I don't think it was until Lakshmi asked me if she was going to the same place as Leah. Then I realized that, all the time, all the treatments—we were just buying time. She wasn't going to be cured, but I didn't think that then [referring to up until the last hospitalization]. Maybe it was just too scary. Or maybe I just didn't want to think that she wouldn't be cured."

Children, like their parents, held on to the possibility of cure (through medical and/or divine intervention), or stabilization, or at the very least a reasonable amount of quality time. And these possibilities were there even in a phase I clinical trial—despite explanations of the trial to the contrary. The parents may have been told that it was a dose escalation trial, without direct medical benefit or curative intent, but saw it otherwise (Bluebond-Langner et al., 2003; Broome, Richards, & Hall, 2001; Deatrick, Angst, & Moore, 2002).

Mutual Pretense

Another obstacle to assessing or eliciting what children know or want is that they may not express it, or express it directly, because they and their parents are acting in a context of mutual pretense.[17] Mutual pretense, where each party in the interaction knows what is going to happen but does not acknowledge it openly to one another, becomes the dominant mode of interaction between parents and children with life-limiting illnesses, especially when cure is not likely. In mutual pretense, difficult issues are evaded, avoided, not met head on. When dangerous topics emerge, such as the unlikelihood of a given trial stopping or shrinking the tumor, care is taken so that neither party breaks down. For example, in response to the physician's remark, "The tumor is growing again," one child responded, looking over to his mother, "Yes, but it grew before, and the chemo helped, so maybe this new medicine [a phase I trial] will work."[18]

While children were aware of the prognosis, they did not always reveal that knowledge directly, especially to their parents (Bluebond-Langner, 1978, 1996;

Bluebond-Langner et al., 2003). Similarly, they did not reveal their awareness that the chances of recovery were minimal to none—in part because they knew how important the new therapy or treatment was to their parents. For example, another child in our study said of a phase I trial of STI-571, "I don't think the drug is working, but I want to try something, and my mom thinks it will work." The children protected their parents from their fears and doubts. They assumed their socially defined roles. They acted as if they would grow up and not die, at least not anytime soon.

Mutual pretense, then, undermines a decision-making process [or guidelines for the decision-making process] that naively assumes that parents, children, and physician can freely discuss protocols, the child's condition, and prognosis. We also found that the children and the parents felt constrained about asking particular questions, or raising or leading into issues such as these when they were all together (Bluebond-Langner et al., 2003).[19] In advance of the meeting, parents sometimes asked physicians to withhold certain kinds information about the child's condition or about the particular clinical trial when the family met.

Societal Roles and Responsibilities

The social roles of parents and children also need to be understood when proposing a role for children in decision making. Being a parent in the United States is of course multifaceted. Most relevant to the question at hand is that parents see their role as one of both nurturing and protecting (Bluebond-Langner, 1978, 1996; Bluebond-Langner et al., 2003). Parents of ill children feel that it is they who are ultimately responsible for the course of their child's life—even, one could say, more responsible than the children themselves (Bluebond-Langner et al., 2003). This means that to varying degrees parents feel that regardless of the competence or awareness of the ill child, the decision of what to do about the child's life belongs to them, not to the child (Bluebond-Langner et al., 2003). Parents' views of their roles can also lead, as in the case presented at the beginning of the chapter, to their limiting the child's access to information about the disease and its treatment. They do so to protect their child from "painful," "harsh," "discouraging" information. This is not to say that parents are insensitive to child's needs or desires or even that they think that children do not understand what is happening to them. As Jeremy's mother said, "Jeremy knows he has cancer, he knows that some people die with cancer. But, we try to have him rely on faith, that you have people praying for you, you pray for yourself, um, and it doesn't necessarily have to mean that. But he knows. . . . I just don't want him to hear anything negative."

In practice, we found that the child was not always present when the physician first told the parents the news, or when the options for further care and treatment were first discussed (Bluebond-Langner et al., 2003). If, as is often the case with children with brain tumors, the knowledge that the tumor had recurred came as a result of a routine scan, the parents were often back at home when the oncologist received the report. When the physician called, it was often left to the parents to decide whether to bring the child with them when they came to review the scans and discuss options for care and treatment. In other cases, the child was in the hospital or in clinic when the results of a scan, laboratory findings, or physical examination indicated a change in the child's condition, which warranted discussion of changes in care and treatment. At such times, the parents may or may not have been offered talking without the child present. Sometimes discussion just got underway without notice or consideration of the child's presence. When parents were offered the option of continuing discussion separately from the child, some chose to have a separate discussion, and others did not. For those who were asked and allowed the child to remain present, it was either because the parents thought the child was too young to understand what would be said, or because the parents had not anticipated what they were going to be told.

In cases where the child was not present, the child often had incomplete information at the time of the signing of the consent and solicitation and acquisition of assent. For example, when Jeremy gave his assent to participate in the phase I trial, he had not been told of the alternatives (e.g., treatment with temozolomide). The physician had not told him, and from the question: "[What] other medicine's?" following his mother's question to Dr. Summer, "If this treatment does not work, does this prevent us from getting other treatments?" one could argue that Jeremy had not been told not only of the other alternatives that had been proposed to his parents (e.g., temozolomide) but also that the "treatment" he was to receive might not arrest or cure his disease.

Consistent with our findings, but working in a different framework, Scherer (1991) found that children are not likely to dissent from a parent-sanctioned decision even when given the opportunity to do so. In the medical setting, children do not want to disappoint or challenge their parents or physician. Both Scherer's (1990) and Susman, Dorn, and Fletcher's (1992) studies found that children's decisions to participate in research were based heavily on their parents' wishes. When questioned about their deference to "parental influence," Scherer's (1990) study participants gave "reasons that fall into four categories: they feel coerced, or that they have no choice; they wish to avoid family tension and conflict with parents; they respect parental judgment and feel that parents know more about these matters; or they feel a need for parental support, emotionally, physically, and/or financially" (p. 443).

Children are socialized to respect the role of parents and other adults as authorities. As Leiken (1993) points out, "Even when [children] have a personal reservation, and the offer is made in a form of request, they may still agree to participate in the research simply because they believe that they should be compliant" (p. 5). According to Leiken (1993), the situation is not very different in preadolescents, albeit for different reasons: "Preadolescents, in order to avoid negative consequences, are prone to defer to authority figures" (p. 4). Leiken (1993) states, "This lack of assertiveness in voicing their authentic choices . . . [raises] serious questions about whether one can justifiably speak of 'assent' when children or young adolescents are concerned" (p. 4). Lest one think that this then precludes children from participating in a meaningful way in the decision-making process, Leiken (1993) takes care to point out that adults defer to social pressures when making decisions regarding care, treatment, and participation in trials. Social and cultural factors are as much a part of decision making involving adults as they are part of those involving children.

In conclusion, current federal regulations protecting children as research subjects direct IRBs to determine which children eligible for a particular protocol should have a role in deciding whether they participate. If deemed able, how they should be involved in the decision making is set out simply and is not in question—the investigator should solicit and acquire the child's assent. On the basis of recent empirical evidence, we would argue that the issue is not which children eligible for a particular study are capable of participating in the decision making. The issues are, How should physicians safely elicit the views of children? And then, how should they put those views into play in a process that gives children a part with which all participants (but especially the children themselves) are comfortable?

Toward a New Approach: Shuttle Diplomacy and Negotiation

We propose an approach for involving these children in decision making that formally recognizes three participants: parents, child-patient, and physician. This approach attempts to address the abilities of children, as well as the reality of their relation to their parents and other adults. In addition, it recognizes what must be explained to parents and children in order for their decision to be informed and meaningful.

We offer this model without proposing a new regulation. Clearly, from the foregoing discussion, we do not regard the giving of assent as the primary goal or measure of an ethical decision-making process with children. The possibility of a sham is too great. Assent can become a sham when a child agrees to participate in a clinical trial when he or she is simply agreeing with a decision of the family. The act can also be a sham when a child feels, or is urged to feel, that the decision is truly his or hers, but in fact will not be allowed to pursue a course that his or her parents do not approve. Parents typically make any number of major decisions concerning their children's lives. Medical decisions need to be consistent with the rest of the child's experience. If important decisions have not been the child's to make in the past, this is not the time to change that by seeking the child's assent. This is not to say that the child does not have a role in the decision-making process, or that his concerns, views, and desires should not be taken account (see below for how this is addressed in the proposed model).

The value of a requirement to seek assent is that it underscores the importance of talking to and listening to a child at a time when it can be extraordinarily difficult to do so. Parents and physicians are, although they typically try to control them, beset by profound feelings of sorrow and grief when there is, as in these cases, only the faintest chance that what is available will extend the child's life, and then only briefly. To explain this to a child, to bring him or her to understand this, to ask the child to make a "choiceless choice," is excruciating for parent and doctor. The pain they feel does not come just from empathy or sympathy. It also derives from their roles as physician and parents—to care for and protect. The directive to seek assent urges physicians to say and hear things that are, to say the least, difficult. It is the value that is implicit in this talking and listening to a child that needs to be preserved and expanded, without the focus on a particular result.

There are several values that need to be respected in the decision-making process with children. One is that it should be conducted without deceit. Second, that participants should be free from coercion. Finally, children, like any other patients, have a right (if they wish to exercise it) to know about the procedures that they undergo. The challenge in creating a role for children in decision making is to balance these values with the social fabric of family life and the rights that are accorded to parents in light of their responsibilities for their children.

A framework for involving children and others in the decision-making process that addresses these requirements is that of shuttle diplomacy and negotiation. Participants in serious negotiations need not be, and often are not, of equal status. The lack of veto power does not render participation ingenuine. What is required is a framework that tries to provide that all the participants are represented and moves toward a resolution that all parties accept. As in any negotiated outcome, trade-offs are made by participants of their individual wants or needs in favor of an overall resolution.

Let us briefly sketch what this diplomatic, negotiated approach might look like in the case of children who at time of recurrence have a less than 30% chance of cure. At the time of recurrence, parents would be told that there will be a family meeting to explore what options are available. The physician-investigator would explain what will be covered in the meeting (e.g., disease status, risks and benefits of what will be offered, prognosis) and ascertain what the parents would be comfortable having said with the child present. For example, parents might indicate a willingness to have a discussion about the various options, even their potential risks and benefits, in front of or with their child, but not the prognosis. Or as in Jeremy's case, the parents might be willing to have the physician explain what the child will be receiving and possible side effects, but would not want the physician to mention the experimental nature of what the child is to receive or the survival rates for children with similar conditions who have been on this study protocol.

It is extraordinarily important as well as beneficial for the physician to pursue with the parents why they do not want particular information shared with the child, and not just because of what is involved in terms of talking to the child. Our study reveals that in talking with parents about what they don't want the child to know the physicians become aware of misunderstandings about various care and treatment options and even the prognosis or other issues in the family that may be effecting choice of care, and even other problems that the parents may be experiencing. In short it is an opportunity not to be missed (Bluebond-Langner et al., 2003).

The physician should open the dialogue by acknowledging that he/she understands where they are coming from. In the course of conversation, the physician might note that from his/her experience the child knows the likely outcome and give some examples of the ways that children indicate either their desire to know more from their parents as well as the cues that children give that indicate what they know and their desire for more information. He/she might ask the parents what they are most afraid of if ——— came up. He/she might suggest that perhaps further discussion with the child, either with them present, or with the physician alone, would be helpful for all of them if not now, then perhaps in the future.

The parents may continue to refuse to have discussions with the child, or to have the physician have discussions with the child that would include the child's prognosis, side effects, or efficacy, for example. However, the groundwork has been laid for further discussions, and insights have been gained that will serve the physician well in other situations as they arise with these parents and their child.

The physician needs to make clear, both in the meetings alone with the child and in the meeting with the parents and child present, that while the child will be listened to by both the parents and the physician and his or her desires taken into account, the decision is not the child's alone to make. This is a collaborative process. Not insignificantly, this also relieves the child of a burden he or she should not have. The child is involved in the process but does not himself or herself determine the outcome.

This does not mean that the child cannot disagree with the parents. The child can, but he or she needs to know just how this dissent will be taken into account;

for we must never forget that from a legal standpoint, if the child is a minor, the ultimate decision is with the adults.

In this shuttle diplomacy framework, there is room for dissent, and there is room for negotiation. If that negotiation fails to bring about a satisfying result, the child has been included in a meaningful way, not set up for something that he or she can not have. The child's inability to determine the outcome has not kept the child from being an active player. And the fact that the child has been told that he or she is not the final or ultimate decision maker may also relieve second thoughts later on.

Of note, the approach and framework we have outlined can be used with adolescents, who can easily become cynical when their desires are solicited but then not acted upon, as well as with children younger than 7 or 8 years, for it acknowledges their understanding and capacity and remains open ended.

In sum, the focus of the child's participation in this framework is not on soliciting the child's willingness to agree to participation—for what does that accomplish in the absence of ability to dissent and have one's decision acceded to? Furthermore, obtaining a child's assent does not guarantee that the child has genuinely participated.

The reality is that decisions will be made with which children do not agree. The guidelines and regulations concerning involving children in the decision-making process must recognize this from the outset. If the child does not agree with a decision, the best one can hope for is that he or she accepts the process by which it was made. To secure this, the other participants, especially the physician, must be honest with the child about the process and how it works.

In conclusion, we recommend an approach for involving children with life-limiting illnesses in the decision to participate in clinical research through a process of shuttle diplomacy, in a negotiated framework, and not turning the process into some watered down consent process (consent has enough of its own problems) with an emphasis on the solicitation and acquisition of assent. Many important decisions in life, decisions that are ethical, have been and are made in a negotiated framework.

Questions for Discussion

1. When the tumor recurred do you think Jeremy should have been told about all three options? If so, what should have been told about each? Who should have discussed them, when, and in what manner?
2. When the tumor recurred Mr. Foster did not want Jeremy involved in the

decision of what to do. Mrs. Foster said that they did not use the words "clinical trial" when they spoke with Jeremy. They also "didn't want him to think of this as some sort of experimental drug that may or may not prove helpful." Mrs. Foster gave several reasons for this position. Do you agree or disagree with the Fosters' position? Why? What right do you think parents, as responsible decision makers for their children's medical care, should have in determining how children should be involved in the decision making process and what they should be told?

3. Mrs. Foster reported that Jeremy directly asked Dr. Sumner, "Well if this tumor doesn't shrink I'm going to die right?" And that Dr. Sumner replied, "No, That is not necessarily so Jeremy. Why are you saying that." Dr. Sumner recalled Jeremy's question. She did not remember the exact words of her reply, but did recall, "that Jeremy and I had talked about his dying. He asked and heard that he would die. He told me that he would be happy in heaven." How would you have replied to Jeremy's question? Why?

4. Federal regulations require that the IRB take into account "age, maturity and psychological state." Do you agree with these criteria? How should maturity and psychological state be assessed? Should there be additional criteria? If so, what should they be?

5. What should physicians or other health care professionals do when they understand that mutual pretense has become the dominant mode of interaction between parents and children with life-limiting illnesses? What are the potential risks and benefits of mutual pretense?

6. Citing the literature, the authors of this chapter suggest that children are not likely to dissent from a parent-sanctioned decision even when given the opportunity to do so. In the medical setting, children do not want to disappoint or challenge their parents or physician. How should these findings impact the regulation of pediatric research, especially in regard to the requirement for assent?

7. According to the authors, "medical decisions need to be consistent with the rest of the child's experience. If important decisions have not been the child's to make in the past, this is not the time to change that by seeking the child's assent." Do you agree with this statement? Why or why not?

8. Do you think that the current regulations regarding assent insure an ethical and meaningful role for children in decisions regarding participation in medical research?

9. The authors propose a framework for involving children and others in the decision-making process that is based on shuttle diplomacy and negotia-

tion. What might be the challenges to implementation? What recommendations would you make?

———

Notes

1. Names and dates have been changed to ensure confidentiality. The timing between events has been preserved.
2. Procarbazine and lomustine (CCNU) are alkylating agents that interfere with the DNA of cancerous cells, thus inhibiting cell growth and proliferation. Vincristine is a vinca alkaloid drug that impedes cancerous cell growth by preventing cell division, a cellular mechanism for cell proliferation (National Cancer Institute, www.cancer.gov/templates/db_alpha.aspx ?expand=p).
3. Thrombocytopenia—a significant and abnormal decline in platelets (Oxford Concise Medical Dictionary, 2002, p. 684).
4. Expressive aphasia—a neurological sensory impairment that results in the inability to express language (e.g., speech impairments such as word-finding difficulties, an inability to write, etc.); these deficits result from brain damage to the temporal lobe, an area of the brain concerned with the expression of language (Medline Plus, www2.merriam-webster.com/cgi-bin/ mwmednlm).
5. Hemiparesis—weakened muscles or partial paralysis on only one side of the body. (Oxford Concise Medical Dictionary, 2002, p. 312)
6. Steppage gait—an abnormal gait associated with neurological damage that prevents normal foot flexion; this disorder is characterized by high lifting of the legs, while toes point downward. (Medline Plus, www2.merriam-webster.com/cgi-bin/mwmednlm?book=medical&va= steppage%20gait)
7. "Family meeting" was the term used by the staff to refer to the formal meetings that took place between the parents and physician(s) and one or more of other assembled staff members (e.g., social worker, nurse practitioner, hospital or clinic staff nurse) outside of in-patient or out-patient clinic visits. The meetings were usually scheduled by the social worker or nurse practitioner at a time convenient for parents and physicians. The purpose of the meeting was to discuss the child's condition and options for care and treatment. Parents would sometimes bring other family members or friends to the meeting. With the exception of infants, children were not usually present at the meetings.
8. Bluebond-Langner was also present. The material used in this case is part of a larger study (Bluebond-Langner et al., 2003). Bluebond-Langner took notes and tape recorded this meeting as well as other conversations and interviews used in this "case study." All tapes were transcribed verbatim.
9. SU5416 is an investigational angiogenesis inhibitor drug that prevents the growth of new blood vessels to cancer cells, thereby starving the mutagenic cells of nutrients and oxygen and additionally preventing waste removal. SU5416 is being studied in a phase I clinical trial— the first step in testing new treatments for humans. This type of study investigates the optimal dose of an experimental drug, typically the maximal dose that can be administered without causing too severe side effects (National Cancer Institute, www.cancer.gov/templates/db _alpha.aspx?expand=p).
10. STI571 (also called Gleevec) is an investigational drug that impedes the growth of certain

cancers by interfering with an oncogene protein (mutagenic oncogenes are one factor in the etiology of cancer). STI571 is being studied in a phase I/II clinical trial (National Cancer Institute, www.cancer.gov/templates/db_alpha.aspx?expand=g)—an intermediate study between phase I and phase II trials when enough research on adults regarding the drug is available to proceed with an investigation of the drug's safety, dosage level, and efficacy (National Cancer Institute, www.cancer.gov/templates/db_alpha.aspx?expand=p).

11. Temozolomide is an alkylating agent that interferes with the DNA of cancerous cells, thereby preventing mutagenic cell division and cell growth (National Cancer Institute, www.cancer .gov/templates/db_alpha.aspx?expand=t).

12. Parents and patients included "second and third line chemotherapies" and phase I or phase I/II trials as disease-directed or cancer-directed therapies. Therapies and medications directed at side effects of treatment or at pain, discomfort, or sequelae (e.g., seizures) were categorized as symptom directed, or palliative care—non-cancer-directed therapies.

13. Administration of SU5416 was to be through a central line. Jeremy did not have one at the time. A central line is a tube surgically placed into a blood vessel for the purpose of giving intravenous fluids or drugs (National Cancer Institute, www.cancer.gov/templates/db_alpha .aspx?expand=c).

14. As part of the study design (see note 9) Bluebond-Langner spoke with parents, patients, and physicians about what happened during the formal encounters (e.g., family meetings, in-patient and out-patient examinations, rounds) in which they each had just participated.

15. Dr. Sumner also recalled this conversation. In her account, "Jeremy and I had talked about his dying. He asked and heard he would die. He told me he would be happy in heaven. But even after this conversation, pretense continued."

16. When queried, the physician said, "What I was trying to say was 'Because you are 14 you have the right to sign the consent. If you choose to be treated but you do not want to sign, if you just want to say it's okay, that's okay, too.' "

17. For further discussion of the concept and its application to children with life-limiting illnesses, see Glaser and Strauss (1965) and Bluebond-Langner (1978).

18. And even in those cases where there was open communication, it was not there at all times in all situations. For example, while one boy and his parents had had a conversation about death, including what they would each like when they died, he did not raise, nor did his parents discuss, death or funeral arrangements when the tumor had progressed and various options for care and treatment were being considered.

19. Olechnowicz, Eder, Simon, Zyanski, and Kodish (2002, p. 813), in a study of the informed consent conference for participation in phase III trials for newly diagnosed patients with leukemia, found that parents asked fewer questions when a patient older than 7 years was present. They also noted that "the patients did very little talking."

References

Bluebond-Langner, M. (1978). *The private worlds of dying children.* Princeton, NJ: Princeton University Press.

Bluebond-Langner, M. (1996). *In the shadow of illness: Parents and siblings of the chronically ill child.* Princeton, NJ: Princeton University Press.

Bluebond-Langner, M., Belasco, J., & Goldman, A. (2003, March). Decision making for children with cancer when cure is not likely: Implications for end-of-life and palliative care. Paper presented at the meeting of the Children's Oncology Group, Atlanta, GA.

Broome, M. E., Richards, D. J., & Hall, J. M. (2001). Children in research: The experience of ill children and adolescents. *Journal of Family Nursing, 7*(1), 32–49.

Children's Hospital Boston. *Child health A to Z: Anaplastic astrocytoma.* Retrieved on 07/26/04 from: http://web1.tch.harvard.edu/cfapps/A2Ztopicsdisplay.cfm?Topic=Anaplastic%20Astro cytoma

Deatrick, J. A., Angst, D. B., & Moore, C. (2002). Parents' views of their children's participation in phase I oncology clinical trials. *Journal of Pediatric Oncology Nursing, 19*(4), 114–121.

Glaser, B., & Strauss, A. (1965). *Awareness of dying: A study of social interaction.* Chicago: Aldine.

Leiken, S. (1993). Minors' assent, consent, or dissent to medical research. *IRB: A Review of Human Subjects Research, 15*(2), 1–7.

Medline Plus. (N/A). Medical Dictionary. Retrieved on July 26, 2004 from www2.merriam -webster.com/cgi-bin/mwmednlm?book=medical&va=steppage%20gait

National Cancer Institute. (N/A). Dictionary of Cancer Terms-C. Retrieved on July 26, 2004 from www.cancer.gov/templates/db_alpha.aspx?expand=c.

National Cancer Institute. (N/A). Dictionary of Cancer Terms-G. Retrieved on July 26, 2004 from www.cancer.gov/templates/db_alpha.aspx?expand=g.

National Cancer Institute. (N/A). Dictionary of Cancer Terms-L. Retrieved on July 26, 2004 from www.cancer.gov/templates/db_alpha.aspx?expand=l.

National Cancer Institute. (N/A). Dictionary of Cancer Terms-P. Retrieved on July 26, 2004 from www.cancer.gov/templates/db_alpha.aspx?expand=p.

National Cancer Institute. (N/A). Dictionary of Cancer Terms-T. Retrieved on July 26, 2004 from www.cancer.gov/templates/db_alpha.aspx?expand=t.

Olechnowicz, J. Q., Eder, M., Simon, C., Zyanski, S., & Kodish, E. (2002). Assent observed: Children's involvement in leukemia treatment and research discussions. *Pediatrics, 109*(5), 806–814.

Oxford University Press. (2002). Oxford Concise Medical Dictionary, 6th ed. Oxford: Oxford University Press.

Scherer, D. (1992). Capacities of minors to exercise voluntariness in medical treatment decisions. *Law and Human Behavior, 15*(4), 431–449.

Susman, E. J., Dorn, L. D., & Fletcher, J. C. (1992). Participation in biomedical research: The consent process as viewed by children, adolescents, young children, and physicians. *Journal of Pediatrics, 121,* 547–552.

Index

abortion, 103
Abuse of Casuistry, 20
academic achievement, influence of teacher
   expectation on, 187
accountability, evading, 69
Ackerson, L., 269
acquiescence, 331. *See also* deference
addiction, 194, 198, 200, 201, 202, 209
adenosine deaminase deficiency, 310
adolescents, 78, 195–196
   capacity of, 78, 85–86, 93–95, 109–112,
      114–115, 195
   decision making by, 206–210, 328
   disagreement with parents, 82
   as fathers, 113
   legal status of, 111–113
   perceptions about heritability, 201, 205
   preferences of, 313
   pregnancy among, 79, 82, 100, 103–105,
      107–109, 113
   reaction to parental permission, 77, 91,
      114
   recruiting at-risk, 103
   responses to interventions, 79
   sexual activity among, 77, 108
   vulnerability of, 86, 89, 111, 195, 199
adverse outcomes
   access to medical care and, 56
   detecting, 37
   identifying rare, 50
   of vaccination, 49
Advisory Committee on Immunization
   Practices (Centers for Disease Control),
   48
advocacy
   child, 286
   groups, 172, 179–180, 271
   role of healthcare professionals, 279
African Americans, bias against, 201
age
   of assent, 13
   capacity and, 84–85
   child status and, 88

as criteria for decision making, 331, 332
   at initiation of sexual activity, 104
   perspective and, 283
   relevance to ethical analysis, 306
   at starting smoking, 198
age of majority, 79–80, 111
aggressive behavior, 189
   children at risk for, 181
   serotonin levels and, 180
AIDS. *See* HIV
air travel, and hypoxia in infants, 29–31, 35–
   36, 38, 39
alcohol addiction, 200
aliens, treatment of, 274, 284
alpha-1 antitrypsin deficiency, 202
   genetic screening for, 126–127
altitude, risk to infants, 38
altruism, 208
American Academy of Pediatrics, 22, 154,
   285
   Committee on Bioethics, 15
   definition of children, 292
   guidelines on placebo use, 300
   policies regarding payment of subjects,
      148–149
American Crop Protection Association, 168
American Medical Association, view of
   mature minor doctrine, 82
American Psychological Association, 189
anaplastic astrocytoma, 323
ancillary services, as participation
   incentives, 285
anesthesia, 156
angiogenesis inhibitors, 341
antidepressants, 297
antitrypsin deficiency, 202
   genetic screening for, 126–127
anxiety, 200
   accompanying genetic screening, 126,
     128, 209
   in parents of at-risk children, 131
aphasia, 323, 341
appearance, concern about, 86, 89, 195